T2-EVX-055

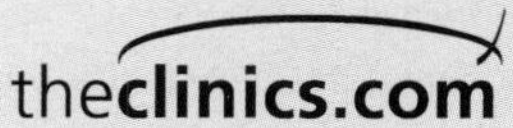

RADIOLOGIC CLINICS OF NORTH AMERICA

Breast Imaging

Guest Editor
EDWARD A. SICKLES, MD

September 2007 • Volume 45 • Number 5

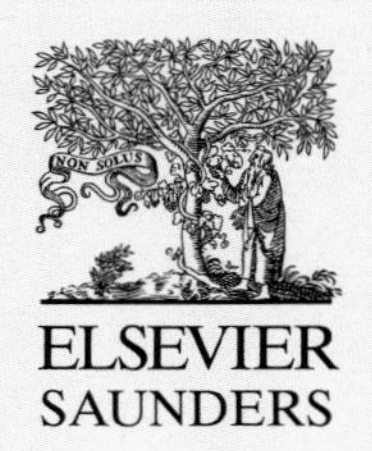

An imprint of Elsevier, Inc
PHILADELPHIA LONDON TORONTO MONTREAL SYDNEY TOKYO

W.B. SAUNDERS COMPANY
A Division of Elsevier Inc.

1600 John F. Kennedy Boulevard • Suite 1800 • Philadelphia, Pennsylvania 19103-2899

http://www.theclinics.com

RADIOLOGIC CLINICS OF NORTH AMERICA Volume 45, Number 5
September 2007 ISSN 0033-8389, ISBN-13: 978-1-4160-5118-3; ISBN-10: 1-4160-5118-X

Editor: Barton Dudlick

Reprints: For copies of 100 or more, of articles in this publication, please contact the Commercial Reprints Department, Elsevier Inc., 360 Park Avenue South, New York, New York 10010-1710. Tel.: (+1) 212-633-3813; Fax: (+1) 212-462-1935; E-mail: reprints@elsevier.com.

Radiologic Clinics of North America (ISSN 0033-8389) is published bimonthly in January, March, May, July, September, and November by Elsevier Inc., 360 Park Avenue South, New York, NY 10010-1710. Business and editorial offices: 1600 John F. Kenedy Boulevard, Suite 1800, Philadelphia, Pennsylvania 19103-2899. Customer Service Office: 6277 Sea Harbor Drive, Orlando, FL 32887-4800. Periodicals postage paid at New York, NY, and additional mailing offices. Subscription prices are USD 259 per year for US individuals, USD 385 per year for US institutions, USD 127 per year for US students and residents, USD 303 per year for Canadian individuals, USD 473 per year of Canadian institutions, USD 352 per year for international individuals, USD 473 per year for international institutions, and USD 171 per year for Canadian and foreign students/residents. To receive student and resident rate, orders must be accompanied by name of affiliated institution, date of term, and the signature of program/residency coordinatior on institution letterhead. Orders will be billed at individual rate until proof of status is received. Foreign air speed delivery is included in all Clinics subscriptionprices. All prices are subject to change without notice. **POSTMASTER:** Send address changes to *Radiologic Clinics of North America,* Elsevier Periodicals Customer Service, 6277 Sea Harbor Drive, Orlando, FL 32887-4800. **Customer Service: 1-800-654-2452 (US). From outside of the US, call (+1) 407-345-4000.**

Radiologic Clinics of North America also published in Greek Paschalidis Medical Publications, Athens, Greece.

Radiologic Clinics of North America is covered in *Index Medicus, EMBASE/Excerpta Medica, Current Contents/Life Sciences, Current Contents/Clinical Medicine, RSNA Index to Imaging Literature, BIOSIS, Science Citation Index,* and *ISI/BIOMED.*

Printed in the United States of America.

BREAST IMAGING

GUEST EDITOR

EDWARD A. SICKLES, MD
Professor Emeritus of Radiology, Department of Radiology, University of California San Francisco School of Medicine, San Francisco, California

CONTRIBUTORS

SOPHIA K. APPLE, MD
Associate Professor of Pathology, Department of Pathology and Laboratory Medicine, David Geffen School of Medicine, University of California Los Angeles, Los Angeles, California

JANET K. BAUM, MD
Director of Breast Imaging, Department of Radiology; and Director of Undergraduate Medical Education, Cambridge Health Alliance, Cambridge; Associate Professor of Radiology, Harvard Medical School, Boston, Massachusetts

LAWRENCE W. BASSETT, MD, FACR
Iris Cantor Professor of Breast Imaging and Director of Breast Imaging, Department of Radiology, David Geffen School of Medicine, University of California Los Angeles, Los Angeles, California

WENDIE A. BERG, MD, PhD, FACR
Breast Imaging Consultant, American Radiology Services, Johns Hopkins Green Spring, Lutherville, Maryland

R. JAMES BRENNER, MD, FACR
Professor of Clinical Radiology and Chief, Breast Imaging Section, University of California, UCSF-Mt. Zion Hospital, San Francisco, California

PETER J. DEMPSEY, MD
Professor of Radiology and Section Chief of Breast Imaging, Division of Diagnostic Imaging, Department of Diagnostic Radiology, The University of Texas M.D. Anderson Cancer Center, Houston, Texas

CARL J. D'ORSI, MD
Professor of Radiology, Hematology, and Oncology, and Director, Breast Imaging Center, Department of Radiology, Emory University Hospital, Atlanta, Georgia

STEPHEN A. FEIG, MD, FACR
Professor of Radiological Sciences, University of California Irvine School of Medicine; and Director, Breast Imaging, UCI Medical Center, Orange, California

MARK HELVIE, MD
Director of Breast Imaging and Professor of Radiology, Department of Radiology, University of Michigan Health System, Ann Arbor, Michigan

JESSICA W.T. LEUNG, MD
Associate Professor in Residence, Department of Radiology, University of California, San Francisco Medical Center, San Francisco, California

MARY C. MAHONEY, MD
Associate Professor of Radiology and Director of Breast Imaging, Department of Radiology, University of Cincinnati Medical Center, Barrett Cancer Center, Cincinnati, Ohio

HELGA S. MARQUES, MS
Biostatistician, Center for Statistical Sciences, Brown University, Providence, Rhode Island

ELIZABETH A. MORRIS, MD
Associate Professor of Radiology and Director of Breast MRI, Memorial Sloan-Kettering Cancer Center, New York, New York

MARY S. NEWELL, MD
Assistant Professor of Radiology, and Assistant Director, Breast Imaging Center, Department of Radiology, Emory University Hospital, Atlanta, Georgia

YURI PARISKY, MD
Director of Medical Imaging, Mammoth Hospital, Mammoth Lakes, California

ETTA D. PISANO, MD
Kenan Professor of Radiology and Biomedical Engineering, Department of Radiology; Department of Biomedical Engineering; University of North Carolina Biomedical Research Imaging Center; University of North Carolina–Linberger Comprehensive Cancer Center; and Vice Dean for Academic Affairs, University of North Carolina School of Medicine, Chapel Hill, North Carolina

ELIZABETH A. RAFFERTY, MD
Instructor of Radiology, Department of Radiology, Harvard Medical School; and Director of Breast Imaging, Avon Comprehensive Breast Cancer, Massachusetts General Hospital, Boston, Massachusetts

EDWARD A. SICKLES, MD
Professor Emeritus of Radiology, Department of Radiology, University of California San Francisco School of Medicine, San Francisco, California

WEI YANG, MD
Associate Professor of Radiology, Division of Diagnostic Imaging, Department of Diagnostic Radiology, The University of Texas M.D. Anderson Cancer Center, Houston, Texas

MARGARITA ZULEY, MD
Associate Professor of Radiology, University of Pittsburgh School of Medicine, Pittsburgh, Pennsylvania

BREAST IMAGING

Volume 45 • Number 5 • September 2007

Contents

The American College of Radiology (ACR) Breast Imaging Reporting and Data System (BI-RADS) is the product of the initial collaboration between various committees of the ACR and several other organizations, such as the American College of American Pathologists and the American College of Surgeons. The impetus to establish a standardized method of reporting and follow-up began as early as 1985 when several of our clinical colleagues made a plea to the ACR to improve the reporting of mammograms. Reports were ambiguous and difficult to interpret, often leaving the clinician without a clear-cut management scenario. Over the years of increasing BI-RADS usage, the BI-RADS committee of the ACR received questions which, when analyzed, focused on specific areas of BI-RADS. A review of these problematic areas, with appropriate guidance, will be presented along with an introduction to the new US and MR imaging lexicons focusing on unique descriptors.

Asymmetry may be the only manifestation of breast cancer on standard mammographic views. The terminology used to describe breast asymmetries changed in 2003 with the publication by the American College of Radiology of the fourth edition of its Breast Imaging Reporting and Data System (BI-RADS). This article describes and illustrates the four types of asymmetry found at mammography (asymmetry, global asymmetry, focal asymmetry, and developing asymmetry). For each type of asymmetry, the article also indicates the frequency of occurrence, likelihood of malignancy, standard imaging work-up, assessment, and management.

FORTHCOMING ISSUES

November 2007

MR Imaging of the Knee

Jeffrey Peterson, MD, *Guest Editor*

January 2008

Current Trends and Future Directions in Genitourinary Tract Imaging

Michael A. Blake, MD,
and Mannudeep K. Kalra, MD, *Guest Editors*

RECENT ISSUES

July 2007

Update on PET/CT

May 2007

Emergency Cross-Sectional Imaging

Vikram S. Dogra, MD, and
Shweta Bhatt, MD, *Guest Editors*

GOAL STATEMENT

The goal of the *Radiologic Clinics of North America* is to keep practicing radiologists and radiology residents up to date with current clinical practice in radiology by providing timely articles reviewing the state of the art in patient care.

ACCREDITATION

The *Radiologic Clinics of North America* is planned and implemented in accordance with the Essential Areas and Policies of the Accreditation Council for Continuing Medical Education (ACCME) through the joint sponsorship of the University of Virginia School of Medicine and Elsevier. The University of Virginia School of Medicine is accredited by the ACCME to provide continuing medical education for physicians.

The University of Virginia School of Medicine designates this educational activity for a maximum of 15 *AMA PRA Category 1 Credits*™. Physicians should only claim credit commensurate with the extent of their participation in the activity.

The American Medical Association has determined that physicians not licensed in the US who participate in this CME activity are eligible for 15 *AMA PRA Category 1 Credits*™.

Credit can be earned by reading the text material, taking the CME examination online at http://www.theclinics.com/home/cme, and completing the evaluation. After taking the test, you will be required to review any and all incorrect answers. Following completion of the test and evaluation, your credit will be awarded and you may print your certificate.

FACULTY DISCLOSURE/CONFLICT OF INTEREST

The University of Virginia School of Medicine, as an ACCME accredited provider, endorses and strives to comply with the Accreditation Council for Continuing Medical Education (ACCME) Standards of Commercial Support, Commonwealth of Virginia statutes, University of Virginia policies and procedures, and associated federal and private regulations and guidelines on the need for disclosure and monitoring of proprietary and financial interests that may affect the scientific integrity and balance of content delivered in continuing medical education activities under our auspices.

The University of Virginia School of Medicine requires that all CME activities accredited through this institution be developed independently and be scientifically rigorous, balanced and objective in the presentation/discussion of its content, theories and practices.

All authors/editors participating in an accredited CME activity are expected to disclose to the readers relevant financial relationships with commercial entities occurring within the past 12 months (such as grants or research support, employee, consultant, stock holder, member of speakers bureau, etc.). The University of Virginia School of Medicine will employ appropriate mechanisms to resolve potential conflicts of interest to maintain the standards of fair and balanced education to the reader. Questions about specific strategies can be directed to the Office of Continuing Medical Education, University of Virginia School of Medicine, Charlottesville, Virginia.

The authors/editors listed below have identified no financial or professional relationships for themselves or their spouse/partner:

Sophia K. Apple, MD; Lawrence W. Bassett, MD, FACR; Janet K. Baum, MD; R. James Brenner, MD, FACR; Peter J. Dempsey, MD; Barton Dudlick (Acquisitions Editor); Stephen A. Feig, MD, FACR; Mark Helvie, MD; Jessica W.T. Leung, MD; Helga S. Marques, MS; Elizabeth A. Morris, MD; Mary S. Newell, MD; Etta D. Pisano, MD; and Edward A. Sickles, MD (Guest Editor).

The authors/editors listed below have identified the following financial or professional relationships for themselves or their spouse/partner:

Wendie A. Berg, MD, PhD, FACR is an independent contractor, a consultant, and is on the speaker's bureau for Naviscan PET Systems, Inc.; is a consultant for Siemens Medical Systems, Inc.

Carl J. D'Orsi, MD is on the Advisory Committee for GE Medical; is on the Advisory Board for and owns stock in Hologic.

Mary C. Mahoney, MD is a consultant and is on the speaker's bureau for Ethicon Eudo-Surgery.

Yuri Parisky, MD is a consultant for Techniscan.

Elizabeth A. Rafferty, MD received a research grant from Hologic, Inc.

Wei Yang, MD is a consultant for Wyeth Pharmaceutical.

Margarita Zuley, MD is a consultant for GE Healthcare and is on the advisory committee for Hologic, Inc.

Disclosure of Discussion of Non-FDA Approved Uses for Pharmaceutical and/or Medical Devices:

The University of Virginia School of Medicine, as an ACCME provider, requires that all authors identify and disclose any "off label" uses for pharmaceutical and medical device products. The University of Virginia School of Medicine recommends that each physician fully review all the available data on new products or procedures prior to clinical use.

TO ENROLL

To enroll in the *Radiologic Clinics of North America* Continuing Medical Education program, call customer service at 1-800-654-2452 or sign up online at http://www.theclinics.com/home/cme. The CME program is available to subscribers for an additional annual fee USD 205.

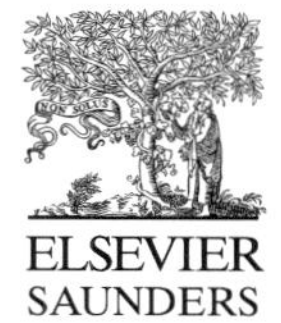

RADIOLOGIC
CLINICS
OF NORTH AMERICA

Radiol Clin N Am 45 (2007) xi

Preface

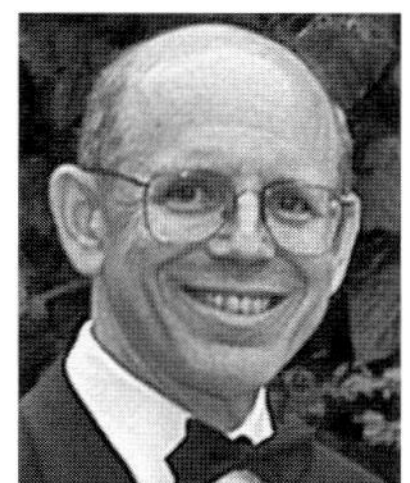

Edward A. Sickles, MD
Guest Editor

Edward A. Sickles, MD
Department of Radiology
University of California San Francisco
School of Medicine
San Francisco, CA 94143-1667, USA

E-mail address:
edward.sickles@ucsfmedctr.org

Breast imaging has come a long way since it first was the subject of an entire issue of *Radiologic Clinics of North America* in March 1983. The widespread use of mammography screening in the United States and many other developed countries has accounted for a substantial portion of the progressive mortality reduction from breast cancer observed over the past decade. Advances in both ultrasound and MR imaging have established these imaging modalities as effective adjuncts to mammography in the detection and diagnosis of breast disease. Add to this a variety of important innovations in interventional breast imaging, particularly those involving percutaneous biopsy techniques, and it is clear that the breast imager now has assumed the principal role among all the players on the breast health care team.

This issue of the *Radiologic Clinics of North America* covers most of the major developments in breast imaging that have taken place in the three years since the last (sixth) breast imaging issue was published in September 2004. Some of the topics are similar but contain substantially updated material; new topics reflect other recent advances in knowledge or technology. The aim of each article is to provide clinically relevant summaries of the state of the art to radiologists both in training and in practice.

I have been most fortunate in recruiting a team of skilled investigators and teachers to write about topics they know so well. These authors actively publish in the peer-review literature on their subjects, teach the subjects extensively, or, in most cases, do both. The result is what I expect will become an important resource for radiologists, for our clinicians, and (indirectly) for our patients.

doi:10.1016/j.rcl.2007.08.001
radiologic.theclinics.com

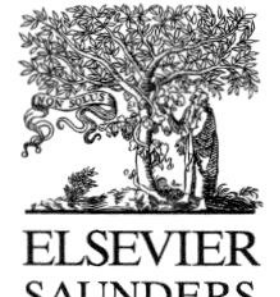

ELSEVIER
SAUNDERS

RADIOLOGIC
CLINICS
OF NORTH AMERICA

Radiol Clin N Am 45 (2007) 751–763

BI-RADS Decoded: Detailed Guidance on Potentially Confusing Issues

Carl J. D'Orsi, MD*, Mary S. Newell, MD

The American College of Radiology (ACR) Breast Imaging Reporting and Data System (BI-RADS) is the product of the initial collaboration between various committees of the ACR and several other organizations, such as the American College of American Pathologists and the American College of Surgeons. The impetus to establish a standardized method of reporting and follow-up began as early as 1985 when several of our clinical colleagues made a plea to the ACR to improve the reporting of mammograms. Reports were ambiguous and difficult to interpret, often leaving the clinician without a clear-cut management scenario.

BI-RADS was always meant to be a dynamic and evolving document that would be able to adapt to changing practice patterns and new scientific data. Some of the initial articles concerning BI-RADS focused on determining the positive predictive value (PPV) of mammographic features and the effect of BI-RADS usage on clinical practice. Orel and colleagues [1] found upon pathologic evaluation of 1312 excised mammographic lesions that the PPV for malignancy was 0% for Category 2 (benign) lesions, 2% for Category 3 (probably benign) lesions, 30% for Category 4 lesions, and 97% for Category 5 lesions. Liberman and colleagues [2] analyzed 492 lesions detected only on mammography with subsequent surgical biopsy; PPVs were 2%, 34%, and 81% for Category 3, 4, and 5, respectively. Thus, the BI-RADS assessment categories seem to be separating breast disease appropriately. Berg and colleagues [3] investigated whether training could lead to observer improvement, with regard to mammographic feature analysis and final assessment when practicing radiologists were compared with the consensus of an expert panel. The expert panel reviewed a test set of cases, agreeing on feature description and analysis. Twenty-three practicing mammographers then reviewed these mammograms before and after a day of training with BI-RADS. There was an improved agreement with the expert consensus after training. Some specific areas, such as calcification distribution, did not show improvement, serving as an early indication that more detailed guidance was required to make successful use of BI-RADS.

Over the years of increasing BI-RADS usage, the BI-RADS committee of the ACR, now a subcommittee of the Breast Cancer Commission of the ACR, received questions which, when analyzed, focused

Breast Imaging Center, Department of Radiology, Emory University Hospital, 1365-C Clifton Road, Suite C1104, Atlanta, GA 30322, USA
* Corresponding author.
E-mail address: carl.dorsi@emoryhealthcare.org (C.J. D'Orsi).

0033-8389/07/$ – see front matter
doi:10.1016/j.rcl.2007.06.003
radiologic.theclinics.com

on specific areas of BI-RADS. A review of these problematic areas, with appropriate guidance, is presented along with an introduction to the new ultrasound and MR imaging lexicons focusing on unique descriptors.

Mammography

Focal asymmetry

One of the most frequently asked questions relates to what constitutes an asymmetry versus a focal asymmetry versus a mass. A soft tissue finding identified only on one view, without matching tissue in a similar location in the contralateral breast, represents an asymmetry. This is in contradistinction to focal asymmetries and masses, both of which are soft tissue findings seen on two views, lying at a comparable depth when one view is compared with another, and showing similar density and shape on those views. Focal asymmetries lack convex outward borders along at least a portion of their periphery on both views, whereas masses display consistent convex margins (Figs. 1 and 2). This distinction may be difficult at times; in general, though, although focal asymmetries may show partial border convexity, this feature usually is not noted in both mammographic views. Focal asymmetries are confined to a small area of the breast (within a quadrant), and may represent a subtle, but important, sign of malignancy (often an infiltrating lobular carcinoma), especially if seen to evolve over time (Fig. 3). Conversely, global asymmetries occupy a large portion of the breast (more than one quadrant). These asymmetries are usually on the basis of normal variation or secondary to the effects of hormone replacement therapy. Note that the term "density" has been removed from the discussion of asymmetries because it is more accurately used as a descriptor of X-ray attenuation.

Calcifications

Detection and management of breast calcifications may be bothersome. Morphologies and distributions that typically are benign and those that are highly suggestive of malignancy usually offer little or no problem for management; however, there are shapes and distributions of calcifications that are difficult to detect, characterize, and manage.

Amorphous, fine pleomorphic, and coarse heterogeneous types of calcification may, at times, be troublesome to separate but can have different prognostic implications. "Fine pleomorphic" calcifications are irregular, small (usually<0.5 mm) calcifications that, together with "fine linear" or "fine, linear branching" calcifications, have the highest probability for malignancy. "Amorphous" calcifications, arguably, may be the most problematic to identify. They also are small (<0.5 mm), irregular calcifications but differ from fine pleomorphic calcification in their conspicuity or density (Fig. 4). Their edges are not defined as sharply as are those in the fine pleomorphic category. They may present with only a slightly higher density than surrounding glandular tissue, accounting for their difficult detection. "Coarse heterogeneous" calcifications are a new addition to the fourth edition of

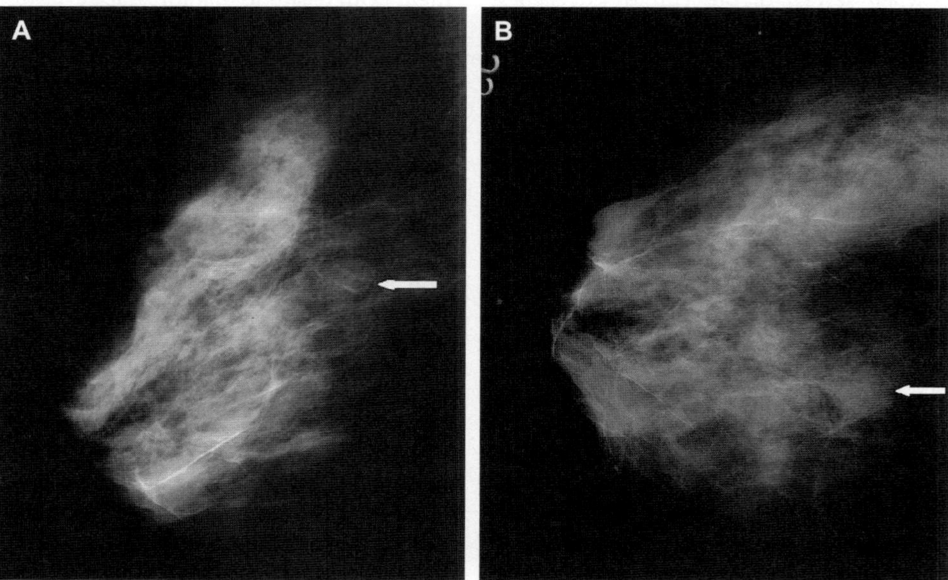

Fig. 1. Mass. Partially circumscribed, partially obscured mass in the mediolateral oblique (*A*) and craniocaudal (*B*) projections. Note the convex outward borders seen on both views (*arrows*).

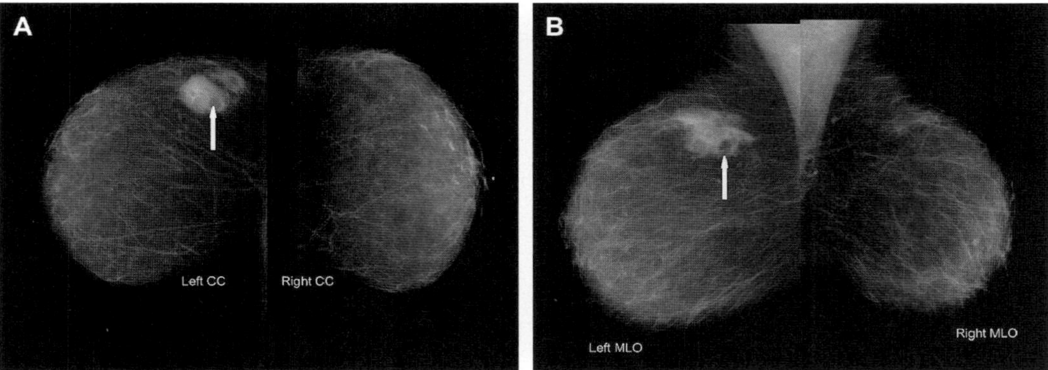

Fig. 2. Focal asymmetry. Asymmetric region seen on craniocaudal (*A*) and mediolateral oblique (*B*) projections with lack of convex outward borders on the MLO view and interspersed fat on both projections (*arrows*).

BI-RADS. These calcifications also are irregular and conspicuous but basically differ from the prior two types in size. They generally are larger than 0.5 mm and are associated most often with benign conditions, such as fibrosis or fibroadenomas, but can be associated with malignancy (Fig. 5). Of the three types of calcifications described, fine pleomorphic are the most suspicious, coarse heterogeneous are the least suspicious, and amorphous are between the former and the latter. Berg and colleagues [4] reviewed 150 lesions that manifested as amorphous calcifications. Twenty percent were malignant and, of these, 90% represented ductal carcinoma in situ (DCIS). As a rule, it is unusual to have calcifications

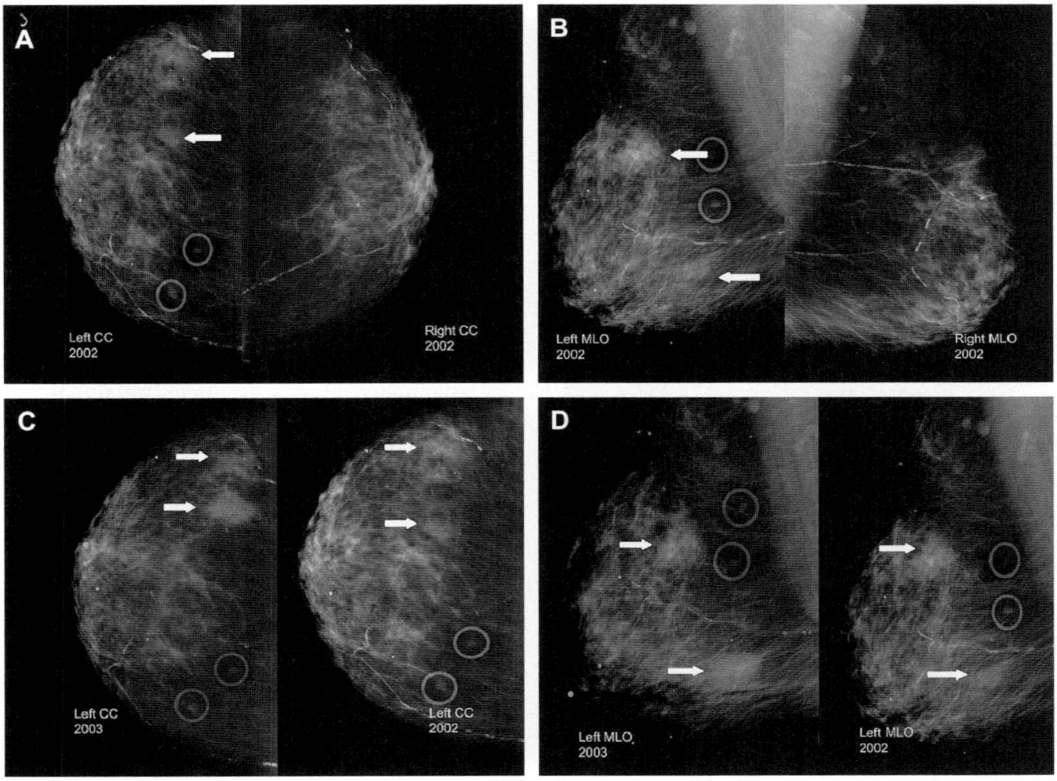

Fig. 3. Developing asymmetry. Two focal asymmetries (*arrows*) are seen in the left craniocaudal (*A*) and mediolateral oblique (*B*) projections. One year later, the more inferior asymmetry has enlarged and has suggestion of spiculations on the craniocaudal (*C*) and mediolateral oblique (*D*) projections compared with the previous examination (*arrows*). Pathology: infiltrating ductal carcinoma.

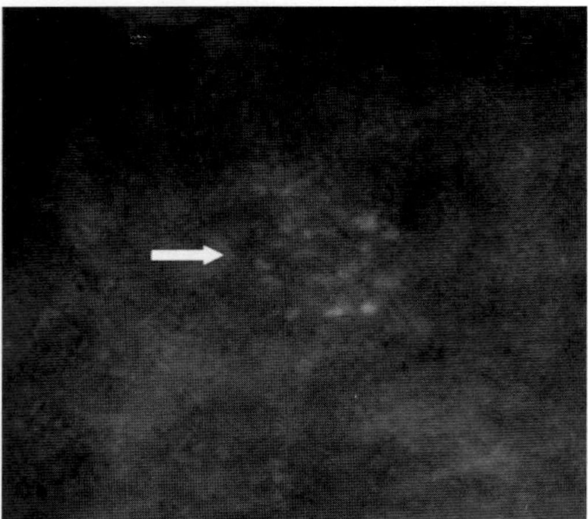

Fig. 4. Amorphous calcifications. A cluster of small, hazy calcifications (*arrow*) without a more specific morphologic classification.

that are exclusively of one shape. Most are mixtures of different forms; however, it is the most worrisome of these forms that should direct subsequent management (Fig. 6).

Although often not given as much attention as shape, the distribution of calcifications within the breast often may allow separation into benign and malignant status with increased accuracy. The terminal duct lobular unit is the anatomic site of origin of most intraductal carcinomas (Fig. 7) [5]. When this concept is kept in mind, calcifications oriented in a "linear" or multiple linear ("segmental") (Fig. 8) orientation assume greater importance, even if the individual calcification shape is of intermediate concern. For example, linear or segmental arrangements of coarse heterogeneous calcifications are more worrisome than a regional distribution of the same calcifications. Grouped or clustered microcalcifications occupy less than 1 cm^3 of tissue and are composed of at least five elements. This distribution is more lobular in nature and does not have the significance of a linear or segmental distribution. A cluster of coarse heterogeneous calcifications is less worrisome than a linear or segmental distribution; however, calcifications in the category of higher probability of malignancy (pleomorphic and fine linear) almost always require tissue diagnosis, regardless of distribution. As the distribution becomes less focal, as in "regional" (>2 cm^3 of breast tissue not conforming to a duct and usually occupying a quadrant or more), or distributed randomly throughout the breast ("diffuse/scattered"), the suspicion for malignancy diminishes; however, one must act on the most worrisome feature or combination of features.

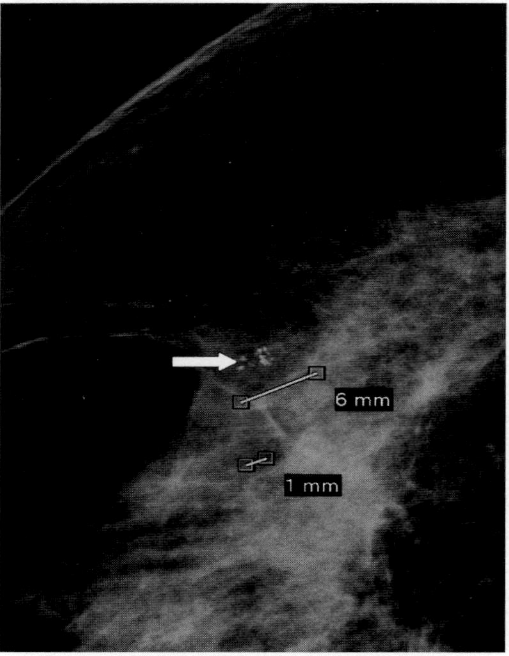

Fig. 5. Coarse, heterogeneous calcifications. A cluster of calcifications (*arrow*), irregular in appearance and larger than 0.5 mm, but not as large as dystrophic calcifications.

Architectural distortion

Another description that requires clarification is architectural distortion. The hallmark of this feature is a series of thin, straight lines or spiculations radiating from an area (Fig. 9) that does not have features of a mass or focal asymmetry; however, these radiating spicules also may be identified from the edge of a mass or focal asymmetry (Fig. 10). In this situation, they become part of the margin description ("spiculated") for the mass or asymmetry. Obviously, there are situations in which it becomes difficult or impossible to determine whether one is dealing with a spiculated mass or architectural distortion; however, the presence of these radially oriented lines, whether originating from a mass, focal asymmetry, or a point, strongly suggest the presence of malignancy.

Assessment categories

The assessment categories are arguably the most important component of the BI-RADS lexicon. Because they are coupled with management options, they categorize the mammogram and direct future management. Lehman and colleagues [6] reviewed the interpretation of 82,620 screening mammograms and compared the assessment categories and accompanying recommendations to determine if they were in accordance with BI-RADS guidelines.

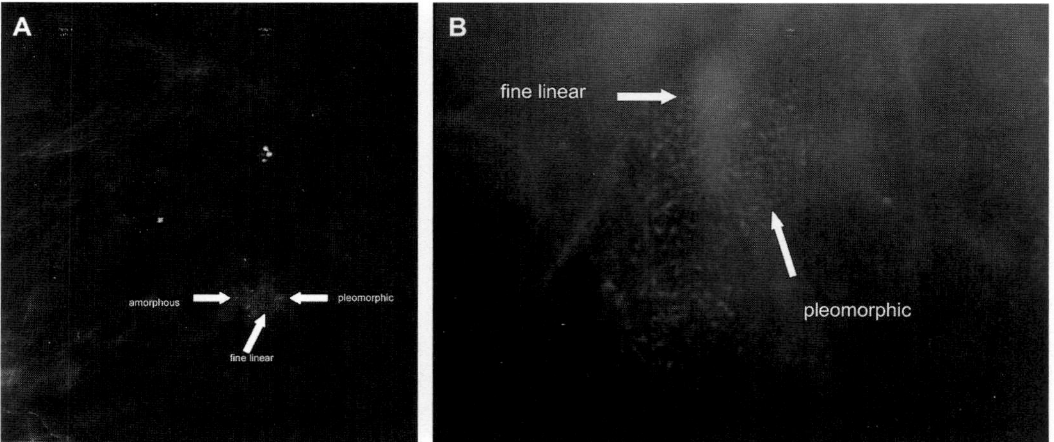

Fig. 6. Clusters of mixed calcification shapes. (*A*) Amorphous, pleomorphic, and a linear form of calcifications seen in the cluster. Pathology: DCIS. (*B*) Fine linear and pleomorphic calcifications in a clustered distribution. Pathology: DCIS.

Overall discordance between category and management was low (3%); however, the assessment category with the highest discordance was "Category 3 – probably benign finding – initial short-term follow-up recommended," at 54%. Thirty three percent of findings placed in Category 3 were managed by normal interval follow-up, 12% were managed with additional views, and 3.5% were managed with biopsy. It is important to underscore two points regarding findings assigned to this category. First, each finding should have less than a 2% chance of malignancy as confirmed by evidence-based literature [7–10]. This category is not the same as an indeterminate ranking that may be given for receiver operating characteristic curve analysis, which implies a relatively equal chance of a finding proving to be benign or malignant. The second important point is to assign findings to this category only after appropriate diagnostic workup. This also is true for Categories 4 and 5. Several studies [7–10] validated the principle of short-term follow-up (Category 3) and demonstrated a malignancy rate ranging from 0.3% to 1.7%. Malignancies discovered subsequently in this category, secondary to change during the follow-up period, still carry a favorable prognosis. All investigators exclude the use of Category 3 for palpable lesions associated with probably benign findings; however, there are recent data [11] to suggest that palpable breast masses, benign in appearance at mammography and ultrasound, can be managed in a fashion similar to nonpalpable Category 3 lesions. In 108 patients with 112 lesions, no malignancy was found after a minimum of 2-year follow-up; however,

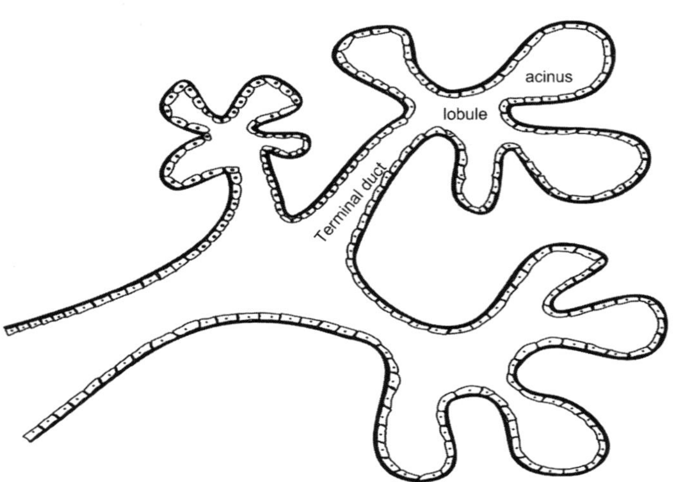

Fig. 7. Terminal ductal lobular unit, composed of the lobule, acini, and the terminal duct, where malignancy originates. Thus, fine linear calcifications or calcifications of other individual morphology in a linear distribution are especially worrisome for malignancy.

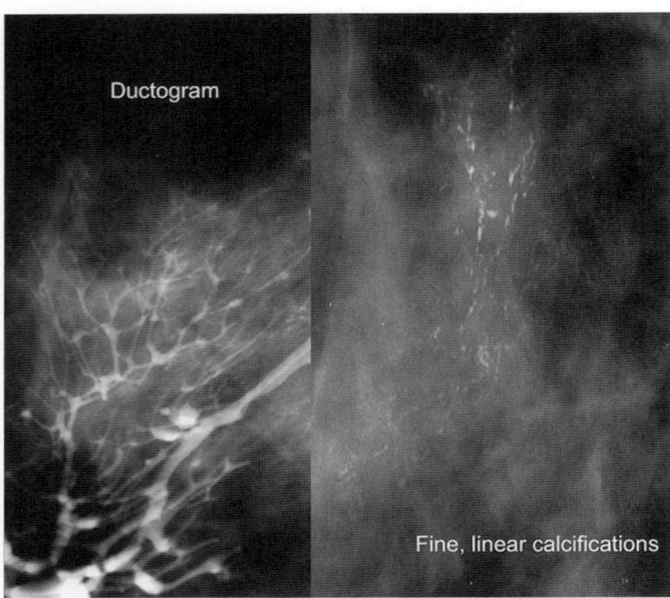

Fig. 8. Segmental distribution. A normal ductogram demonstrating the arborization of the ductal system. This appearance is closely mimicked by the segmental distribution of the fine linear calcifications. Pathology: DCIS.

these data must be validated with a larger series of patients.

The reassignment of a finding from a probably benign category to a benign category requires more than the initial 6-month follow-up. Sickles [7] described a follow-up protocol for these findings that extended 3 to 3.5 years from initiation of an initial short-term follow-up. He found that all but one of the cancers was discovered by change that occurred within 2 years of follow-up (Fig. 11). A finding that is stable upon 2 years of follow-up is unlikely to represent a cancer, and at that time, the patient can be returned to Category 2 status. Because the experience and expertise of readers varies greatly, a finding placed into Category 3 by one

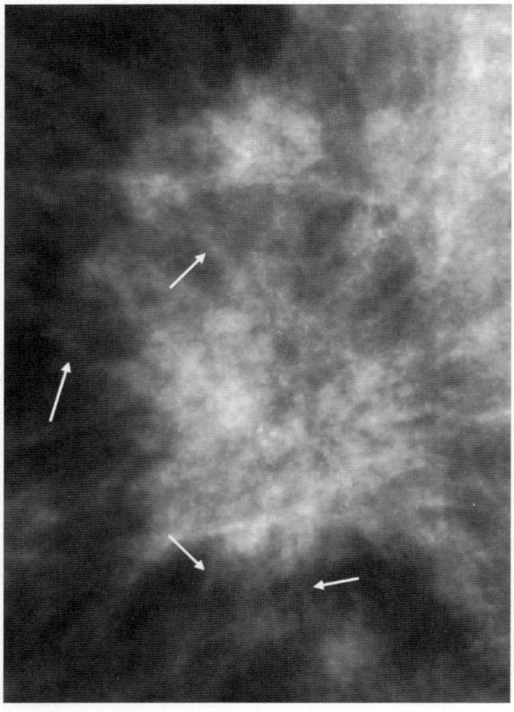

Fig. 9. Architectural distortion. Multiple radiating spicules (*arrows*) that do not converge to the edge of a definable mass.

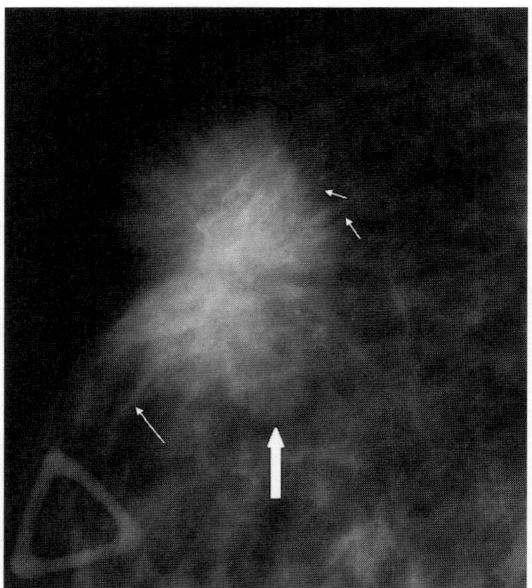

Fig. 10. Spiculated mass. Radiating spicules (*small arrows*) are seen to diverge for the edge (*large arrow*) of a mass.

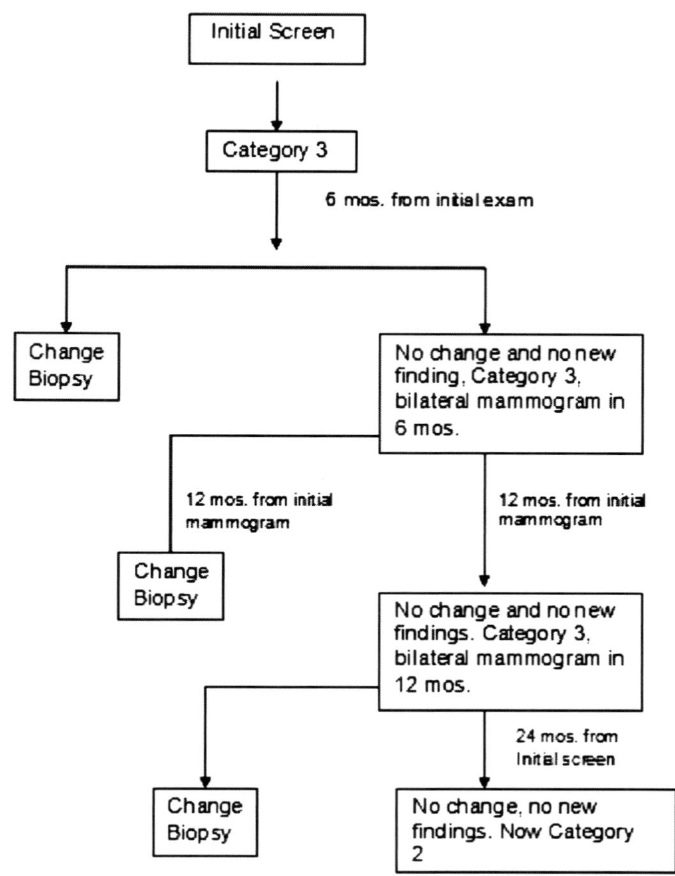

Fig. 11. Algorithm for follow-up of findings placed in "Category 3, short-term follow-up."

reader may be changed to a Category 2 or 4 by a more experienced reader before the 2 years of follow-up.

Category 0 originally was meant to indicate a recall from a screening mammogram for women requiring further imaging analysis; however, software vendors may include the request for a prior examination or a technical recall as Category 0. It is imperative to realize that these latter "recalls" should not be entered into an audit as a recall. Many users have questioned the use of Category 0 to request prior examinations. The request for prior examinations is not always required, especially when there are no findings of concern. In a study by Bassett and colleagues [12], prior films changed clinical management in approximately 3% of cases, showing little effect on cancer detection, but having a bigger impact on avoiding unnecessary recalls. In a more recent article by Roelofs and colleagues [13], the presence of prior mammograms helped in the analysis of questionable findings but had no effect on initial detection. This reinforces the request for prior studies only when the radiologist deems it necessary. Some users may prefer not to dictate a case for which prior films are required, but rather wait until they are received or not received in a predetermined time frame. This obviates separating this Category 0 from the audit; however, one must keep track of these cases to ensure that the report is sent out by the 30-day US Food and Drug Administration (FDA) limit, whether prior films are reviewed or not. Others prefer to dictate a report using Category 0 to indicate a request for prior films, which can be awkward when the software generates a clinical report; however, these studies are now entered into a mammography module and are easily tracked. If prior films are received, an additional "no charge" request can be made and another report generated indicating comparison to prior examinations. If no prior films are received, again a "no charge" request can be generated and appropriate findings can be evaluated with a second Category 0 assigned, which now relates to the need for a diagnostic workup rather than a request for prior examinations. With the advent of the MR imaging and ultrasound lexicons, Category 0 also may be used in a diagnostic setting, although this is done infrequently. One scenario may involve a screen/diagnostic center with no ultrasound or MR imaging capabilities. A finding may be evaluated fully by mammography but still require an MR imaging or ultrasound. This examination, although diagnostic, would receive a Category 0 for further imaging.

Categories 4, 5, and 6 are fairly straightforward but deserve some clarification. Category 4 may be subdivided into 4a (low suspicion for malignancy; Fig. 12), 4b (intermediate suspicion for malignancy; Fig. 13), and 4c (moderate concern but not classic for malignancy; Fig. 14). This new set of subdivisions addresses the fact that Category 4 encompasses a broad variety of findings, from complicated cysts at one extreme to irregular indistinct masses at the other extreme, with a consequent uncomfortably broad range in likelihood of malignancy (3% to 94%). By subdividing Category 4, internal audits will be more precise, research is facilitated, and clinically, physicians will understand that these subdivisions deliver different rates of malignancy and are not surprised if biopsy of a Category 4a finding yields a benign diagnosis. In a recent publication by Lazarus and colleagues [14], validation of the subdivisions was demonstrated. Ninety-four lesions were analyzed, and a pathologic diagnosis was available for all. The PPV for Category 4a, 4b, 4c, and 5 were 6%, 15%, 53%, and 91%, respectively. One important caveat to remember is the unofficial nature of these subdivisions. These are suggested and are for internal use only. If you wish to include them on the official report, the FDA mandates that the standard Category 4 language be present ("suspicious abnormality – biopsy should be considered"); however, it may be amended by the previously mentioned subdivisions. For example, if a complicated cyst is recommended for aspiration, the assessment may properly state: "Category 4 – suspicious abnormality – biopsy should be considered, 4a – low suspicion for malignancy." The report, however, may not read "Category 4a – low suspicion for malignancy – cyst aspiration recommended." Although the latter assessment may make more sense, it will take up to

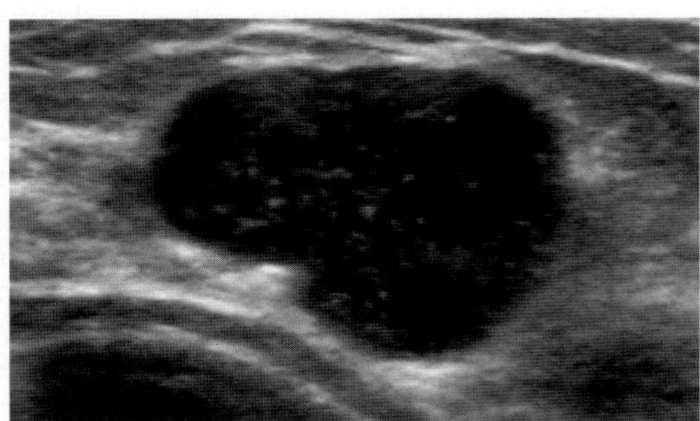

Fig. 12. Category 4A – low suspicion. Circumscribed mass, with moving internal echoes identified at real-time investigation, compatible with a complicated cyst.

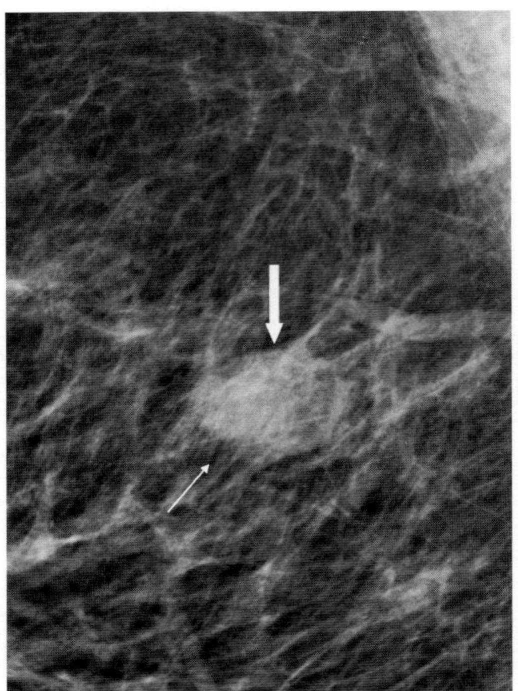

Fig. 13. Category 4B – intermediate suspicion. Partially circumscribed (*large arrow*) and partially indistinct (*small arrow*) solid mass.

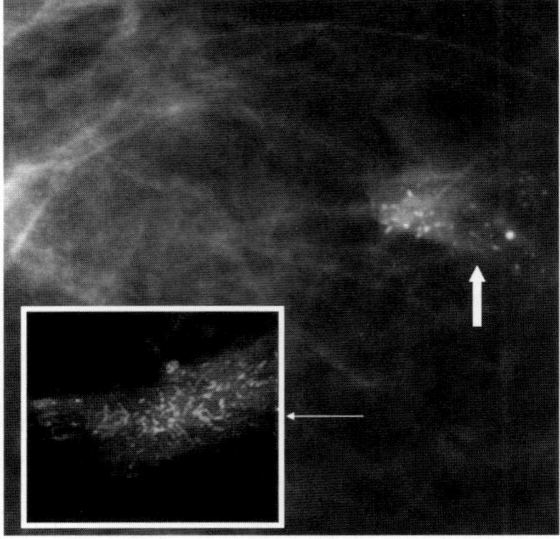

Fig. 14. Category 4C – Moderate suspicion, but not classic for malignancy. Cluster of pleomorphic calcifications (*large arrow*). Compare with inset (*small arrow*) of a segmental arrangement of predominantly fine linear calcifications, which should be placed in "Category 5 – highly suggestive of malignancy."

3 to 4 years to undergo the FDA approval process to incorporate these subdivisions into regulation.

At first, Category 5 seems to be redundant. This category was developed at the request of surgical members of the first BI-RADS committee and was meant to define lesions with at least a 95% chance of malignancy, for which a one-stage surgical procedure without prior biopsy could be considered. This category should be reconsidered at this point, because the original intent of its inclusion may not be as widely applicable today.

Category 6 is reserved for biopsy-proven malignancy before definitive therapy and is not used for audit purposes. If a facility performs a study for a second opinion that has a biopsy-proven malignancy but an additional finding requiring further imaging is identified, this case should receive a BI-RADS 0 and not a BI-RADS 6 assessment. If the only finding on the second-opinion examination is the known biopsy-proven malignancy, then a BI-RADS Category 6 assessment is appropriate.

The BI-RADS committee is actively discussing management and coding issues not covered directly in the fourth edition of BI-RADS. One question that many users have identified is "Which BI-RADS category should be assigned when a palpable mass is present but imaging is negative?" BI-RADS is an imaging lexicon and if imaging is negative, even in the face of a clinical finding, the examination should be coded as "Category 1 – negative." Obviously, direction regarding further management of the clinical finding should be included in the report. For example, a notation that the area of clinical concern should be dealt with independently from the mammogram may be included. The scenario becomes a little more complicated when a palpable and imaging finding coincide. The imaging finding should drive the management category. Thus, if a simple cyst is seen at the site of a clinical finding, it would be a Category 2 for imaging; however, the clinician may opt to aspirate the cyst clinically.

Another problematic area concerning coding and management is detection of findings that are not part of the breast, but are seen on breast-imaging studies. For example, one may detect bilateral axillary adenopathy. How is this coded? Is it ignored? The BI-RADS committee is in the process of discussing the options available, ranging from an additional assessment category to use of existing categories. For example, using existing categories, if there is a known benign reason for the adenopathy (eg, sarcoid, rheumatoid arthritis), this may be coded as a BI-RADS Category 2. If further imaging is required (eg, ultrasound, MR imaging), this may be a Category 0. If biopsy is needed, a Category 4 can be used; if the woman has a known lymphoma or leukemia, a Category 6 can be used. With this scenario, the coding depends much more on the combination of the history and the imaging findings.

The BI-RADS committee also is discussing breast density. There is evidence in the literature that mammographic accuracy may range from 98% in fatty breasts to as low as 64% to 70% in dense breasts [15–17]. To provide a better sense of the amount of fat and glandular tissue present, which affects sensitivity and is an independent risk factor for malignancy, consideration of using more precisely defined percentages of fibroglandular tissue, within the current broad density categories, is under consideration. "Almost entirely fat" would be up to and including 10% density, instead of the current range of 0% to 25%. "Scattered fibroglandular densities" might then range from 11% to 50% density but could be subdivided into two categories: 11% to 25% density might be described as "few scattered areas" and 26% to 50% as "moderate scattered areas." "Heterogeneously dense" currently is defined as 51% to 75% glandular, but modifiers may be added to describe where the densest area resides (eg, dense tissue located anteriorly or in the upper outer quadrants). "Extremely dense" would remain at 76% to 100%. Although these changes may be construed as unnecessary, the relative amounts of fibroglandular tissue and fat define mammographic sensitivity, may be helpful in the medicolegal arena, and may facilitate research concerning the risk for malignancy related to mammographic density.

This exercise may not be necessary after the widespread adoption of digital mammography. Computer programs are being developed that are able to analyze pixel gray levels and then determine the percentage of fibroglandular tissue by dividing the number of dense pixels by the total number of pixels. This technique was used to compare radiologists' estimates of breast density with that of a computer [18]. The computer-generated estimate compared favorably with the radiologists' estimates of percent-density; however, more interesting and important was the superior reproducibility of the computer program with little overlap of the categories, as occurred with the qualitative assessment of the radiologists.

Audit

Although the audit section is fairly straightforward, some points of clarification deserve mention. The major metrics used for a breast audit (sensitivity, specificity, and PPV) all use true positive (TP), false positive (FP), true negative (TN), and false negative (FN) terminology. A positive mammogram is one that receives BI-RADS 0, 4, or 5, whereas a negative mammogram is one coded as 1, 2, or 3. Note again that Category 6 and Category 0 for prior studies or technical reasons are omitted for audit purposes. If cancer is found within a year from the mammogram, this is proof of malignancy; when no cancer is found in that same period, this constitutes no evidence for malignancy. Thus, BI-RADS 0, 4, or 5 with confirmation of cancer within the year represents a TP; lack of discovery of cancer is a FP. A BI-RADS assessment of 1, 2, or 3 with no cancer found within the year is a TN; if cancer is found, this is an FN. This is the foundation for all of the metrics described for auditing a practice.

Addition to the fourth edition of BI-RADS

An ultrasound and MR imaging lexicon have been added to the fourth edition of BI-RADS. With the advent of multiple lexicons, which may be used for a single patient, the features most associated with malignancy should influence the BI-RADS category chosen. Because most, if not all, radiologists involved with breast imaging are using a computer-based dedicated tracking module, it is important to realize the hierarchy of the assessments as they relate to immediate, intermediate, or routine action. This understanding will be helpful when using all three lexicons within a computer-based breast-imaging module. Categories 5, 4, and 0 require immediate action and will be ordered from the most to least chance of malignancy in computer modules (ie, 5, 4, 0). Category 3 indicates intermediate action (6-month initial short-term follow-up) and Categories 1 and 2 are routine. Thus, the hierarchy that all of the lexicons will use is 5, 4, 0, 3, 2, and 1, from the highest to the lowest possibility for malignancy and from findings requiring immediate action to examinations needing only routine action. Although there may be many scenarios that could arise when intertwining the lexicons on a single patient, some examples may help to clarify this association. A woman may come for a diagnostic mammogram because of the presence of a palpable mass; the mammogram workup views are negative, but the ultrasound done on the same day shows an irregular solid mass. When using all of the lexicons, the final code would be "Category 4, biopsy suggested." This would be the patient's final management category and would appear on the report, whether or not the palpable mass coincides with the ultrasound finding. If there is no imaging finding in the area of clinical concern this can be handled by a statement indicating that the area of clinical concern should be managed independently of the imaging examinations. Thus, even though a Category 1 assessment would be appropriate for the mammogram because these modules are hierarchical in nature, only the most worrisome would be coded for that patient (ie, Category 4 for the ultrasound instead of Category 1 for the mammogram).

A problem arises when an imaging examination is negative but another imaging examination is needed. For example, a diagnostic mammogram for a woman with implants demonstrates a contour change on an implant. This should be a "0" and perhaps ultrasound requested to determine if there is capsular rupture not identified on the mammogram. If the ultrasound examination is negative, it should be given a Category 1; however, MR imaging would be the next logical imaging examination. This can be handled in the body of the report by stating that although ultrasound is negative, an MR imaging is more precise to identify intracapsular rupture. In this way, correct imaging codes are given, and the additional imaging is recommended in the report. The problem here is because Category 1 is entered with the ultrasound examination, there is no way to record or remind the patient and clinician of the requested MR imaging examination. We could use Category 0 for the ultrasound and request MR imaging. In this way, it would be recorded in the computer and reminders could be sent out automatically until the outstanding "0" is closed by the assessment from the MR imaging examination; however, the ultrasound examination is negative and does not fit with the associated recommendation. These points are being addressed actively by the BI-RADS committee. For the present, it is probably better to assess such examinations based on their imaging findings and explain in the report the need for any other imaging examination.

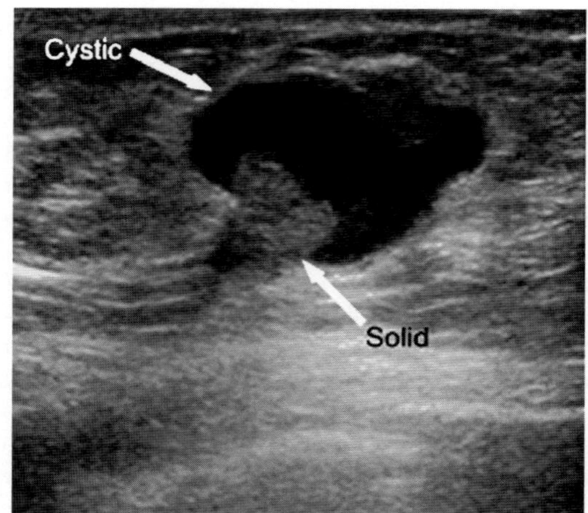

Fig. 15. Complex mass. Circumscribed mass with solid and cystic components (*arrows*). Pathology: intracystic papillary carcinoma.

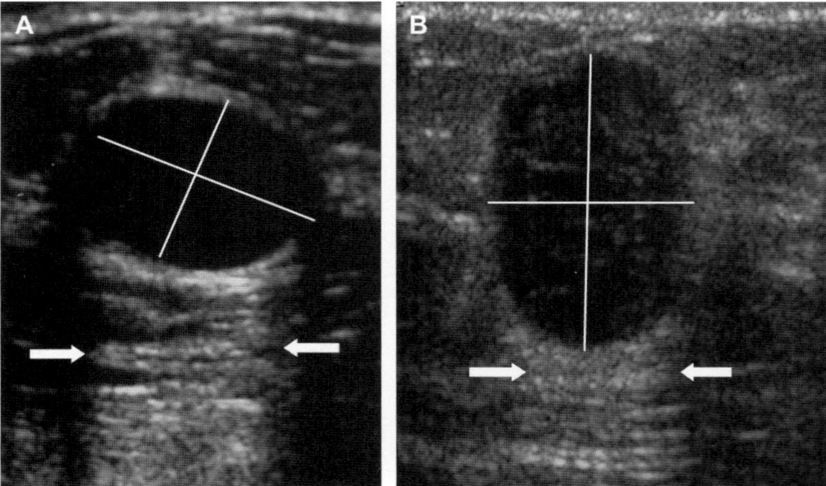

Fig. 16. Ultrasound mass orientation. (*A*) Anechoic circumscribed mass with parallel orientation (wider than tall). Simple cyst. (*B*) Hypoechoic mass with abrupt transition and nonparallel orientation (taller than wide). Mucinous carcinoma. Note the acoustic enhancement posterior to the simple cyst and present, to a lesser extent, behind the mucinous carcinoma (*arrows*).

Ultrasound/MR imaging lexicons

This final section focuses on some of the features that are unique to ultrasound and MR imaging.

"Background echotexture" is the sonographic term that best corresponds to mammographic density. A homogeneous echotexture may be composed almost entirely of fat lobules or echogenic tissue (ie, fibroglandular). A heterogeneous echotexture is a mixture of these echogenicities. Echogenicity is described using fat in the subdermal layer of the breast as an internal reference and as the midpoint between hypo- and hyperechoic. Findings with greater echogenicity are hyperechoic, those with a similar echogenicity are isoechoic, and those with less echogenicity are hypoechoic. Findings with no echogenicity are anechoic. In general, anechoic and hyperechoic masses are benign, whereas hypoechoic masses may represent benign or malignant findings. Masses that contain anechoic and fixed (hyper- or hypo-) echogenic components are termed complex masses (Fig. 15). Masses with a mixture of movable internal echoes and interspersed anechoic areas are termed complicated cysts. At times, it may be difficult to differentiate a complicated cyst from a hypoechoic mass.

The ultrasound properties posterior to a mass, as well as its orientation, are important to realize and comment upon. If there is an increase in echogenicity directly posterior to a mass compared with the adjacent posterior tissues, this is an indication that the energy of the sound beam has been maintained passing through the mass, producing posterior acoustic enhancement. This is seen frequently in cystic lesions. The reverse is true when the sound beam passes through a solid mass with many energy-absorbing interfaces, producing a weaker beam behind the mass, which is displayed as acoustic shadowing. A mass that is taller than it is wide is more suspicious than one that is wider than it is tall (nonparallel versus parallel orientation) (Fig. 16).

Breast MR imaging adds physiologic information in the form of vascular flow to that of morphology. Basically, MR-sensitive contrast agents are used to enhance T1-weighted signals. This enhancement is

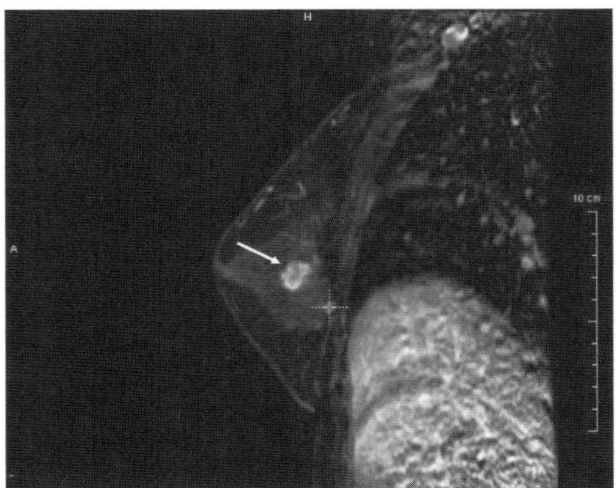

Fig. 17. MR mass enhancement. Rim-enhancing mass (*arrow*), suggestive of malignancy. Pathology: infiltrating ductal carcinoma. Cursor overlies synchronous cancer.

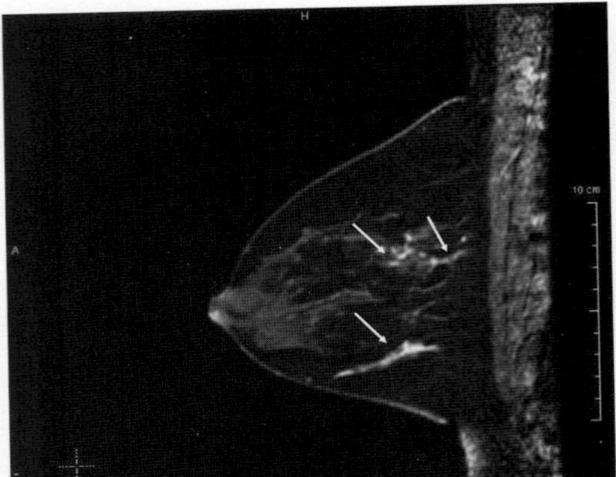

Fig. 18. Nonmass-like enhancement, linear. Arrows demonstrate separate areas of linear enhancement. Both areas were biopsy-proven DCIS.

in proportion to the increased vessel density and leakage of contrast from abnormal tumor vessels, which do not contain all of the layers of normal vessels. Thus, the unique terminology here relates to signal enhancement after the use of contrast agents. The enhancement within a mass may be homogenous (uniform enhancement) or heterogeneous (nonuniform). Within the heterogeneous group, there is mass enhancement that may be preferentially in the periphery (rim) (Fig. 17) or have nonenhancing septations, or have central enhancement. Enhancement also may be nonmass-like, with a distribution terminology similar to that of calcification distributions. A focal area of enhancement occupies less than 25% of a quadrant. Linear enhancement is enhancement in a line but not definitely in a ductal distribution (Fig. 18), whereas ductal enhancement also is linear but points toward the nipple and may have branching. Segmental

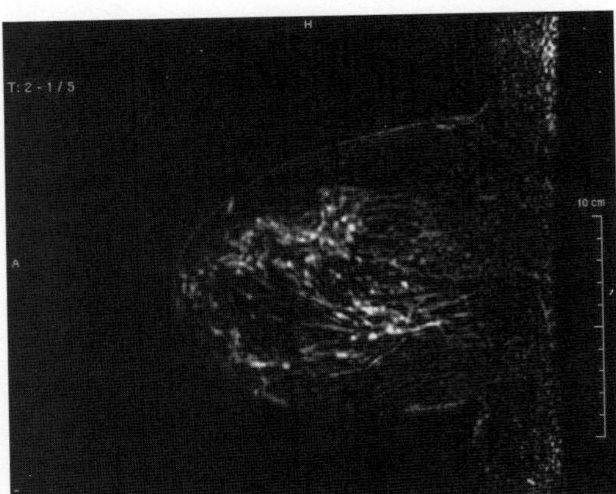

Fig. 19. Nonmass-like enhancement, diffuse stippled. Multiple scattered small foci of enhancement. Benign parenchymal tissue.

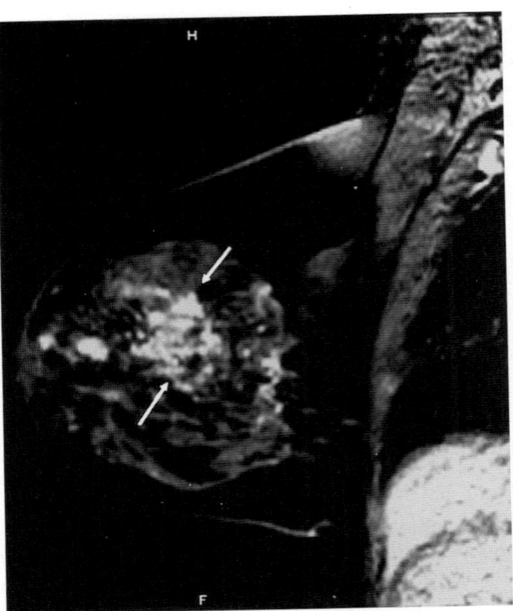

Fig. 20. Nonmass-like enhancement, regional. Clumped "cobblestone" appearance of enhancing areas (*arrows*). Pathology: extensive infiltrating lobular carcinoma.

enhancement is triangular in shape, with its apex pointing toward the nipple. Regional enhancement involves a large volume, whereas diffuse or scattered enhancement is distributed uniformly throughout the breast. The enhancement within these distributions may be homogeneous, stippled (small punctate) (Fig. 19), clumped (cobblestone-like) (Fig. 20), or reticular (strandlike).

Another unique enhancement feature relates to the intensity of enhancement of a mass or region over time. The faster the enhancement of a mass or area and the faster that the increased signal later disappears (washout), the more worrisome is the finding for malignancy.

Thus, proper understanding and use of the ACR BI-RADS will promote the generation of standardized, clear, clinically useful reports and will facilitate breast-imaging research by allowing reproducible comparison of nationally and internationally collected data.

References

[1] Orel SG, Kay N, Reynolds C, et al. BI-RADS categorization as a predictor of malignancy. Radiology 1999;211:845–50.

[2] Liberman L, Abrams AF, Squires FB, et al. The breast imaging reporting and data system: positive predictive value of mammography features and final assessment categories. AJR Am J Roentgenol 1998;171:35–40.

[3] Berg WA, D'Orsi CJ, Jackson VP, et al. Does training in the breast imaging reporting and data system (BI-RADS) improve biopsy recommendation or feature analysis agreement with experienced breast imagers at mammography? Radiology 2002;224:871–80.
[4] Berg WA, Arnoldus CL, Teferra E, et al. Biopsy of amorphous breast calcifications: pathologic outcome and yield at stereotactic biopsy. Radiology 2001;221:495–503.
[5] Rosen PP. Rosen's breast pathology. 2nd edition. New York: Lippincott, Williams and Wilkins; 2001.
[6] Lehman C, Holt S, Peacock S, et al. Use of the American College of Radiology BI-RADS guidelines by community radiologists. AJR Am J Roentgenol 2002;179:15–20.
[7] Sickles EA. Periodic mammographic follow-up of probably benign lesions: results in 3,184 consecutive cases. Radiology 1991;179:463–8.
[8] Varas X, Leborgne F, Leborgne JH. Nonpalpable, probably benign lesions: role of follow-up mammography. Radiology 1992;184:409–14.
[9] Vizcaino I, Gadea L, Andreo L, et al. Short-term follow-up results in 795 nonpalpable probably benign lesions detected at screening mammography. Radiology 2001;219:475–83.
[10] Varas X, Leborgne F, Leborgne JH, et al. Revisiting the mammographic follow-up of BI-RADS category 3 lesions. AJR Am J Roentgenol 2002;179:691–5.
[11] Graf O, Helbich T, Fuchsjaeger M, et al. Follow-up of palpable circumscribed noncalcified solid breast masses at mammography and US: can biopsy be averted? Radiology 2004;233:850–6.
[12] Bassett LW, Shayestehfar B, Hirbawi I. Obtaining previous mammograms for comparison: usefulness and costs. AJR Am J Roentgenol 1994;163:1083–6.
[13] Roelofs AAJ, Karssemeijer N, Wedekind MS, et al. Importance of comparison of current and prior mammograms in breast cancer screening. Radiology 2007;242:70–7.
[14] Lazarus E, Mainiero MB, Schepps B, et al. BI-RADS lexicon for ultrasound and mammography: interobserver variability and positive predictive value. Radiology 2006;239:385–91.
[15] Kerlikowske K, Grady D, Barclay J, et al. Effect of age, breast density, and family history on the sensitivity of first screening mammography. JAMA 1996;276(1):22–38.
[16] Kolb T, Lichy J, Newhouse J. Comparison of the performance of screening mammography, physical examination, and breast ultrasound and evaluation of factors that influence them: an analysis of 27,825 patient evaluations. Radiology 2002;225:165–75.
[17] Berg WA, Gutierrez L, Ness Aiver MS, et al. Diagnostic accuracy of mammography, clinical examination, ultrasound, and MR imaging in preoperative assessment of breast cancer. Radiology 2004;233:830–49.
[18] Martin KE, Helvie MA, Zhou C, et al. Mammographic density measured with quantitative computer-aided method: comparison with radiologists' estimates and BI-RADS categories. Radiology 2006;240:656–65.

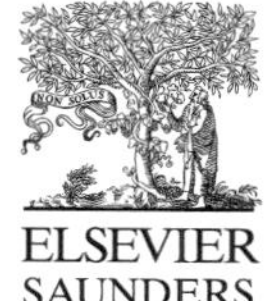

ELSEVIER
SAUNDERS

RADIOLOGIC
CLINICS
OF NORTH AMERICA

Radiol Clin N Am 45 (2007) 765–771

The Spectrum of Breast Asymmetries: Imaging Features, Work-Up, Management

Edward A. Sickles, MD

Right and left breast mammograms traditionally are displayed back-to-back, projection for projection, to facilitate the perception of areas of asymmetry (Fig. 1). This detection is advantageous because occasionally asymmetry may be the only manifestation of breast cancer on standard mammographic views [1–8]. The terminology used to describe breast asymmetries changed in 2003 with the publication by the American College of Radiology of the fourth edition of its Breast Imaging Reporting and Data System, commonly known as BI-RADS [9].

Types of asymmetry

There are four types of breast asymmetry (Table 1), all of which represent areas of fibroglandular-density tissue that is more extensive in one breast than the other. Asymmetry usually is distinguished from mass in that it demonstrates concave-outward rather than the convex-outward contours typical of a mass and is interspersed with fat rather than appearing denser in the center than at the periphery, as is typical of a mass.

Asymmetry (formerly called "density") is an area of fibroglandular-density tissue that is visible on only one of the two standard mammographic views (Fig. 2). Summation artifact, which accounts for approximately 80% of cases of one-view-only asymmetry, is caused by the superimposition of normal fibroglandular breast structures on a given mammographic projection [3,10]. Therefore this finding is not visible on additional views taken in different projections, although in many cases one can characterize an asymmetry as summation artifact reliably without the need for additional mammographic views [3]. It is important to distinguish summation artifact from the other types of asymmetry described later, because it never represents breast cancer and never should be subjected to biopsy.

Global asymmetry (formerly called "asymmetric breast tissue") represents a substantially greater volume of fibroglandular tissue in one breast than in the corresponding location in the opposite breast, occupying at least one quadrant of the breast, without an associated mass, microcalcifications, or architectural distortion (Fig. 3) [9]. It has been reported to occur in approximately 3% of mammography examinations [11]. It almost always represents a normal variant, but occasionally it may indicate the presence of an underlying breast cancer

Department of Radiology, University of California San Francisco School of Medicine, University of California San Francisco Medical Center, Box 1677, San Francisco, CA 94143-1667, USA
E-mail address: edward.sickles@ucsfmedctr.org

0033-8389/07/$ – see front matter
doi:10.1016/j.rcl.2007.06.002
radiologic.theclinics.com

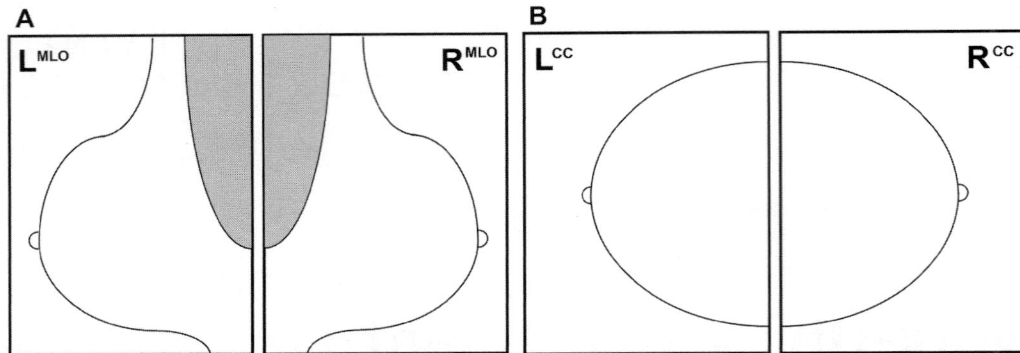

Fig. 1. Line drawings of standard mammographic views displayed back-to-back to facilitate the perception of areas of asymmetry. (*A*) Mediolateral oblique views. (*B*) Craniocaudal views. It is a matter of personal preference whether paired images are displayed with the right breast facing right (as shown) or with the right breast facing left.

if it corresponds to a palpable abnormality [11]. In this latter clinical setting, the radiologist usually recalls the patient for additional imaging evaluation.

Focal asymmetry (formerly called "focal asymmetric density") is a smaller asymmetry of fibroglandular-tissue density, visible on at least two different mammographic projections but lacking the convex-outward contours and conspicuity of a mass (Fig. 4). By definition, it occupies a volume of less than one quadrant of the breast, to distinguish it from global asymmetry [9]. A focal asymmetry usually represents an island of normal dense breast tissue, but its lack of specific benign characteristics may warrant further evaluation, especially if it is not interspersed with fat. The frequency of occurrence of focal asymmetry at screening mammography is less than 1% [4–8]. In a retrospective study of 300 consecutive nonpalpable breast cancers, 3% were identified as focal asymmetries [2]. The likelihood of malignancy among findings characterized as focal asymmetry (without associated mass, calcifications, architectural distortion, sonographic abnormality, or palpable correlate), for which previous mammograms are not available to assess for stability, is less than 1% [4–8].

Developing asymmetry (formerly called "developing density" or "neodensity") is a focal asymmetry that is new, larger, or denser on current examination than previously (Fig. 5). To identify such a lesion, prior mammograms must be available for comparison. There is little difficulty distinguishing developing asymmetry from the increase in dense breast tissue seen in postmenopausal women undergoing hormone therapy, because developing asymmetry

***Table 1:* The four types of breast asymmetry identified at mammography**

Type of asymmetry	Description[a]	Frequency	Likelihood of malignancy	References
Asymmetry	Visible on only one standard view	2023/61,273 (3.3%)	36/2023 (1.8%)[b]	[3]
Global asymmetry	At least one breast quadrant	221/8048 (2.7%)	Nonpalpable: 0/181 (0%) Palpable: 3/40 (7.5%)[c]	[11]
Focal asymmetry	Less than one breast quadrant	741/85,188 (0.87%)	5/741 (0.67%)	[4–8]
Developing asymmetry	New, increasing, or more dense	292/180,801 (0.16%)	36/281 (12.8%)[d]	[14]

[a] See text for complete description.
[b] Although the overall likelihood of malignancy for a one-view asymmetry is slightly less than 2%, such findings should not be assessed as probably benign (BI-RADS category 3). Approximately 80% of such findings are readily and reliably identified as summation artifact either at screening mammography or at recall for diagnostic mammography; hence, these findings do not require short-interval follow-up [3]. The likelihood of malignancy for the remaining (real) lesions is 36/350 (10.3%). This percentage is far greater than the upper limit of 2% that is appropriate for probably benign lesions [9].
[c] In palpable global asymmetry lesions that are biopsied, the frequency of malignancy is reported to be 3/20 (15%) [11].
[d] The likelihood of malignancy of developing asymmetry at diagnostic mammography is reported to be 8/30 (26.7%) [14].

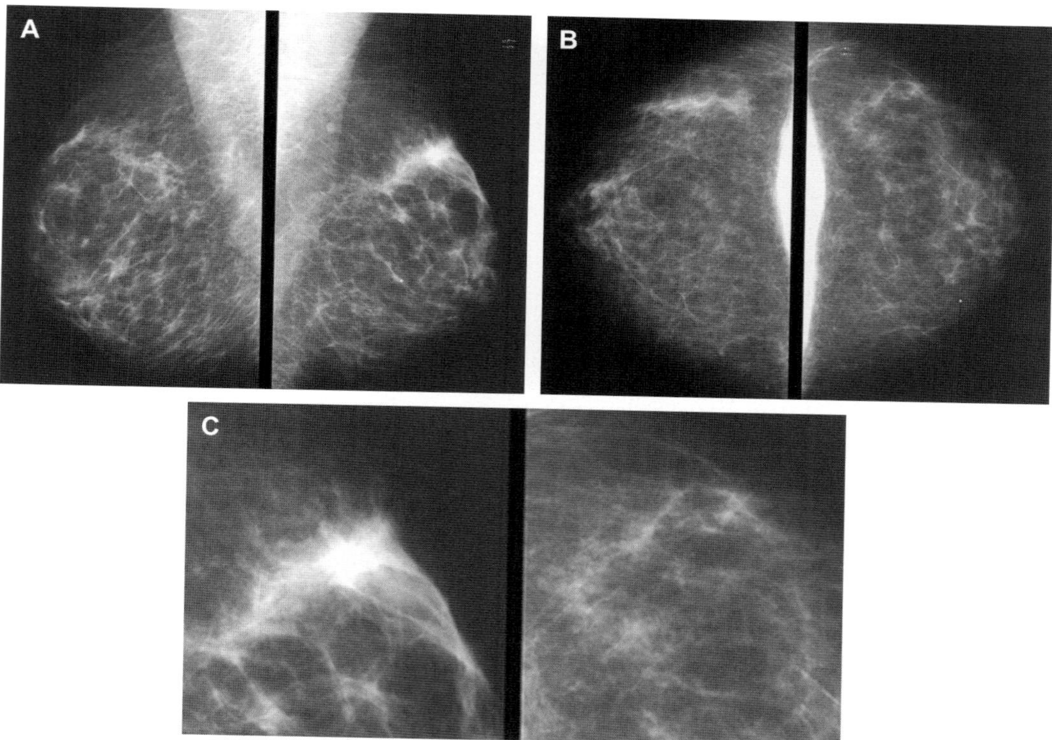

Fig. 2. Asymmetry. (*A*) Paired mediolateral oblique views. (*B*) Paired craniocaudal views. (*C*) Enlarged areas of the superior and lateral aspects of the breast facing right. Note the area of asymmetric dense fibroglandular tissue in the superior aspect of one breast, seen only on the mediolateral oblique view. Because this finding is seen only on one of the two standard mammographic views, it is properly termed an asymmetry.

is unilateral and focal, whereas hormone therapy–related change usually is bilateral and global [12,13]. Developing asymmetry is an uncommon mammographic finding, reported as occurring in less than 1% of examinations [14]. In the same retrospective study of 300 consecutive nonpalpable breast cancers, however, 6% were identified as developing asymmetry [2]. The likelihood of malignancy among findings characterized as developing asymmetry ranges from 13% to 27%, depending on whether the lesion is identified at screening mammography or at diagnostic mammography [14].

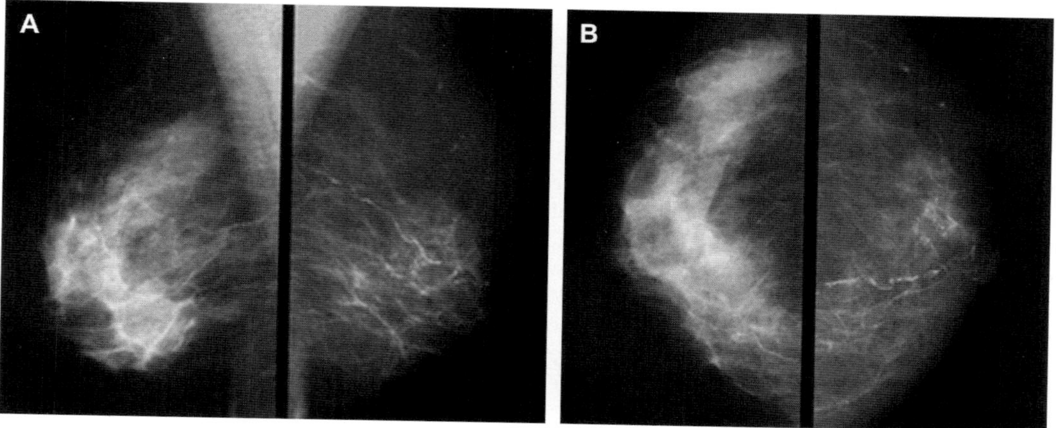

Fig. 3. Global asymmetry. (*A*) Paired mediolateral oblique views. (*B*) Paired craniocaudal views. The breast facing left is substantially denser than the breast facing right. Basic to the definition of global asymmetry is that the difference in asymmetric dense fibroglandular tissue involves a volume occupying at least one quadrant of the breast. In addition, as seen in this case, there is no associated mass, microcalcifications, or architectural distortion.

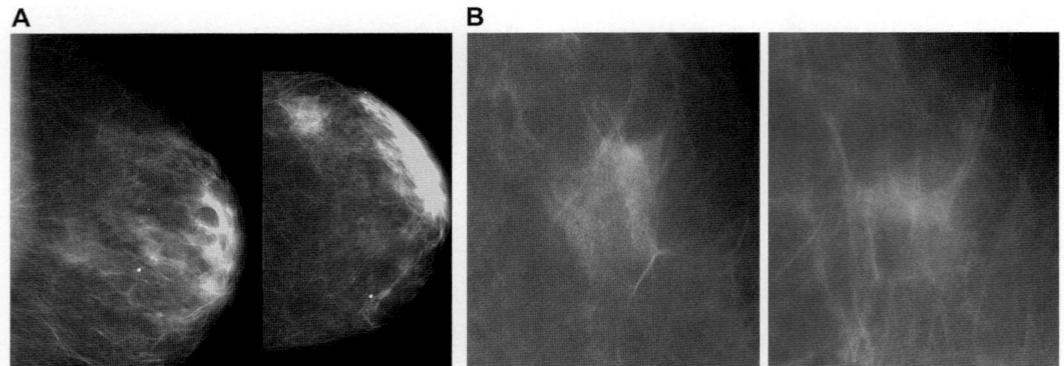

Fig. 4. Focal asymmetry. (*A*) Mediolateral oblique and craniocaudal views. There is an area of asymmetric dense fibroglandular tissue in the posterior third of the lower outer quadrant (lateral to nipple level on craniocaudal view, at nipple level on mediolateral oblique view, and hence triangulated to be located below nipple level if a mediolateral view were obtained). No similar finding was visible in the contralateral breast (not shown). Basic to the definition of focal asymmetry is that the difference in asymmetric dense fibroglandular tissue involves a volume occupying less than one quadrant of the breast. (*B*) Enlarged areas of mediolateral oblique and craniocaudal views of a different focal asymmetry. Note the concave-outward contours of the focal asymmetry and that it is interspersed with fat. These typical features of focal asymmetry also are apparent for the focal asymmetry illustrated in panel A.

Medical history

The presence of a palpable correlate to a global asymmetry, focal asymmetry, or developing asymmetry raises concern that breast cancer may account for some (perhaps all) of the asymmetric dense tissue seen at mammography. Therefore, the radiologist should check the medical history form (intake sheet) completed by the patient or technologist and the request for service provided by the referring clinician to search for the report of a palpable lesion in the same or similar location as the mammographic finding. If such a palpable correlate is reported, or if the technologist places a radiopaque marker over a palpable finding that corresponds to the asymmetry, the radiologist usually recalls the patient for additional imaging evaluation.

Assessment at screening mammography

In addition to the presence of a palpable correlate, several associated mammographic findings raise concern that breast cancer may underlie a global asymmetry, focal asymmetry, or developing asymmetry. These findings include microcalcifications, architectural distortion, and mass. If even one of these associated mammographic findings is visible at screening mammography within or adjacent to the asymmetry, the radiologist usually recalls the patient for additional imaging evaluation.

In some cases, it is possible to assess an area of asymmetric dense fibroglandular tissue confidently as representing summation artifact. This assessment usually takes place when (1) the area of asymmetric dense tissue is visible on only one of the two standard mammographic views; (2) the area of asymmetric dense tissue is sufficiently anterior to the chest wall (as seen on the view on which it is visible) that it must be included in the image field on the other standard view; and (3) the breast is sufficiently fatty in content that, on the standard view not showing an asymmetry, there is no concern about substantial additional dense tissue obscuring the asymmetry. If the radiologist can confidently characterize an asymmetry as representing summation artifact at screening mammography, the examination should be assessed as negative (BI-RADS category 1), with a recommendation for routine mammographic screening in 1 year. Using this approach to screening mammography interpretation, the examination displayed in Fig. 2 may be assessed as negative without the need for additional mammographic views.

Global asymmetry should not be confused with summation artifact because it always is visible on both standard mammographic views (by definition it is so large that it occupies at least a quadrant, and portions of each breast quadrant are included in the image field of both standard mammographic views). The definition of global asymmetry also excludes any associated mammographic findings (microcalcifications, architectural distortion, mass). Therefore, it is exceedingly unlikely that a nonpalpable global asymmetry represents breast cancer, because a malignancy so large as to occupy an entire quadrant should be palpable either as a mass or large area of thickening. This near-zero likelihood of malignancy is the reason uncomplicated

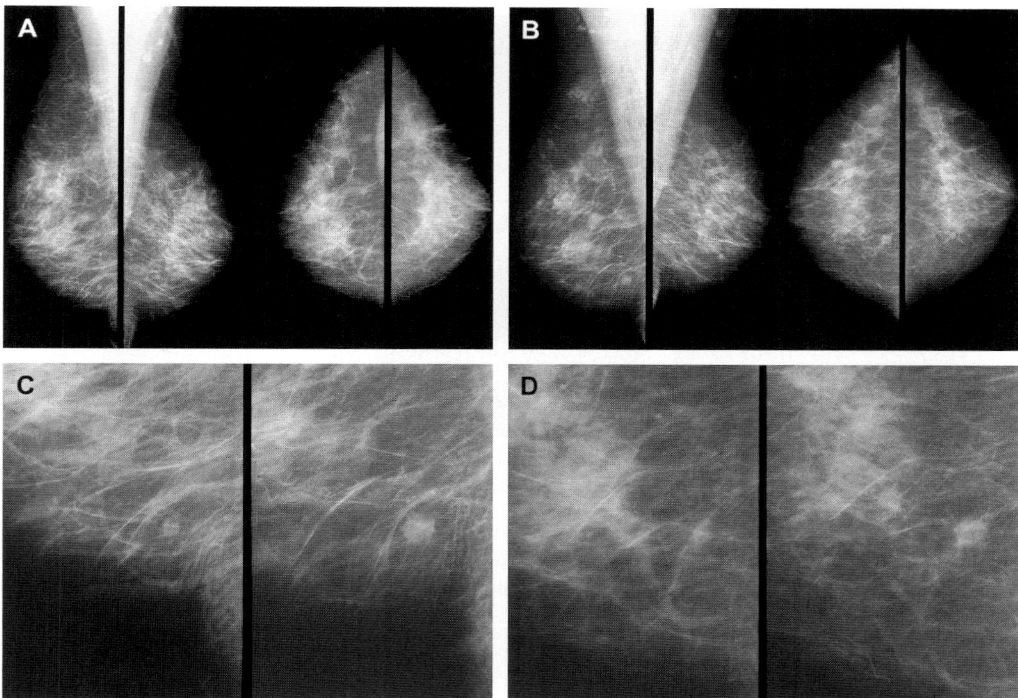

Fig. 5. Developing asymmetry. (*A*) Paired mediolateral oblique and paired craniocaudal views of a previous mammography examination. (*B*) Paired mediolateral oblique and paired craniocaudal views of the current mammography examination. (*C*) Enlarged areas of the mediolateral oblique views of the previous and current examinations of the breast facing left. (*D*) Enlarged areas of the craniocaudal views of the previous and current examinations of the breast facing left. There is a developing asymmetry (enlarging focal asymmetry) in the posterior third of the lower inner quadrant of the breast facing left. Note the concave-outward contours and interspersed fat that distinguish this developing asymmetry from an enlarging mass.

global asymmetry usually is regarded as a normal variant and does not require recall for additional imaging evaluation.

Additional imaging evaluation

If additional imaging evaluation is performed to assess an asymmetry further, the first step should be to differentiate between summation artifact and true lesion. If the asymmetry is no longer seen on repeat images taken in the same or similar mammographic projections (including shallow oblique views or roll views, with or without spot compression and/or magnification) to those on which it was initially visible, the radiologist can make a confident diagnosis of summation artifact, render a negative assessment (BI-RADS category 1), and recommend routine mammographic screening in one year (Fig. 6).

For findings that prove to be real, the next step should be to triangulate the three-dimensional location precisely on orthogonal (usually craniocaudal and 90° lateral) mammographic views. This measure permits accurate placement of a spot-compression paddle for additional standard or magnification views, to define more clearly the morphology of the underlying lesion and specifically to search for the associated findings of microcalcifications, architectural distortion, or an underlying mass. Precise triangulation also permits targeted breast ultrasound examination in search for a sonographic or palpable correlate to the mammographic finding.

A role for MR imaging of breast asymmetries has not yet been established, but the major strength of MR imaging is its high sensitivity in identifying malignancy, whereas its major limitation is relatively low specificity, a substantial limitation given the low likelihood of malignancy among all types of asymmetry (see Table 1).

Management of asymmetry after full imaging evaluation

Unless a definitive benign diagnosis (eg, simple cyst as seen at ultrasound) can be given for a palpable asymmetry, the standard recommendation is tissue diagnosis, because of the considerably greater than

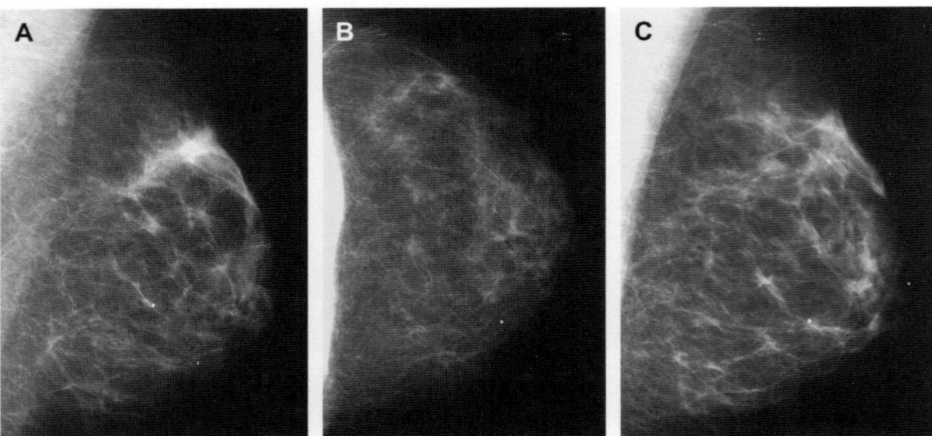

Fig. 6. Asymmetry demonstrated to be summation artifact (same case as shown in Fig. 2). (*A*) Mediolateral oblique view shows a noncalcified asymmetry in the superior aspect of the breast. (*B*) No corresponding finding is seen on the craniocaudal view of the same breast. (*C*) Repeat mediolateral oblique view obtained at a slightly different angle of obliquity (48° instead of 46°) no longer shows the asymmetry. Disappearance of an asymmetry on a shallow-oblique view establishes the finding as a summation artifact. Also note that, as discussed in the text, the asymmetry in this case could have been assessed as a summation artifact without the need for an additional mammographic view.

2% frequency of underlying breast cancer. If percutaneous biopsy is performed instead of surgical excision for palpable lesions smaller than 2 cm, imaging guidance may be helpful in maximizing the likelihood that the target lesion is actually sampled.

If the presence of associated microcalcifications, architectural distortion, or an underlying solid mass raises some suspicion of malignancy at either diagnostic mammography or ultrasound of a nonpalpable lesion, the standard recommendation also is tissue diagnosis; in this case the likelihood of underlying breast cancer is even greater. Imaging-guided biopsy usually targets the most suspicious imaging feature of the lesion.

If no one area of an asymmetry is more suspicious for malignancy than any other, biopsy should involve a representative sampling of the entire lesion, if not complete excision. Especially because a benign diagnosis is more likely than that of malignancy, the radiologist should be familiar with concordant benign diagnoses at percutaneous biopsy. These diagnoses include fibrocystic change, focal fibrosis, pseudoangiomatous stromal hyperplasia, and fibroadenoma [14–16].

The remaining cases involve nonpalpable focal asymmetries with no associated mammographic or sonographic abnormalities. If no previous mammograms are available for comparison, these lesions often are assessed as probably benign (BI-RADS category 3), with a recommendation for periodic mammographic surveillance, including one short-interval (6-month) follow-up examination [4–8,15–18]. When previous mammograms are available for comparison, demonstration of short-term (1-year) stability eliminates the need for short-interval follow-up but usually requires annual follow-up until 2-year or 3-year stability is shown. Demonstration of lesion stability for at least 2 or 3 years or demonstration of lesion regression justifies a definitively benign assessment (BI-RADS category 2), whereas lesion progression effectively establishes the diagnosis of developing asymmetry, which is assessed as suspicious (BI-RADS category 4) and managed by tissue diagnosis.

Summary

In the absence of palpability or associated suspicious findings at diagnostic mammography or ultrasound, the assessment of asymmetries usually is straightforward. One easy method is to take note of the numerical sequence in which the four types of asymmetries are presented in this article and use the sequence number to indicate the appropriate BI-RADS assessment category:

1. Uncomplicated asymmetry (summation artifact) is assessed as negative, BI-RADS category 1.
2. Uncomplicated global asymmetry is assessed as benign, BI-RADS category 2.
3. Uncomplicated focal asymmetry (no prior examinations available for comparison) is assessed as probably benign, BI-RADS category 3.

4. Uncomplicated developing asymmetry (not a simple cyst at ultrasound) is inherently suspicious, BI-RADS category 4.

References

[1] Sickles EA. Mammographic features of "early" breast cancer. AJR Am J Roentgenol 1984; 143(3):461–4.
[2] Sickles EA. Mammographic features of 300 consecutive nonpalpable breast cancers. AJR Am J Roentgenol 1986;146(4):661–3.
[3] Sickles EA. Findings at mammographic screening on only one standard projection: outcomes analysis. Radiology 1998;208(2):471–5.
[4] Helvie MA, Pennes DR, Rebner M, et al. Mammographic follow-up of low-suspicion lesions: compliance rate and diagnostic yield. Radiology 1991;178(1):155–8.
[5] Sickles EA. Periodic mammographic follow-up of probably benign lesions: results in 3,184 consecutive cases. Radiology 1991;179(2):463–8.
[6] Varas X, Leborgne F, Leborgne JH. Nonpalpable probably benign lesions: role of follow-up mammography. Radiology 1992;184(2):409–14.
[7] Vizcaíno I, Gadea L, Andreo L, et al. Short-term follow-up results in 795 nonpalpable probably benign lesions detected at screening mammography. Radiology 2001;219(2):475–83.
[8] Varas X, Leborgne JH, Leborgne F, et al. Revisiting the mammographic follow-up of BI-RADS category 3 lesions. AJR Am J Roentgenol 2002; 179(3):691–5.
[9] American College of Radiology. Breast imaging reporting and data system (BI-RADS). 4th edition. Reston (VA): American College of Radiology; 2003.
[10] Sickles EA. Lesion seen on only one standard mammographic projection. In: Sickles EA, editor. Breast disease (second series): test and syllabus. Reston (VA): American College of Radiology; 1993. p. 20–35.
[11] Kopans DB, Swann CA, White G, et al. Asymmetric breast tissue. Radiology 1989;171(3):639–43.
[12] Stomper PC, Van Voorhis BJ, Ravnikar VA, et al. Mammographic changes associated with postmenopausal hormone replacement therapy: a longitudinal study. Radiology 1990;174(2): 487–90.
[13] Cyrlak D, Wong CH. Mammographic changes in postmenopausal women undergoing hormonal replacement therapy. AJR Am J Roentgenol 1993;161(6):1177–83.
[14] Leung JWT, Sickles EA. Developing asymmetry identified on mammography: correlation with imaging outcome and pathologic findings. AJR Am J Roentgenol 2007;188(3):667–75.
[15] Piccoli CW, Feig SA, Palazzo JP. Developing asymmetric breast tissue. Radiology 1999; 211(1):111–7.
[16] Samardar P, de Paredes ES, Grimes MM, et al. Focal asymmetric densities seen at mammography: US and pathologic correlation. Radiographics 2002;22(1):19–33.
[17] Sickles EA. Management of probably benign breast lesions. Radiol Clin North Am 1995; 33(6):1123–30.
[18] Sickles EA. Focal asymmetric density. In: Bassett LW, editor. Breast disease (third series): test and syllabus. Reston (VA): American College of Radiology; 2000. p. 65–70.

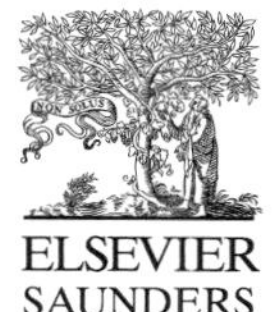

RADIOLOGIC
CLINICS
OF NORTH AMERICA

Radiol Clin N Am 45 (2007) 773–789

The Probably Benign Assessment

Jessica W.T. Leung, MD*, Edward A. Sickles, MD

The term "probably benign" is widely recognized and accepted in breast imaging. Earlier descriptors included "low suspicion" [1] and "minimally suspicious," [2] but, because of concern that the pejorative nature of such terms might prompt unintended biopsy, "probably benign" was substituted [3]. An assessment of probably benign is clinically helpful when used for a lesion that is not definitely benign and that can be followed safely with short-term imaging surveillance rather than biopsy. Indeed, this term has been incorporated into the Breast Imaging Reporting and Data System (BI-RADS) as assessment category 3 [4–6].

The probably benign assessment was introduced and popularized in the early 1990s, once screening mammography had become widely implemented. The major goal of screening mammography is the detection of early-stage, favorable-prognosis cancers, but to detect such cancers, false-positive biopsy recommendations are occasionally necessary. The primary rationale behind probably benign assessments is to reduce false-positive recommendations for biopsy substantially while maintaining an acceptably high detection rate of early-stage cancer. This goal is accomplished by defining as probably benign those lesions that carry a less than 2% likelihood of malignancy (lesions for which at least 50 biopsies are needed to identify one cancer) and by observing during periodic imaging surveillance that (1) these lesions demonstrate interval increase only infrequently and (2) those few lesions later found to be malignant are almost always still early-stage cancers, even though diagnosis was delayed until interval progression prompted biopsy. The costs and morbidity of false-positive biopsies thus can be reduced, enhancing the cost effectiveness and efficacy of screening mammography. Before the introduction of the probably benign assessment, the biopsy costs for mammographic abnormalities or palpable masses constituted half the total costs of screening programs [7]. The proper use of probably benign assessments can reduce

Supported in part by grants from the American Roentgen Ray Society and the Society of Breast Imaging.
Department of Radiology, University of California San Francisco Medical Center, 1600 Divisadero Street, Room C-250, San Francisco, CA 94115, USA
* Corresponding author.
E-mail address: jessica.leung@ucsfmedctr.org (J.W.T. Leung).

0033-8389/07/$ – see front matter doi:10.1016/j.rcl.2007.06.008
radiologic.theclinics.com

the costs associated with false-positive biopsies and increase the positive predictive value of biopsy [2].

Robust data from diverse sources support the use of the probably benign assessment in mammography. It has stood the test of time, even after percutaneous core biopsy, with reduced cost and morbidity, was introduced as an alternative to surgical biopsy [8]. Recently BI-RADS has added probably benign assessments to the interpretation of breast ultrasound [5] and MR imaging examinations [6]. This article examines in depth the use of the probably benign assessment: which lesions should be assessed as probably benign, the published evidence supporting such use, pitfalls in misuse, and areas of potentially expanded use that currently are under investigation.

Inclusion criteria

Three types of mammographic lesions can be assessed confidently as probably benign: a circumscribed mass, clustered round (punctate) or oval calcifications, and a focal asymmetry. Additional miscellaneous types of lesions have been described as probably benign, although relatively few cases of each of these lesion types have been reported.

Mass

A mammographic mass is a space-occupying lesion, seen on at least two different mammographic projections, denser in the center than at the periphery, and characterized by convex outer margins. Ultrasound may be used to establish the diagnosis of a cyst, which is a definitively benign mass. Other than demonstrated location in the skin or depiction of internal fat, there are no characteristically benign mammographic features for a mass. Therefore, to be considered benign at mammography, a mass should have morphologic features suggestive of benignity as well as a minimum of 2-year stability [9]; the shape of the mass should be round, oval, or lobular, and its margins should be circumscribed. A probably benign mass is one that is noncalcified and circumscribed (Fig. 1) but lacks the requisite 2-year stability [3]. Not infrequently, portions of the margins of a mass are obscured by adjacent isodense fibroglandular tissue. In this circumstance, at least 75% of the margins of the mass should be deemed circumscribed to qualify as probably benign; none of the margins may be indistinct or spiculated (Fig. 2A, B). Diagnostic mammography views (such as those using spot compression with or without magnification) often can help in displacing adjacent obscuring tissues and reducing geometric blur to assist in margin assessment (see Fig. 2A, B; Fig. 3A, B) [10].

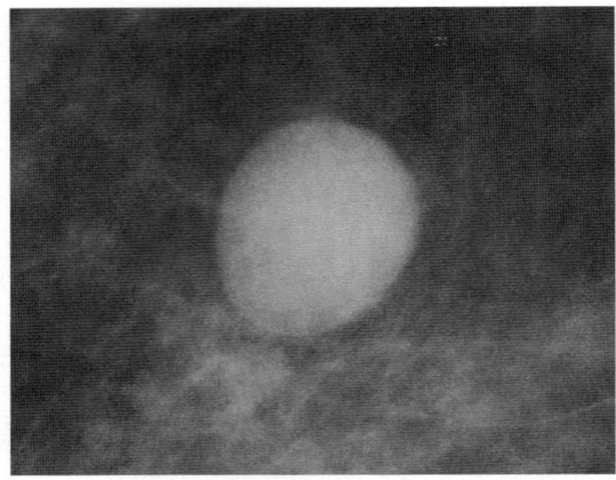

Fig. 1. Mammogram showing a circumscribed oval mass. In the absence of a suspicious sonographic correlate or sonographic demonstration of a simple cyst, this mass is associated with a probability of malignancy of less than 2%. Therefore, it may be assessed as probably benign and managed with periodic mammographic surveillance that begins with short-interval follow-up.

Calcifications

A cluster (defined as five or more particles per cubic centimeter) of tiny round or oval calcifications (Fig. 4) may be considered probably benign [3]. BI-RADS uses two descriptors for round calcifications; those tiny enough to be probably benign (< 0.5 mm) are termed "punctate," and those that are larger and more characteristically benign are simply termed "round" [4]. Spot-compression magnification mammography usually is required to provide sufficient resolution to portray the round shapes of probably benign calcifications. Note that calcifications that are amorphous in shape (Fig. 5) (too small or too indistinct to be considered round) are associated with a sufficiently high probability of malignancy (20%) that they should not be assessed as probably benign [11]. Although uncommon, tiny round calcifications that are linear or segmental in distribution also are considered suspicious (Fig. 6), based on limited anecdotal experience indicating a likelihood of malignancy substantially higher than 2%.

Focal asymmetry

A focal asymmetry is a space-occupying lesion, seen on at least two different mammographic projections, occupying less than a quadrant of the breast. It differs from a mass in that its margins are concave-outward, and it usually is seen interspersed with fat (Fig. 7A–D). In the absence of palpability or associated findings more suspicious for malignancy, as seen at fine-detail mammography or ultrasound, a focal asymmetry may be considered

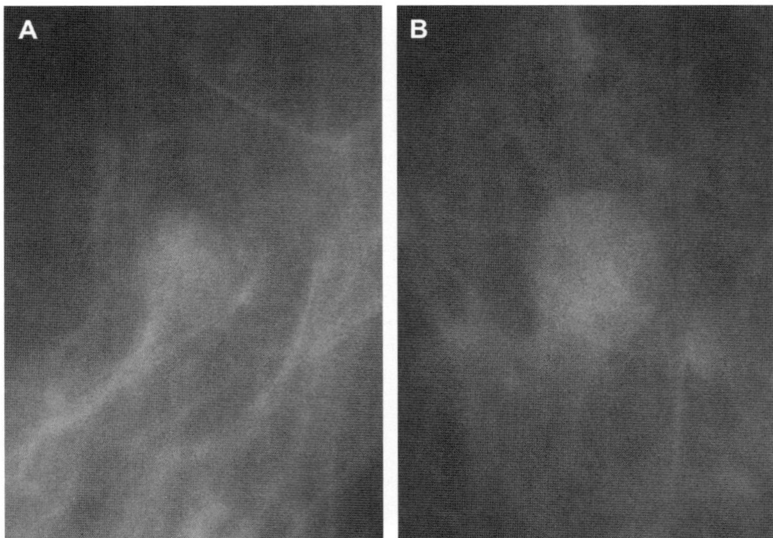

Fig. 2. Spot-compression magnification mammography revealing the circumscribed margins of a mass that was obscured and indistinct at screening. Because this mass is circumscribed, it may be assessed as probably benign and managed with periodic mammographic surveillance that begins with short-interval follow-up. Diagnostic imaging allowed the probably benign assessment to be made with confidence. (*A*) Screening mammogram showing a partially obscured mass with somewhat indistinct margins. (*B*) Spot-compression magnification mammogram displacing adjacent dense tissues so that the mass margins are less obscured and are depicted in finer detail. The mass now is seen to be circumscribed over at least 75% of its contour, supporting a probably benign assessment. (*From* Sickles EA. Breast masses: mammographic evaluation. Radiology 1989;173:297–303; with permission.)

probably benign and managed with short-interval follow-up [3]. If a focal asymmetry is seen to have increased in size or conspicuity, it should be termed a "developing asymmetry" (Fig. 8A, B). A recent study reported the probability of malignancy in developing asymmetries identified at screening and diagnostic mammography to be 12.8% and 26.7%, respectively [12]. Because these frequencies

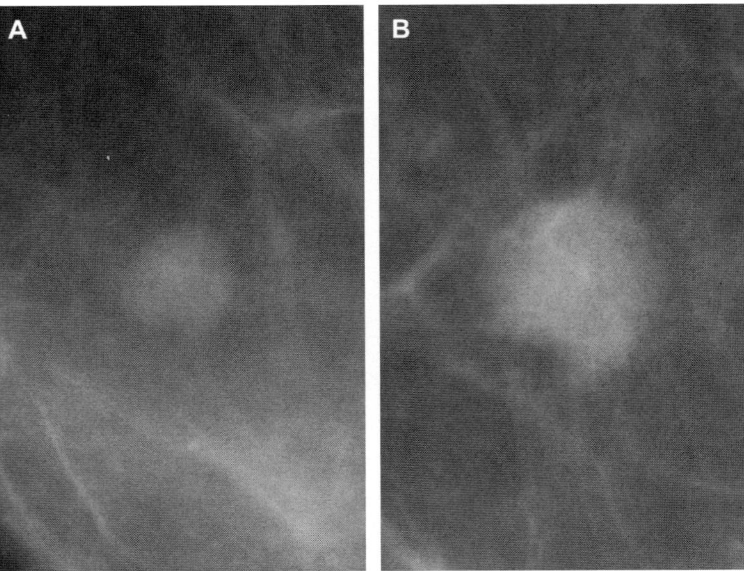

Fig. 3. Spot-compression magnification mammography revealing the indistinct margins of a mass that appeared to be circumscribed at screening. Because this mass has indistinct margins, it should be assessed as suspicious rather than probably benign, and biopsy should be recommended. Because of the findings at diagnostic imaging, biopsy was performed promptly, and delayed cancer diagnosis was avoided. (*A*) Screening mammogram showing a primarily circumscribed mass. (*B*) Spot-compression magnification mammogram depicting the margins of the mass in finer detail. The mass now is seen to be irregular in contour and to have indistinct margins, supporting assessment as suspicious rather than probably benign. (*From* Sickles EA. Breast masses: mammographic evaluation. Radiology 1989;173:297–303; with permission.)

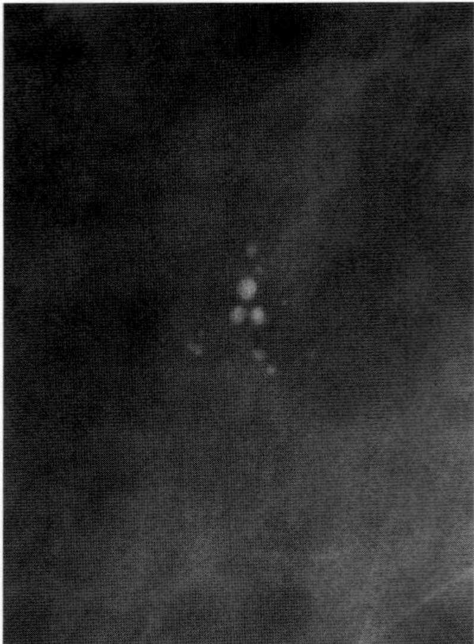

Fig. 4. Spot-compression magnification mammogram showing a cluster of round (punctate) calcifications. These calcifications are associated with a probability of malignancy of less than 2%. Therefore, they may be assessed as probably benign and managed with periodic mammographic surveillance that begins with short-interval follow-up. (*From* American College of Radiology (ACR). Breast (2nd edition). American College of Radiology; 1993. Reprinted with permission of the American College of Radiology. No other representation of this material is authorized without expressed, written permission from the American College of Radiology.)

are considerably greater than the ceiling of a 2% probability of malignancy accepted for probably benign lesions, a developing asymmetry should be assessed as suspicious, and biopsy should be recommended.

Miscellaneous

Other findings that have been described as probably benign and followed with short-interval follow-up include solitary dilated duct (Fig. 9), subtle areas of architectural distortion occurring at known surgical biopsy sites (Fig. 10), and grouped calcifications suggestive of but not diagnostic for fat necrosis (partial rim calcification with central fat) (Fig. 11). Only anecdotal experience supports the characterization of these miscellaneous findings as probably benign. As yet unpublished data from the University of California, San Francisco (UCSF) indicate that the likelihood of malignancy for cases of solitary dilated duct may be too high to justify a probably benign assessment (Natalya Lvoff, MD, personal communication, 2007).

Fig. 5. Spot-compression magnification mammogram showing a cluster of amorphous calcifications. These calcifications are associated with a sufficiently high probability of malignancy that they should be assessed as suspicious rather than probably benign. Biopsy should be recommended rather than periodic mammographic surveillance.

Supporting evidence

The published evidence on the probably benign assessment is robust and plentiful, indicating that radiologists in diverse practices working in different countries can use this assessment prospectively to

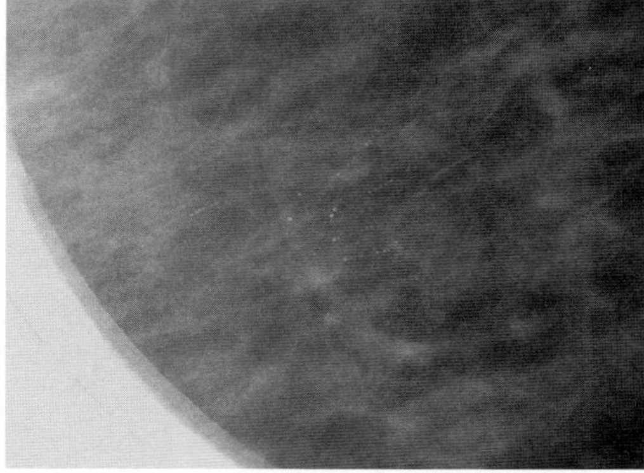

Fig. 6. Spot-compression magnification mammogram showing round (punctate) calcifications in linear distribution. Although the morphology of the calcifications is consistent with a probably benign assessment, the linear distribution is suspicious for malignancy. Therefore, these calcifications should be assessed as suspicious rather than probably benign. Prompt biopsy showed ductal carcinoma in situ.

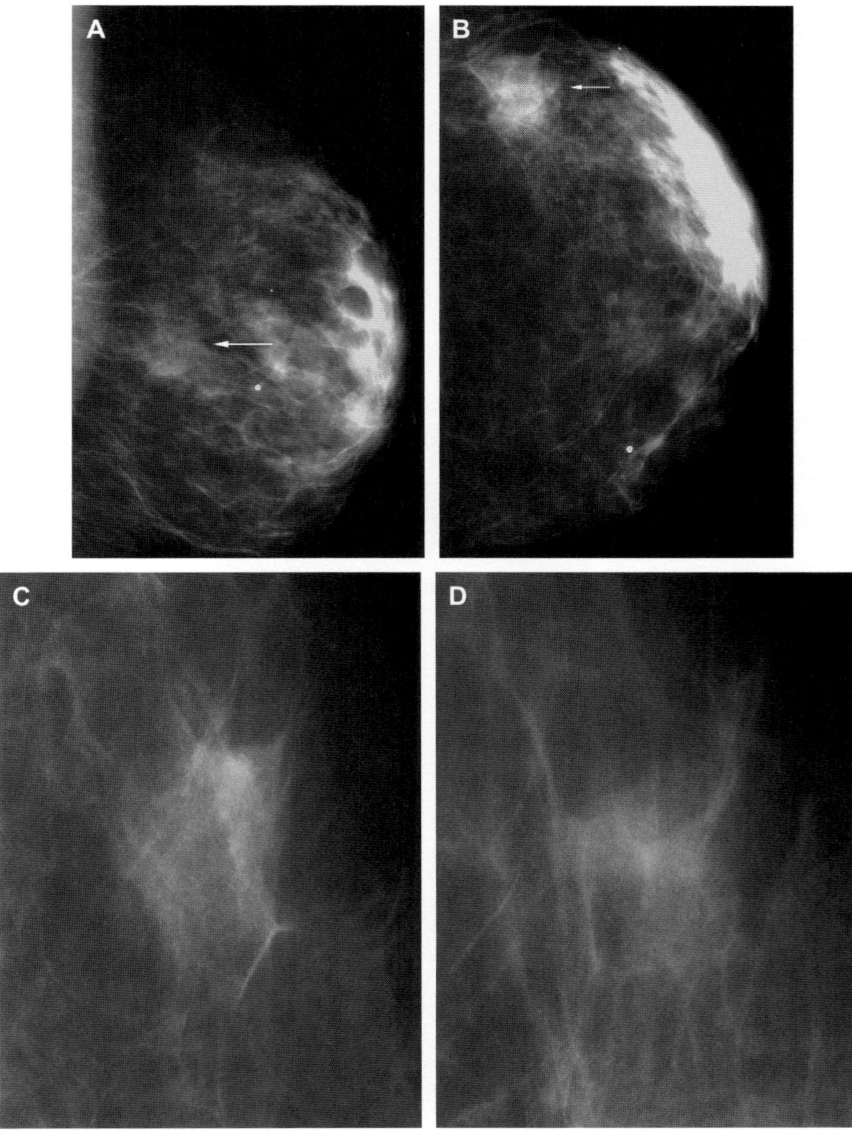

Fig. 7. Mammograms showing a focal asymmetry. In the absence of an underlying mass or other suspicious mammographic or sonographic features, this finding may be assessed as probably benign and managed with periodic mammographic surveillance that begins with short-interval follow-up. (*A*) Mediolateral oblique projection mammogram showing a focal asymmetry (*arrow*). (*B*) Craniocaudal projection mammogram showing a focal asymmetry (*arrow*). (*C*) Spot-compression magnification mediolateral mammogram demonstrating a focal asymmetry, with no underlying mass or associated architectural distortion or calcifications. (*D*) Spot-compression magnification craniocaudal mammogram demonstrating a focal asymmetry, with no underlying mass or associated architectural distortion or calcifications.

identify lesions for which the likelihood of malignancy is less than 2% [3,13–23]. The evidence also demonstrates that only about 5% of followed lesions change sufficiently under surveillance to require biopsy (almost always such change is detected at imaging while the lesion is still nonpalpable), and that almost all identified cancers are still early-stage, good-prognosis lesions [3,16,22,23].

Initial studies suggested that a subset of mammographic lesions might be followed without compromising the diagnosis of early-stage, favorable-prognosis cancers [1,2,24]. The strongest data legitimizing the use of the probably benign assessment, however, come from two large-scale prospective longitudinal studies, similar in design, published in 1991 [3] and 1992 [16]. The major

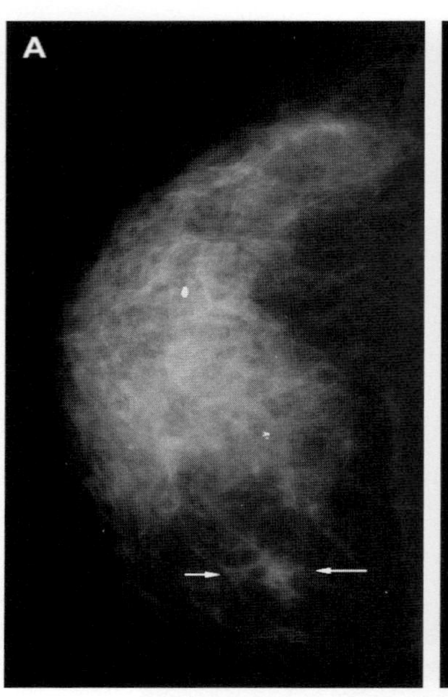

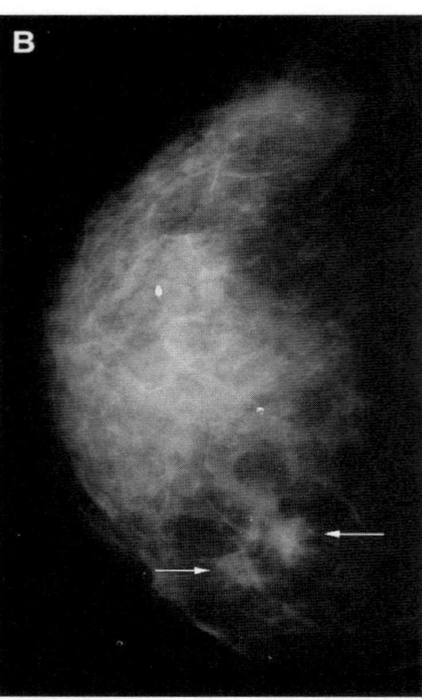

Fig. 8. Mammograms showing a developing asymmetry. In the setting of interval increase in size or conspicuity, this finding should be assessed as suspicious rather than probably benign. Biopsy should be recommended rather than periodic mammographic surveillance. (*A*) Craniocaudal projection mammogram at baseline, showing an asymmetry in the medial aspect of the breast (*arrows*). (*B*) Craniocaudal projection mammogram 3 years later. The lesion now should be described as a developing asymmetry because it has increased in size and conspicuity (*arrows*).

difference between these two studies is that Sickles [3] included patients who had scattered bilateral tiny round or oval microcalcifications (Fig. 12), whereas Varas and colleagues [16] did not.

Of 28,458 consecutive screening mammography examinations, Sickles [3] at UCSF prospectively assessed 3184 nonpalpable lesions as probably benign after recalling the subjects for diagnostic imaging. Among these lesions, 842 were masses (26.4%), 1853 were calcification lesions (58.2%), and 449 were focal asymmetries (14.1%). Rather than biopsy, these lesions were prospectively assigned to follow-up mammography. The total surveillance period was 3 to 3.5 years. During follow-up, 161 cases (5.1%) were biopsied. The 19 lesions

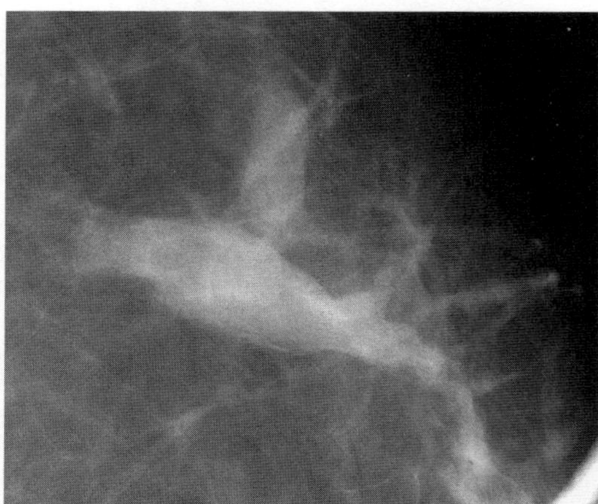

Fig. 9. Spot-compression magnification mammogram showing a solitary dilated duct. Previous reports, based on few cases rather than robust data, indicate that this finding may be assessed as probably benign. Ongoing research, however, suggests that this finding may be associated with a greater than 2% probability of malignancy and hence more appropriately assessed as suspicious.

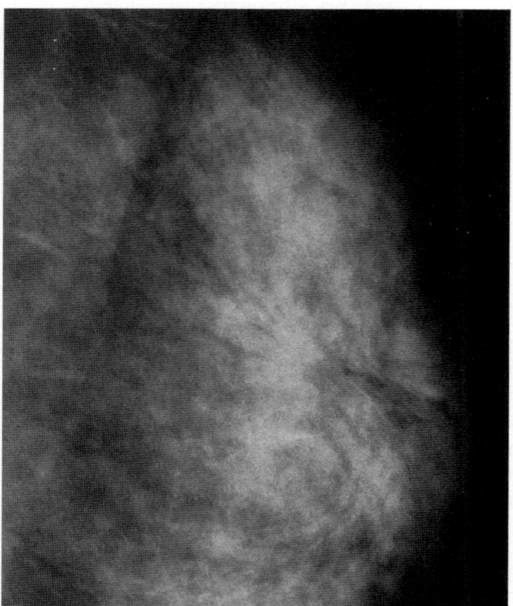

Fig. 10. Mammogram showing architectural distortion at a known site of surgical biopsy. Although previous reports, based on few cases rather than robust data, indicate that this finding may be assessed as probably benign, this is not an established indication for probably benign assessment.

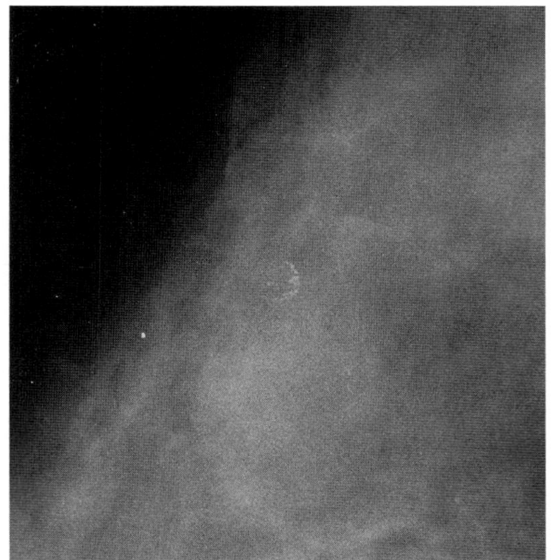

Fig. 11. Spot-compression magnification mammogram showing a cluster of partial rim calcifications suggestive of fat necrosis. Although previous reports, based on few cases rather than robust data, indicate that this finding may be assessed as probably benign, this is not an established indication for probably benign assessment.

that were biopsied because of patient preference (12 at initial time of probably benign assessment and 7 after imaging follow-up showing no interval change) all yielded benign findings. One hundred thirty-one biopsies (4.1%) were performed because of interval change at mammographic surveillance, with 15 cancers diagnosed. Twelve lesions became palpable and were biopsied without concurrent mammographic evaluation, with two cancers diagnosed at 7 and 10 months.

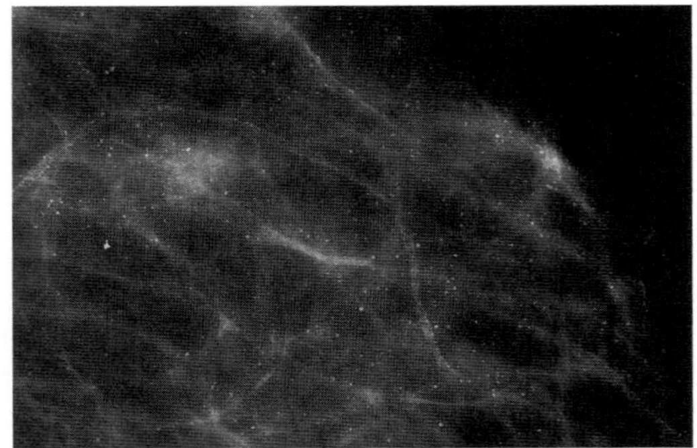

Fig. 12. Mammogram showing scattered and occasionally grouped, mostly round (punctate) calcifications. When calcifications such as these are distributed throughout both breasts, and no one area of calcifications is different from all other areas, the examination may be assessed as benign, with a recommendation for routine mammographic screening.

Altogether, the overall probability of malignancy in the study group of probably benign lesions was 0.5% (17 of 3184). Twelve of the 17 cancers were solitary, noncalcified, circumscribed solid masses. In this subgroup, the probability of malignancy was 2.0% (12 of 589), in part giving rise to the often-quoted upper value of a 2% malignancy rate for probably benign lesions.

All 17 cancers were small in size, early in stage (stage 0 or 1), and favorable in prognosis, similar to those identified in the general screening population at UCSF [25]. Pathologic analysis showed ductal carcinoma in situ (DCIS) in 2 cases, invasive ductal carcinoma in 14, and invasive lobular carcinoma in 1. The two cases of DCIS were 8 and 14 mm in size. The invasive cancers ranged in size from 5 to 18 mm (median size, 13 mm). No cases with systemic metastasis were identified. In 2 of 17 cancers (12%), a single axillary node was positive for metastasis. No tumor recurrence was identified at follow-up (median, 60 months; range, 33–119 months). Subsequent long-term observation of these cancer cases showed no evidence of tumor recurrence, with follow-up now ranging from 19 to 26 years; three women subsequently have died from other causes (Edward A. Sickles, personal communication, 2007).

Similarly, Varas and colleagues [16] studied 21,855 consecutive screening mammography examinations at Hospital Pereira Rossell in Montevideo, Uruguay. Among these, 558 (2.6%) were prospectively assigned to mammographic surveillance for nonpalpable probably benign findings. Twenty-three patients (4%) were lost to follow-up, so the study consisted of 535 patients. Nine cancers were identified, resulting in a probability of malignancy of 1.7%. All nine cancers were detected through progression at follow-up imaging, and no cancer was diagnosed as a result of biopsy performed at the preference of referring physician or patient. There were seven invasive carcinomas and two cases of DCIS. All cancers were either stage 0 or 1. Only two of nine patients (22%) had axillary nodal involvement, and only one patient (staged T_1, N_0 at diagnosis) showed distant metastases at follow-up (mean interval, 23 months).

An independent study by the same authors 10 years later again concluded that the use of probably benign assessments is a safe and efficacious practice [23]. Of 18,435 consecutive screening mammography examinations performed in 1996, 454 (3.0%) were prospectively assessed as probably benign. Thirty patients were lost to follow-up, and three died of causes other than breast cancer. The remaining 511 patients constituted the study. Two cancers were diagnosed, resulting in a probability of malignancy of 0.4%. Both cancers in this study were diagnosed because of mammographic interval progression (follow-up of 11 and 17 months, respectively). There was no recurrence at 30 and 36 months of follow-up. The association of mammographic progression and malignancy was statistically significantly ($P = .0009$).

Comparing Varas' initial and subsequent studies, the likelihood of malignancy in a probably benign assessment decreased from 1.7% to 0.4%, and the positive biopsy yield increased from 48% to 60%. The authors believed that technologic advances in breast imaging, better quality assurance requirements, and increased experience contributed to these improved outcomes.

In recent years, several additional reports have supported the use of periodic mammographic surveillance for probably benign lesions. A prospective study of 13,790 women from Valencia, Spain involved 795 patients (5.8%) who underwent mammographic follow-up [22]. Two cancers were diagnosed: one DCIS with microinvasion, and one 7-mm invasive ductal carcinoma with no nodal involvement. Both cancers were detected because of progression at imaging follow-up. The probability of malignancy was 0.3%. The Women's Health Initiative involved a prospective study of 68,126 postmenopausal women at 40 centers in the United States [26]. In this study, the probability of malignancy associated with probably benign mammographic lesions was 1.0%.

Use of the probably benign assessment also was studied in the recently published Digital Mammographic Imaging Screening Trial (DMIST) [27]. This study involved 49,528 asymptomatic women who underwent mammography screening using both screen-film and digital technologies. The use of the probably benign assessment category by 178 radiologists at 33 academic and private practices was studied. There were 1138 patients (2.3%) assigned to short-interval follow-up. Twelve cancers were detected, for a malignancy rate of 1.1%. As in previous studies, all 12 cancers were of early stage and favorable prognosis; there were six cases of DCIS and six T_1 invasive cancers.

Patient compliance and follow-up protocols

Successful application of the probably benign assessment hinges on appropriate recommendation for imaging follow-up and patient compliance. If the patient cannot be relied upon to return for imaging follow-up, or if imaging follow-up is not feasible (eg, because of pregnancy or expectation of pregnancy, augmentation or reduction surgery, travel to locations where imaging would not be available, or extreme patient anxiety), prompt biopsy may be the more appropriate management, regardless of the imaging findings [6].

As a first step in ensuring that the patient returns for follow-up imaging, it is important that short-interval follow-up is the initial management recommended when a probably benign assessment is made. Poplack and colleagues [28] studied the mammography practice patterns in a community network of 53,803 women. They found that discordant management recommendations were most frequent for mammograms assessed as probably benign. Short-interval follow-up imaging of less than 270 days was recommended in only 63.1% of screening and 64.1% of diagnostic mammographic examinations that were assessed as probably benign. Other investigators also have observed substantial discordance between assessment and management recommendations for probably benign lesions [29,30].

The rate of patient compliance in returning for follow-up imaging for probably benign lesions varies depending on the population studied. A low compliance rate of 40% was reported in the National Breast and Cervical Cancer Early Detection Program [31], and a high compliance rate of 88% was reported in the single-institution study by Helvie and colleagues [1]. Patient compliance increased from 76% in the first study by Varas and colleagues [23] to 83% in their second study ($P = .003$). Sickles [3] found that patient compliance decreased progressively with the duration of follow-up. Of the 3184 patients initially recommended for follow-up, 92% returned at 6 months, 89% at 12 months, 82% at 24 months, and 65% at 36 months.

In the DMIST trial, in which 1138 patients were recommended for short-interval follow-up, only 802 (70%) returned for the short-interval follow-up [27]. Furthermore, among the remaining 336 patients, only 228 (68%) returned for annual mammography. In other words, patient compliance was limited, even in a selected population that consented to participate in a clinical trial.

The ideal follow-up protocol should optimize patient compliance, cost effectiveness, and early cancer detection. The several prospective studies of probably benign assessments involved somewhat different surveillance protocols, however. There is no established standard-of-care protocol.

Homer [32] studied the timing of follow-up studies in a national survey. More than 90% of the respondents reported that they recommended that the first follow-up imaging examination take place within 3 to 6 months, and more than half followed probably benign lesions for at least 2 years. In clinical practice, most radiologists interpret "short-interval" as 6-month follow-up. Of the several follow-up examinations, the initial 6-month follow-up examination is the most important, so that rapidly growing cancers can be diagnosed without further delay.

At UCSF, the follow-up strategy first described by Sickles is used [3]: unilateral mammography at 6 months and bilateral mammography at 12, 24, and 36 months. Using this protocol, only one additional 6-month mammography examination (after the initial rendering of a probably benign assessment) is added to otherwise routine annual mammography. The probably benign finding is followed until stability is documented for a total of 3 years. The most recent edition of BI-RADS includes a follow-up algorithm that duplicates this UCSF follow-up protocol, except that it acknowledges that many radiologists prefer to shorten the total follow-up interval to 2 years [4]. Note that the BI-RADS algorithm suggests continuing to render probably benign assessments but recommends yearly (rather than short-interval) follow-up after the first year of surveillance. Thus, the BI-RADS management associated with probably benign assessments is periodic imaging surveillance beginning with 1 year of short-interval follow-up, not short-interval follow-up throughout the surveillance period.

Some investigators have questioned the need for the initial 6-month follow-up examination [33]. Although only 16% of cancers are identified at this initial follow-up examination, there is indirect evidence that these cancers are more rapidly growing tumors that may benefit substantially from the earlier detection provided at 6 (rather than 12) months [20].

Short-term follow-up versus percutaneous biopsy

The concept of following probably benign lesions rather than performing biopsy originated before the advent of percutaneous core or fine-needle aspiration biopsy, when tissue diagnosis necessarily involved surgery. Despite the considerably lesser cost and morbidity of percutaneous biopsy, probably benign assessment continues to be the much more cost-effective management in the United States [6,17].

The relative costs of mammographic surveillance and percutaneous biopsy are substantially different in some other countries. For example, in the United Kingdom, where routine mammography screening is performed every 3 years instead of yearly, the periodic surveillance protocol would involve three additional mammography examinations (6 months, 12 months, and 24 months after initial probably benign assessment) instead of one additional examination 6 months after initial probably benign assessment. Moreover, the cost of percutaneous fine-needle aspiration in the United Kingdom is much less than the cost of core biopsy in the United States. The net result is that percutaneous biopsy actually may be a more cost-effective approach in the United Kingdom, at least partially accounting for the infrequent use of periodic surveillance there [34,35].

Periodic mammographic surveillance also is associated with less stress than core biopsy or fine-needle aspiration biopsy. In a retrospective study, surveys were mailed to 80 patients who were assigned to follow-up (probably benign assessment) and 58 patients for whom core biopsy was recommended (suspicious or highly suggestive of malignancy assessment) [36]. The patients in the follow-up group reported less stress than those in the core biopsy group. On a scale of 1 to 5 (1 representing "not at all stressful" and 5 being "extremely stressful"), the patients in the core biopsy group reported a mean score of 2.74, whereas the patients in the follow-up group reported a mean score of 2.13 ($P < .001$). Even when only the core biopsy patients who had a lower likelihood of malignancy (ie, those assessed as suspicious rather than highly suggestive of malignancy) were analyzed, the reported stress was higher than in the follow-up group ($P < .025$).

Proper use of the probably benign assessment

As important as it is not to miss an early breast cancer, it also is important not to overuse the probably benign assessment. Characteristically benign lesions, such as simple cysts and intramammary lymph nodes diagnosed at ultrasound, should be interpreted as benign with routine (not short-interval) follow-up recommended. Other typically benign lesions identified at mammography include milk-of-calcium within tiny benign cysts, skin calcifications, calcified fibroadenomas, vascular calcifications, dystrophic calcifications, secretory calcifications, and entirely or partially fatty masses, including some intramammary lymph nodes [9,37]. Multiple and bilateral circumscribed (or partially circumscribed) similar-appearing masses also should be interpreted as benign and not as probably benign (Fig. 13A, B) [38]. Leung and Sickles [38] studied a cohort of 1440 such multiple-mass cases and reported an interval cancer rate of only 0.14%, which was lower than the age-matched United States incident cancer rate of 0.24%. Among the 76 cases of "multiple, noncalcified sharply marginated masses" included in the 1992 study of probably benign lesions by Varas

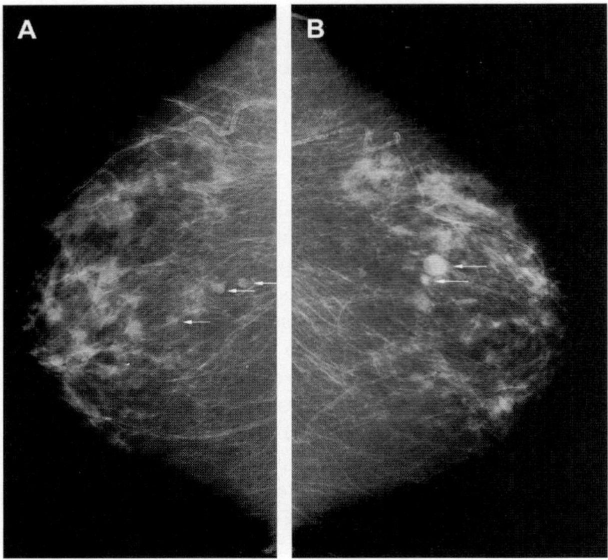

Fig. 13. Mammograms showing multiple bilateral, similar-appearing, circumscribed or partially circumscribed noncalcified masses, consistent with cysts. Such cases may be assessed as benign with a recommendation for routine mammographic screening, accompanied by the caveat that aspiration should be considered if clinical breast examination raises concern for a particular mass. (*A*) Craniocaudal projection mammogram of one breast showing multiple masses (*arrows*). (*B*) Craniocaudal projection mammogram of the other breast showing multiple masses (*arrows*).

and colleagues [16], not a single cancer was found at follow-up. Similarly, the generalized finding of bilateral scattered and occasionally grouped similar-appearing calcifications can be safely assessed as benign rather than probably benign (Edward A. Sickles, MD, personal communication, 2007).

According to standard mammography auditing practice, the probably benign assessment is considered "negative," in that biopsy is not recommended [4]. Hence, inappropriately broadening the imaging criteria for rendering probably benign assessments (either by failing first to perform a full diagnostic imaging evaluation or, alternatively, by including low-suspicion lesions) may raise the false-negative rate, because some otherwise detectable cancers may be missed. In the community practice setting, Poplack and colleagues [28] found that 27 (46%) of the 59 interval cancers in their geographic region had been assessed as probably benign.

Rosen and colleagues [39] studied 51 cancers at their institution that were initially assessed as probably benign. Among these cancers, there were 23 calcification lesions (45%), 12 masses (24%), 12 developing asymmetries (24%), and 4 cases of architectural distortion (8%). There were 35 invasive carcinomas (69%), 15 DCIS (29%), and 1 primary breast lymphoma (2%). In retrospect, none of the 51 lesions fulfilled the established imaging criteria for probably benign assessment. Most notably, 47 (92%) of the 51 cancers already had shown interval progression at the time of initial assessment as probably benign. Additionally, many did not meet the morphologic criteria for a probably benign lesion. None of the 23 cases of calcifications had punctate or oval calcific particles, and only 1 of 12 masses had circumscribed margins. Rosen and colleagues [39] hypothesized that the desirable outcomes associated with the probably benign assessment were not achieved because individual radiologists used criteria based on their own individual training and experience rather than relying on evidence-based criteria when assessing lesions as probably benign. In review, specific lesions that should not have been assessed as probably benign included enlarging or new lesions, subtle architectural distortions, and clusters of amorphous or pleomorphic microcalcifications.

Interval change

Interval progression increases the probability of malignancy for any mammographic lesion [40]; hence change versus stability must be considered when assessing a lesion as probably benign. If a mammographic finding already has demonstrated interval progression, even if slight, it should not be assessed as probably benign (Fig. 14A–D). Similarly, any lesion that appears new since the prior examination should be viewed as demonstrating interval progression and should not be assessed as probably benign. Indeed, the very basis of the probably benign assessment is that the few cancers occurring in this category can be identified through interval progression at follow-up imaging. During the follow-up of a probably benign lesion, either increase in size or suspicious change in morphology should prompt the recommendation for biopsy.

In their 1992 study, Varas and colleagues [16] suggested the following criteria as prompting biopsy of a lesion previously assessed as probably

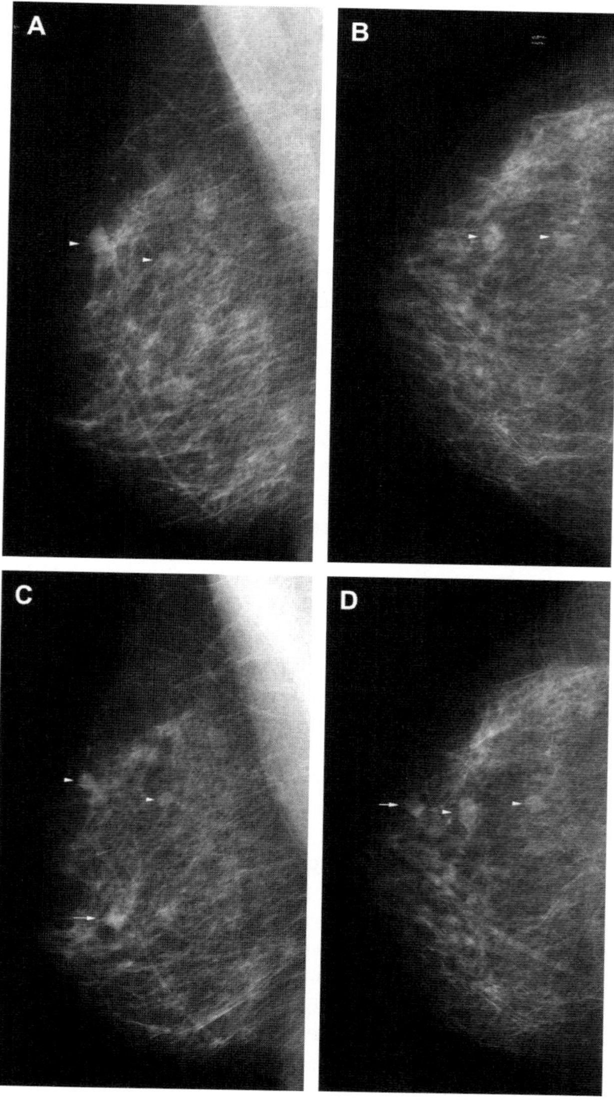

Fig. 14. Mammograms showing interval appearance of a circumscribed mass. Although the margins of this lobular mass are primarily circumscribed, the examination should not be assessed as probably benign because this mass was not present previously. A hypoechoic (solid) circumscribed mass was identified at ultrasound (not shown), and ultrasound-guided core biopsy revealed invasive ductal carcinoma. (*A*) Mediolateral oblique projection baseline mammogram. Two simple cysts, characterized as such at ultrasound, are visible (*arrowheads*). (*B*) Craniocaudal projection baseline mammogram. Two simple cysts, characterized as such at ultrasound, are visible (*arrowheads*). (*C*) Mediolateral oblique projection mammogram 1 year later. A new circumscribed lobular mass is seen (*arrow*), whereas the two known cysts (*arrowheads*) are unchanged. (*D*) Craniocaudal projection mammogram 1 year later. A new circumscribed lobular mass is seen (*arrow*), whereas the two known cysts (*arrowheads*) are unchanged.

benign: "increase in mass size, loss of distinct borders, increase in the number of microcalcifications, new forms of calcifications, a newly appeared mass within microcalcifications, and a palpable lump." In their 2002 study, Varas and colleagues [23] determined that mammographic progression has a statistically significantly association with malignancy ($P = .0009$). Several other studies showed that interval increase in size is a suspicious change, even if probably benign morphology is maintained [1,3,16,22].

In the study by Rosen and colleagues [39] of 51 cancers that initially were assessed as probably benign, 47 (92%) either were new or had increased when compared with a prior examination. Progression was noted in the original radiology report in 41 (80%) of these 47 cases, and progression was identified in the other six cases by retrospective review. Rather than any suspicious morphologic feature, "temporal instability" was most predictive of malignancy. Of note, the cancers in this series were larger and more aggressive than those previously published for probably benign lesions. For example, when compared with the study by Sickles [3], the range of cancer size was considerably larger (0.2–3.8 cm versus 0.4–1.8 cm). Also, 8 (16%) of the 51 cancers were stage 2, whereas all the cancers in the Sickles series were either stage 0 or 1. In other words, not only was the false-negative rate unacceptably high, but the cancers that were found were of relatively late stage. Hence, interval progression should preclude a lesion from being assessed as probably benign.

In a different study, 27 (84%) of 32 interval (false-negative) cancers were prospectively assessed as probably benign, even though many of them already had shown progression at the time of the probably benign assessment [41]. Nearly one third of these cancers were termed "developing densities." Recent data show that all developing asymmetries are associated with a sufficiently high probability of malignancy to warrant biopsy rather than imaging follow-up [12].

Whenever a probably benign assessment is contemplated, and previous mammograms are not available at the time of interpretation for comparison, the previous studies should be obtained for comparison. In almost all circumstances the presence (and availability) of at least one previous mammographic examination will avert the use of the probably benign assessment. If the mammographic finding of concern has regressed, it will be assessed as benign; if the mammographic finding is stable, short-interval (6-month) follow-up no longer will be needed; and if the mammographic finding has progressed, it should undergo biopsy. Thus, because fewer than 10% of mammography examinations are baseline examinations, the frequency of probably benign assessments now is reported to be considerably less than 5%.

Interval change may be difficult to assess if there are sufficient technical differences between the two studies. The current examination should be performed with a technique similar to that of the previous study [39]. For example, if spot-compression magnification views were not obtained at prior examination, then comparison should be made between the current standard views and the prior standard views. If the lesion was not visible on the previous study because of deep location (not included or only partially included in the image field) or limited technique (such as motion blur), the current study simply should be interpreted without consideration of stability (because there is no comparable prior study for comparison).

Full diagnostic work-up

Although all published data indicate that interval progression should prompt biopsy rather than follow-up, controversy exists as to whether a probably benign assessment might be made from standard screening views alone, or whether the patient always should be recalled for additional diagnostic imaging before rendering a probably benign assessment [3,18,21,42]. All the prospective studies involving probably benign assessment involve cases that first underwent full diagnostic imaging work-up [1,3,16,22,23]. It is widespread clinical practice, however, occasionally to make probably benign assessments directly from screening examinations [29]. Kerlikowske and colleagues [43] studied data from seven mammography registries that comprise the Breast Cancer Surveillance Consortium (BCSC). The study consisted of 119,199 first screening examinations and 1,052,593 subsequent screening examinations. They found that probably benign assessments were made based only on screening views (rather than diagnostic imaging at recall) in 86.2% of first screens and in 77.5% of subsequent screens. This finding differed dramatically from that in the DMIST trial, in which the great majority of probability benign assessments were based on diagnostic imaging at recall rather than on screening views alone (1034 versus 104 examinations, respectively) [27]. The primarily general radiology–based practices that contribute data to the BCSC seem to make probably benign assessments directly from screening examinations much more commonly than the primarily breast imaging specialist–based practices that contributed data to the DMIST trial.

Sickles [3,18] has advocated that the probably benign assessment should be rendered only after full diagnostic imaging work-up and not made based only on screening views. At diagnostic imaging, definitively benign lesions such as cysts or benign types of calcifications may be identified with confidence. In these cases, the appropriate assessment would be benign rather than probably benign, and annual screening rather than short-interval follow-up would be indicated. In some other cases, fine-detail mammography and/or ultrasound may identify features of malignancy that were not evident on standard screening views (see Fig. 3A, B) [3,10,18]. Recall imaging, therefore, should aid in reducing the numbers of both definitively benign and suspicious findings misinterpreted as probably benign. Furthermore, the diagnostic views obtained at recall imaging provide a fine-detail baseline to facilitate determination of stability or change at subsequent follow-up examinations.

In addition to specialized mammographic views, diagnostic imaging commonly includes ultrasound. Ultrasound has been shown to have significant utility in evaluating cases of mass and focal asymmetry [44]. In the study by Rosen and colleagues [39], 5 (18%) of 18 noncalcified cancers were assessed with ultrasound, and solid lesions were detected in all five cases. In other words, ultrasound should be used to identify potentially malignant lesions at the outset, minimizing the false-negative assessment of cancers as probably benign. A suspicious finding at ultrasound, despite the presence of probably benign mammographic features, would indicate the need for biopsy. Currently, MR imaging does not seem to be useful in the evaluation of probably benign lesions [45]. MR imaging was performed in a study of 56 mammographic lesions that were assessed as probably benign [45]. A low positive predictive value was observed, and clinical management was not significantly affected.

Debate on the use of probably benign assessments directly from screening examinations occurs most often when an apparently probably benign screen-detected mammographic finding is seen in a fatty breast [46]. That is, are there common circumstances when recall imaging is not likely to contribute additional diagnostic information affecting clinical management? The BCSC study by Kerlikowske and colleagues [43] helps answer this question. This large-scale study reports that recall imaging significantly increases the identification of definitively benign lesions (thus promptly establishing benignity, reducing anxiety, and avoiding unnecessary short-interval follow-up imaging); results of the study also suggest that recall imaging contributes to the early diagnosis of some aggressively growing cancers by identifying these tumors promptly, when they are smaller and more likely to be node-negative, rather than 6 months later at initial short-interval follow-up [43].

The American College of Radiology, in BI-RADS, indicates that there are many approaches to the work-up of a lesion before assessment as probably benign and describes that the work-up approach is often "intuitive," but it summarizes the discussion with the recommendation that "it is inadvisable to render [a probably benign assessment] when interpreting a screening examination" [4]. In particular, it is inappropriate to use probably benign assessments (instead of recall examinations) at screening mammography as an interpretation strategy designed to reduce the observed recall rate artificially.

Palpability

The prospective longitudinal studies on probably benign lesions were conducted on screen-detected lesions in nominally asymptomatic women. In other words, the robust data on the efficacy of probably benign assessments were acquired by examinations limited to nonpalpable lesions [18]. Given that both nonpalpable and palpable fibroadenomas appear probably benign at mammography and ultrasound, it seems reasonable that one may safely follow the subset of palpable noncalcified circumscribed solid masses instead of recommending biopsy. At this time, however, there is no large-scale evidence supporting this practice. Indeed, standard practice is to biopsy a solid mass if it is palpable, even if probably benign imaging criteria have been met otherwise [47–49]. Whether or not palpability excludes a lesion from being assessed as probably benign is currently an area of active investigation.

Graf and colleagues [50] reported outcomes of 157 palpable lesions in 152 women that otherwise met the mammographic and sonographic criteria for probably benign lesions. To qualify for this assessment, the lesions were circumscribed, noncalcified masses with a round, oval, or lobular contour at mammography. At ultrasound, the masses were solid, with round, oval, or macrolobulated shape, circumscribed margins, and orientation with long axis parallel to the skin. Of the 152 patients, 108 (71%) chose periodic imaging follow-up, and 44 (29%) preferred tissue diagnosis. There were 45 lesions among the patients who selected biopsy: 43 fibroadenomas, 1 adenomyoepithelioma, and 1 benign fibrocystic change. For patients who accepted imaging surveillance, follow-up was done for a minimum of 2 years and for a mean of 4.1 years (range, 2–7 years), so that lesions not biopsied were assumed to be benign. Lesions in six patients (5.6%) increased in size during follow-up and were excised. A seventh patient underwent surgical excision for calcifications that were unrelated to the solitary palpable mass being followed. Fibroadenoma was diagnosed at excision in all seven cases. No patient underwent biopsy because of suspicious changes at clinical follow-up. Although palpable lesions generally are associated with greater probability of malignancy than nonpalpable lesions [51], no cancers were found among the 157 palpable probably benign lesions. Note that this study was limited to circumscribed masses and did not evaluate other probably benign lesions, such as focal asymmetries. Hence, any conclusions that are drawn should apply only to masses. Furthermore, validation of these results at other institutions and with larger numbers of cases will be needed before palpable lesions can be reliably assessed as probably benign.

Age and size considerations

Caplan and colleagues [31] found that younger women are statistically more likely to be given a probably benign assessment than older women. In part this finding results from the much larger number of fibroadenomas and complicated cysts seen in younger women. Furthermore, the likelihood of breast cancer is known to increase with advancing patient age and increasing lesion size [16]. Therefore, biopsy (rather than periodic imaging surveillance) may be recommended for some probably benign lesions simply because they occur in women older than a given threshold age or because they are larger than a given threshold size.

In a study of 1403 nonpalpable, solid, noncalcified masses that were interpreted prospectively as probably benign, however, Sickles [52] did not find a threshold age or size beyond which the likelihood of malignancy is unacceptably high. Patient age ranged from 28 to 94 years (mean, 52.7 years; median, 50 years). Lesion size ranged from 4 to 32 mm (mean, 10.1 mm; median, 9 mm). Only very small increases in likelihood of malignancy were found with increasing patient age and lesion size, no given cohort had a likelihood of malignancy greater than 2%. Thus, neither age nor size thresholds seem to be appropriate in deciding on whether to render probably benign assessments.

Ultrasound

In 1995 Stavros and colleagues [53] proposed a set of sonographic imaging features to define probably benign breast lesions that may be managed by periodic surveillance instead of prompt biopsy. To be appropriate for follow-up, a solid mass should have an ellipsoid shape (Fig. 15) or fewer than four gentle lobulations and display a thin echogenic pseudocapsule; alternatively it should display intense homogeneous hyperechogenicity. In addition, such a mass must not display any of several suspicious sonographic features (spiculation, taller-than-wide orientation, angular margins, marked hypoechogenicity, shadowing, punctate calcifications, duct extension, branch pattern, or microlobulation). Using these imaging criteria to characterize 424 probably benign masses in a patient population heavily weighted with young women, these investigators reported a very high negative predictive value of 99.5%. In the primarily young patient population (mean age, 47 years), however, the probability of prior malignancy was considerably lower than expected for women undergoing routine screening (338 studied lesions were fibroadenomas), thereby limiting the clinical applicability of the reported high negative predictive value. Furthermore, the reproducibility of the Stavros criteria has been shown to be variable [54], which may further limit the validity of the criteria in general clinical use. Finally, given that ultrasound is an operator-dependent study, lesion follow-up using ultrasound is subject to both interobserver and intraobserver variability [55].

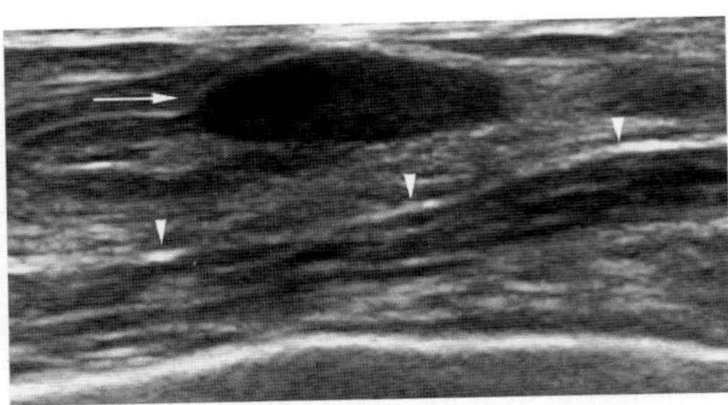

Fig. 15. Sonogram showing hypoechoic circumscribed oval mass (*arrow*) with orientation parallel to the skin and chest wall (*arrowheads*). Such a lesion probably is a fibroadenoma, but if it is visible only at ultrasound (hence not demonstrated to be probably benign at mammography), current data are not robust to support a probably benign assessment and management with periodic sonographic surveillance that begins with short-interval follow-up. Ongoing research may clarify the appropriate management of such lesions.

The American College of Radiology Imaging Network (ACRIN) is conducting a large-scale multi-institution prospective study of the utility of bilateral whole-breast ultrasound in breast cancer screening [56]. In the trial, the following sonographic findings are considered probably benign:

1. An oval, hypoechoic, circumscribed mass with orientation parallel to skin and no or minimal posterior acoustic enhancement, ranging from a solitary mass to multiple bilateral masses
2. A hyperechoic mass with central hypoechoic to anechoic components (consistent with fat necrosis)
3. A hypoechoic oval mass with homogeneous low-level internal echoes (consistent with complicated cyst)
4. Clustered microcysts with or without layering microcalcifications
5. Probable artifactual posterior shadowing at the interface of a fat lobule
6. Architectural distortion related to post-surgical scarring

Patient accrual in this trial has been completed, and periodic imaging surveillance is currently being obtained.

Although probably benign imaging criteria have been validated for noncalcified, circumscribed, solid masses seen at both mammography and ultrasound [1,3,16,22,23], there has been no such validation for lesions seen at ultrasound but obscured at mammography by adjacent isodense fibroglandular tissue. This distinction is pertinent, especially when considering the clinical acceptability of screening ultrasound, at which numerous mammographically occult lesions are found for which biopsy yield may be unacceptably low. Because of the large number of patients enrolled in the ACRIN trial, it is expected that results will provide valuable insight into the clinical validity of probably benign assessments for lesions that are visible only at ultrasound. Specifically, robust data are expected on frequency of occurrence and subsequent biopsy, likelihood of malignancy, and whether subsequently diagnosed cancers (those that progress during follow-up) remain early in stage.

MR imaging

MR imaging of the breast is a highly sensitive but only moderately specific imaging modality for the detection of breast cancer [57]. Thus, there necessarily will be false-positives. To avoid too high a biopsy rate, and because of the technical challenges in performing MR imaging–guided biopsies, it is clinically important to render probably benign MR imaging assessments for which imaging surveillance rather than biopsy is recommended. Currently, there are very limited data on the use of probably benign assessments for lesions seen on MR imaging [58]. This situation is acknowledged in the MR imaging section of BI-RADS, which states that for probably benign assessments "at the present time, most approaches are intuitive" [6].

Liberman and colleagues [59] retrospectively examined the records of 367 asymptomatic high-risk women who had negative mammography and underwent baseline-screening MR imaging examinations. A probably benign assessment was rendered in 89 (24%) of the MR imaging examinations. MR imaging lesions that were considered probably benign included (1) bilateral areas of stippled or regional enhancement (Fig. 16); (2) multiple unilateral areas of stippled or regional enhancement; (3) multiple (bilateral or unilateral, scattered) smooth subcentimeter masses; and (4) localized mass or non–mass-like enhancement that probably represented benign findings, such as lymph nodes or patches of benign parenchyma. Of the 89 probably benign MR imaging assessments, visual inspection of kinetics data showed plateau enhancement in 71 (80%), progressive (currently termed "persistent" enhancement in 16 (18%), and washout in 2 (2%). The two cases demonstrating washout kinetics were multiple, smooth masses that were thought to represent benign lymph nodes. At follow-up, six cancers (7%) were detected because of progression of the MR imaging finding previously identified as probably benign. An additional three cancers were identified in areas initially interpreted as probably benign but for which the patients did not undergo follow-up MR imaging. Hence, the overall probability of malignancy was 10% (9 cancers in 89 lesions). There were five cases of DCIS and four cases of invasive ductal carcinoma. The median size of the invasive cancers was 0.6 cm (range, 0.2–0.9 cm), and micrometastases were detected in two patients on sentinel node sampling.

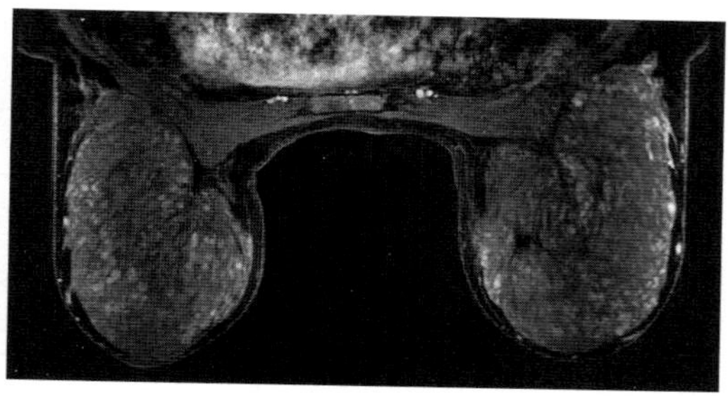

Fig. 16. Three-dimensional, contrast-enhanced, gradient-echo with fat saturation MR image of both breasts in the axial plane, demonstrating multiple areas of stippled enhancement in both breasts. Such a finding on MR imaging probably is benign because of bilaterality and extensive multiplicity. Most radiologists recommend short-interval imaging follow-up even though current data are not robust to support a probably benign assessment. Ongoing research may clarify the appropriate management of such lesions.

In another study, Sadowski and Kelcz [60] retrospectively reviewed reports of 473 patients who underwent breast MR imaging for evaluation of indeterminate mammographic lesions, local staging of known cancers, or assessment of breast symptoms such as breast pain or nipple discharge. Probably benign MR imaging findings were identified in 72 (15%) of the 473 patients. Lesions assessed on MR imaging as probably benign in this study included lesions that showed focal or diffuse mild to moderate enhancement (with benign enhancement kinetics) that corresponded to the mammographic finding of concern and incidental enhancing lesions showing progressive (currently termed "persistent") enhancement and lacking a mammographic correlate. Three cancers (4%) were found in these 72 cases: 3-mm and 10-mm invasive ductal carcinomas and a 2.7-cm low-grade intracystic papillary carcinoma. All three lesions were identified at imaging follow-up at 14 to 18 months.

In these two studies the reported rate of malignancy among probably benign MR imaging lesions is higher than the 2% upper limit established for probably benign lesions assessed at mammography and ultrasound [3,16,22,23,26,27,50] and is higher than the 2% upper limit for probably benign lesions as defined by BI-RADS [4]. Therefore, the constellation of MR imaging findings considered to be probably benign in these studies may require revision. Also of concern is the very high frequency (range, 15%–24%) of probably benign assessments reported for MR imaging findings. Finally, it has yet to be demonstrated in large-scale studies whether subsequently diagnosed cancers (the probably benign findings on MR imaging that progress during follow-up) remain early in stage. Thus, the use of the probably benign assessment for findings on MR imaging awaits validation by more robust data.

Summary

The probably benign assessment has been demonstrated to be a safe and effective approach to reducing the financial costs, morbidity, and patient anxiety associated with false-positive biopsies, thereby increasing the cost effectiveness of screening mammography. This assessment also is well accepted by patients. Its use in mammography has been substantiated by robust data, which show that it is associated with a less than 2% probability of malignancy. The few cancers in this category are of early stage and favorable prognosis and are detected through interval change at imaging follow-up. The authors believe that no newly apparent or enlarging lesion should be assessed as probably benign and that all screen-detected lesions should undergo full diagnostic imaging evaluation before being assessed as probably benign. Preliminary data suggest that some palpable lesions may be managed safely with periodic imaging surveillance, if strict imaging criteria for a probably benign mass are met. Use of the probably benign assessment for lesions visible only at ultrasound or MR imaging is much less well established, and further investigation is needed.

Acknowledgment

The authors thank Yelena Borodina and Renante Ramos for their assistance in manuscript preparation.

References

[1] Helvie MA, Pennes DR, Rebner M, et al. Mammographic follow-up of low-suspicion lesions: compliance rate and diagnostic yield. Radiology 1991;178(1):155–8.

[2] Hall FM, Storella JM, Silverstone DZ, et al. Nonpalpable breast lesions: recommendations for biopsy based on suspicion of carcinoma at mammography. Radiology 1988;167(2):353–8.

[3] Sickles EA. Periodic mammographic follow-up of probably benign lesions: results in 3,184 consecutive cases. Radiology 1991;179(2):463–8.

[4] American College of Radiology. Breast imaging reporting and data system—mammography (BI-RADS—mammography). 4th edition. Reston (VA): American College of Radiology; 2003.

[5] American College of Radiology. Breast imaging reporting and data system—ultrasound (BI-RADS—US). 1st edition. Reston (VA): American College of Radiology; 2003.

[6] American College of Radiology. Breast imaging reporting and data system—magnetic resonance imaging (BI-RADS—MRI). 1st edition. Reston (VA): American College of Radiology; 2003.

[7] Cyrlak D. Induced costs of low-cost screening mammography. Radiology 1988;168(3):661–3.

[8] Brenner RJ, Sickles EA. Surveillance mammography and stereotactic core breast biopsy for probably benign lesions: a cost comparison analysis. Acad Radiol 1997;4(6):419–25.

[9] Sickles EA. Breast masses: mammographic evaluation. Radiology 1989;173(2):297–303.

[10] Sickles EA. Combining spot-compression and other special views to maximize mammographic information [letter]. Radiology 1989;173(2):571.

[11] Berg WA, Arnoldus CL, Teferra E, et al. Biopsy of amorphous breast calcifications: pathologic outcome and yield at stereotactic biopsy. Radiology 2001;221(2):495–503.

[12] Leung JWT, Sickles EA. Developing asymmetry identified on mammography: correlation with imaging outcome and pathologic findings. AJR Am J Roentgenol 2007;188(3):667–75.

[13] Jackson FI. Acceptability of periodic follow-up as an alternative to biopsy for mamographically detected lesions interpreted as probably benign. Radiology 1989;173(2):580–1.

[14] Hall FM. Follow-up as an alternative to biopsy for mammographically detected lesions interpreted as probably benign. Radiology 1989;173(1):284–5.

[15] de Waal JČ. Periodic mammographic follow-up of probably benign lesions [letter]. Radiology 1991;181(2):608.

[16] Varas X, Leborgne F, Leborgne JH. Nonpalpable probably benign lesions: role of follow-up mammography. Radiology 1992;184(2):409–14.

[17] Sickles EA. Management of probably benign lesions of the breast. Radiology 1994;193(2):582–3.

[18] Sickles EA. Management of probably benign breast lesions. Radiol Clin North Am 1995;33(6):1123–30.

[19] Duijm LE, Zaat JO, Guit GL. Nonpalpable, probably benign breast lesions in general practice: the role of follow-up mammography. Br J Gen Pract 1998;48(432):1421–3.

[20] Sickles EA. Probably benign lesions: when should follow-up be recommended and what is the optimal follow-up protocol? Radiology 1999;213(1):11–4.

[21] Hall FM. Follow-up of probably benign breast lesions. Radiology 2000;217(1):303–5.

[22] Vizcaino I, Gadea L, Sandreo L, et al. Short-term follow-up results in 795 nonpalpable probably benign lesions detected at screening mammography. Radiology 2001;219(2):475–83.

[23] Varas X, Leborgne JH, Leborgne F, et al. Revisiting the mammographic follow-up of BI-RADS category 3 lesions. AJR Am J Roentgenol 2002;179(3):691–5.

[24] Wolfe JN, Buck KA, Salane M, et al. Xeroradiography of the breast: overview of 21,057 consecutive cases. Radiology 1987;165(2):305–11.

[25] Sickles EA, Ominsky SH, Sollitto RA, et al. Medical audit of a rapid-throughput mammography screening practice: methodology and results of 27,114 examinations. Radiology 1990;175(2):323–7.

[26] Yasmeen S, Romano PS, Pettinger M, et al. Frequency and predictive value of a mammographic

recommendation for short-interval follow-up. J Natl Cancer Inst 2003;95(6):429–36.
[27] Baum JK, Mahoney MC, Conant EF, et al. Use of BI-RADS 3: probably benign in the American College of Radiology Investigative Network (ACRIN) Digital Mammography Screening Trial (DMIST). Radiology 2006;241(P):226.
[28] Poplack SP, Tosteson AN, Grove MR, et al. Mammography in 53,803 women from the New Hampshire mammography network. Radiology 2000;217(3):832–40.
[29] Taplin S, Ichikawa L, Kerlikowske K, et al. Concordance of Breast Imaging Reporting and Data System assessments and management recommendations in screening mammography. Radiology 2002;222(2):529–35.
[30] Lehman C, Holt S, Peacock S, et al. Use of the American College of Radiology BI-RADS guidelines by community radiologists: concordance of assessments and recommendations assigned to screening mammograms. AJR Am J Roentgenol 2002;179(1):15–20.
[31] Caplan LS, Blackman D, Nadel M, et al. Coding mammograms using the classification "probably benign finding—short interval follow-up suggested". AJR Am J Roentgenol 1999;172(2):339–42.
[32] Homer MJ. Nonpalpable mammographic abnormalities: timing the follow-up studies. AJR Am J Roentgenol 1981;136(5):923–6.
[33] Rubin E. Six-month follow-up: an alternative view. Radiology 1999;213(1):15–8.
[34] Wilson R. Management of probably benign breast lesions [letter to editor]. Radiology 1995;194(3):912.
[35] Sickles EA. Management of probably benign breast lesions [reply to letter to editor]. Radiology 1995;194(3):912.
[36] Lindfors KK, O'Connor J, Acredolo CR, et al. Short-interval follow-up mammography versus immediate core biopsy of benign breast lesions: assessment of patient stress. AJR Am J Roentgenol 1998;171(1):55–8.
[37] Sickles EA. Breast calcifications: mammographic evaluation—state of the art. Radiology 1986;160(2):289–93.
[38] Leung JW, Sickles EA. Multiple bilateral masses detected on screening mammography: assessment of need for recall imaging. AJR Am J Roentgenol 2000;175(1):23–9.
[39] Rosen EL, Baker JA, Soo MS. Malignant lesions initially subjected to short-term mammographic follow-up. Radiology 2002;223(1):221–8.
[40] Hermann G, Keller RJ, Tartter P, et al. Interval changes in nonpalpable breast lesions as an indication of malignancy. Can Assoc Radiol J 1995;46(2):105–10.
[41] Ganott MA, Harris KM, Klaman HM, et al. Analysis of false-negative cancer cases identified with a mammography audit. Breast J 1999;5(3):166–75.
[42] Hall FM. Malignancy in BI-RADS category 3 mammographic lesions. Radiology 2002;225(3):918–9.
[43] Kerlikowske K, Smith-Bindman R, Abraham LA, et al. Breast cancer yield for screening mammographic examinations with recommendation for short-interval follow-up. Radiology 2005;234(3):684–92.
[44] Mendelson EB. Problem-solving ultrasound. Radiol Clin North Am 2004;42(5):909–18.
[45] Gokalp G, Topal U. MR imaging in probably benign lesions (BI-RADS category 3) of the breast. Eur J Radiol 2006;57(3):436–44.
[46] Hall FM. Probably benign breast nodules: follow-up of selected cases without initial full problem-solving imaging. Radiology 1995;194:305.
[47] Donegan WL. Evaluation of a palpable breast mass. N Engl J Med 1992;327(13):937–42.
[48] Sickles EA, Parker SH. Appropriate role of core breast biopsy in the management of probably benign lesions. Radiology 1993;188(2):315.
[49] Dawson AE, Mulford DK, Taylor AS, et al. Breast carcinoma in women age 35 years and younger: mammography and diagnosis by fine-needle aspiration cytology. Cancer 1998;84(3):163–8.
[50] Graf O, Helbich TH, Fuchsjaeger MH, et al. Follow-up of palpable circumscribed noncalcified solid breast masses at mammography and US: can biopsy be averted? Radiology 2004;233(3):850–6.
[51] Kopans DB, Swann CA, White G, et al. Asymmetric breast tissue. Radiology 1989;171(3):639–43.
[52] Sickles EA. Nonpalpable, circumscribed noncalcified solid breast masses: likelihood of malignancy based on lesion size and age of patient. Radiology 1994;192(2):439–42.
[53] Stavros AT, Thickman D, Rapp CL, et al. Solid breast nodules: use of sonography to distinguish between benign and malignant lesions. Radiology 1995;196(1):123–34.
[54] Rahbar G, Sie AC, Hansen GC, et al. Benign versus malignant solid breast masses: US differentiation. Radiology 1999;213(3):889–94.
[55] Baker JA, Kornguth PJ, Soo MS, et al. Sonography of solid breast lesions: observer variability of lesion description and assessment. AJR Am J Roentgenol 1999;172(6):1621–5.
[56] ACRIN 6666 protocol, pages 31–2. November 20, 2006. Available at: http://www.acrin.org/6666_protocol.html. Accessed May 1, 2007.
[57] Kuhl CK, Schild HH. Dynamic image interpretation of MRI of the breast. J Magn Reson Imaging 2000;12(6):956–74.
[58] Orel SG, Kay N, Reynolds C, et al. BI-RADS categorization as a predictor of malignancy. Radiology 1999;211(3):845–50.
[59] Liberman L, Morris EA, Benton CL, et al. Probably benign lesions at breast magnetic resonance imaging: preliminary experience in high-risk women. Cancer 2003;98(2):377–88.
[60] Sadowski EA, Kelcz F. Frequency of malignancy in lesions classified as probably benign after dynamic contrast-enhanced breast MRI examination. J Magn Reson Imaging 2005;21(5):556–64.

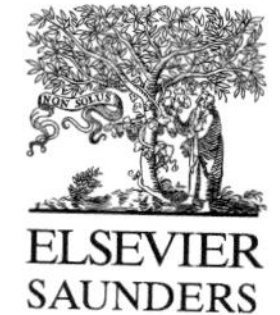

ELSEVIER
SAUNDERS

RADIOLOGIC CLINICS OF NORTH AMERICA

Radiol Clin N Am 45 (2007) 791–800

Auditing and Benchmarks in Screening and Diagnostic Mammography

Stephen A. Feig, MD, FACR[a,b,*]

- Surrogate markers
- Requirements for a screening test
- Detection rates
- Recall rates
- Positive predictive values
- Ductal carcinoma in situ
- Minimal carcinoma
- Desirable goals for surrogate measures of screening outcomes
- Breast Cancer Surveillance Consortium benchmarks
- Benchmarks for screening mammography
- Setting goals for screening recall rates and positive biopsy rates
- Benchmarks for diagnostic mammography
- Comparison of screening outcomes among radiology practice groups
- Current and proposed audit requirements of the Mammography Quality Standards Act
- Summary
- References

Randomized clinical trials conducted in the United States and Europe have demonstrated the ability of screening mammography to reduce breast cancer deaths among women age 40 years and older by up to 32% [1–3]. These trials compared cumulative breast cancer mortality rates in study populations offered screening with otherwise comparable control group populations that were not offered screening. Following the general success of these trials, several European countries offered screening mammography as a public health initiative. These service screening studies estimate the effect of mammography on breast cancer mortality after adjustment for potential biases such as age, self-selection, and historical trends. They found that application of periodic screening mammography to the general population reduced breast cancer deaths by as much as 45% [4–10]. In the United States, screening mammography has led to a substantial downstaging of breast cancer since 1980 (Table 1). Today women who have invasive cancer are 39% less likely to die from their disease than were their counterparts in the early 1980s [4].

Surrogate markers

There is good evidence that radiologists can predict the ability of their screening practice to reduce breast cancer mortality by using combined assessment of outcome measures such as tumor size and stage, node positivity, and detection rates. Demonstration of adequate values for these surrogate measures suggests that a mammography screening program will be effective in lowering

[a] University of California, Irvine School of Medicine, Orange, CA, USA
[b] University of California, Irvine Medical Center, 101 The City Drive South, Route 140, Orange, CA 92868-3298, USA
* University of California Irvine Medical Center, 101 The City Drive South, Route 140, Orange, CA 92868-3298.
E-mail address: sfeig@uci.edu

radiologic.theclinics.com

doi:10.1016/j.rcl.2007.07.001

Table 1: **Breast cancer stage at diagnosis: a 20-year retrospective in the United States**

Stage	1980 (%)	2001 (%)	5-Year Relative Survival
Ductal carcinoma in situ	3	21	100
Stage I	25	42	98
Stage II	45	25	80
Stage III, IV	14	7	25
Unknown	13	5	56

Data from National Cancer Institute. SEER: surveillance epidemiology and end results. Available at: http://www.seer.cancer.gov. Accessed November 15, 2004.

breast cancer deaths [11–13]. Years before decreased mortality was found among screened women in the Kopparberg Sweden Trial, Tabar and colleagues [14] were able to predict the subsequent appearance of this benefit on the basis of an initial decrease in the proportion of advanced (stage II and higher) cancers in the study population compared with the control population, followed in the second and third round of screening by a significant decrease in the absolute number of these advanced cancers in the study population relative to the control population. By comparison, the lack of reduction in tumor size in the National Breast Screening Study of Canada explains why that study was the only randomized trial that failed to demonstrate any mortality reduction through screening [15]. Thus, surrogate markers may serve as a harbinger of the benefit (or lack of benefit) to come.

Requirements for a screening test

In 1968, the World Health Organization proposed guidelines for the implementation of any given modality for screening for early disease. Among these requirements were a high level of sensitivity and specificity, demonstration of a net benefit (versus risks) to the target population, and justification of resources expended in terms of net benefits [16]. To meet the requirements for a practical screening test, adverse consequences to the patient such as excessive recalls of screenees for supplementary mammographic views, breast ultrasound, breast MR imaging, excessive recommendations for short-interval (American College of Radiology Breast Imaging and Reporting Data System [ACR BI-RADS] 3) follow-up, excessive false-positive biopsy rates, and costs also must be limited [17]. On a national level, the limited number of breast-imaging radiologists, technologists, and equipment must not be overextended by performing unnecessary procedures [18].

With these considerations in mind, the Agency for Health Care Policy and Research (AHCPR), now renamed the Agency for Health Care Research and Quality, in 1994 published a table of desirable goals for screening mammography outcomes [19]. These goals were endorsed by the ACR and may be found in the 1998 and 2003 editions of the BI-RADS *Atlas* [20,21]. The goals include detection rates, recall rates, positive predictive values, and levels for ductal carcinoma in situ (DCIS), minimal carcinoma, and higher stages of disease.

Detection rates

The AHCPR and BI-RADS guidelines recommend the use of multiple outcome measurements. The term "cancer detection rates" refers to the number of cancers detected per thousand women screened. For any size population, detection rates are higher on initial (prevalence) screen than on a subsequent (incidence) screen unless the screens are many years apart [22]. Detection rates also depend on screening frequency, patient age, and risk status of the population [23]. For these reasons, acceptable detection rates are provided as a range of values.

Interval cancers refer to these cancers which are missed at screening, and surface clinically before the next screen. Internal cancer rates equal the number of interval cancers divided by the sum of screen-detected and interval cancers. Interval cancer rates are higher in younger women than in older women [19,21,23].

Recall rates

The term "recall rates" refers to the percentage of screenees asked to return for additional imaging work-up, such as supplementary mammographic views or ultrasound after batch interpretation of their screening mammograms. Batch reading is much faster and less expensive to perform than on-line interpretation of screening mammography and is preferable because of limited staffing and low reimbursement rates. Batch interpretation can be performed successfully only when recall rates are maintained within acceptable limits. Recall rates that are too high result in inconvenience and anxiety for the patient and unnecessary costs and inefficiency for the medical care system. If recall rates are too low, some subtle cancers may be missed, and some benign lesions may undergo unnecessary biopsy because further imaging work-up could have established their lack of suspicious features. Recall rates will be higher on initial (incidence) screening than on subsequent (prevalence) screening because comparison with previous screening mammography showing a finding usually will reduce the need for further evaluation.

Positive predictive values

The term "positive predictive value" (PPV) may refer to one of three different measures. PPV_1 is the percentage of all positive screening examinations (BI-RADS categories 0, 4, and 5) that result in a tissue diagnosis of cancer within 1 year. For BI-RADS category 0, additional imaging is required. BI-RADS categories 4 and 5 are suspicious for malignancy and highly suggestive for malignancy, respectively. PPV_1 equals the true positives (TP) divided by the number of positive screening examinations (TP plus false positives [FP]): $PPV_1 = TP/(TP + FP_1)$.

PPV_2 (biopsy recommended) is the percentage of all screening or diagnostic examinations recommended for biopsy or surgical consultation (BI-RADS categories 4 and 5) that resulted in a tissue diagnosis of cancer within 1 year. PPV_2 equals the number of screening or diagnostic examinations recommended for biopsy divided by the number of TP and FP examinations: $PPV_2 = TP/(TP + FP_2)$.

PPV_3 (biopsy performed) is the percentage of all known biopsies done as a result of a positive screening or diagnostic examination or additional imaging evaluations of positive screening examinations (BI-RADS categories 4 and 5) that resulted in a tissue diagnosis of cancers within 1 year. PPV_3 also is known as the "biopsy yield of malignancy" or the "positive biopsy rate." $PPV_3 = TP/(TP + FP_3)$.

An FP examination must have no known tissue diagnosis of cancer within 1 year of a positive screening examination (FP_1), or a recommendation for biopsy (FP_2) or surgical consultation, or a benign tissue diagnosis within 1 year after a recommendation for biopsy (FP_3).

Ductal carcinoma in situ

DCIS refers to breast cancer confined by the basement membrane with little or no invasion into the parenchyma. A substantial body of evidence indicates that detection of DCIS prevents the development of invasive carcinoma. Several compelling studies have been published since the author's last analysis of the literature on this topic in 2001 [24]. In a 30-year follow-up of Page's series, of 28 women who had low-grade DCIS treated by excisional biopsy alone, 11 developed invasive breast cancer in the same breast, and 1 developed recurrent DCIS [25]. Five of these 11 women died of metastatic disease. Among women who had no subsequent invasive cancer, complete removal of DCIS by excision or nonprogression of DCIS is assumed. Thus, even low-grade DCIS has been shown to have a lethal progression. In another retrospective series of 13 women whose biopsy specimens with DCIS originally were diagnosed as benign, the odds ratio for development of invasive cancer in the ipsilateral breast was 13.5 compared with women who had nonproliferative lesions [26]. Although these 13 women had DCIS of all nuclear grades, none exhibited comedonecrosis.

Progressive DCIS is defined as DCIS that has the propensity to progress to invasive disease. Nonprogressive DCIS is defined as DCIS that could not have progressed to invasive disease if left untreated. Applying a mathematical Markov chain model to empiric observations from five screening programs, Yen and colleagues [27] estimated that among cases of DCIS detected at prevalence (initial) screening, 63% were progressive, and 37% were nonprogressive. At incidence (subsequent) screenings, 96% of detected cases of DCIS were progressive, and 4% were nonprogressive. The authors conclude that although there may be an element of overdiagnosis of DCIS in breast cancer screening, the phenomenon is small in both relative and absolute terms.

Further insight into the natural history of DCIS has been derived by McCann and colleagues [28] from the United Kingdom National Health Services Screening Programe, which screened women age 50 to 64 years. As found by other screening studies, detection rates of breast cancer are higher than the expected natural incidence, especially for the first several years after women enter the program, because screening detects cancers that ordinarily would not surface clinically until later when they had grown to the clinical threshold size. After women leave the program at age 65 years, the incidence of breast cancer is actually lower than the expected natural incidence of the disease because there is a deficit of larger palpable cancers. This deficit gradually recedes, and after several more years there is a return to the expected age-related incidence for nonscreened women. The key finding of this study was that earlier detection of invasive cancer at screening was not sufficient to account for all the decreased incidence of invasive cancer after cessation of screening. Fully 25% of the decreased incidence of invasive cancer and prevented deaths resulted from the increased detection of DCIS during the screening years. The authors concluded, "cancer for cancer, there is as much benefit from detection and treatment of DCIS as from detection and treatment of invasive cancer."

Minimal carcinoma

The concept of minimal cancer originated from the seminal research of Gallager and Martin [29–31] in the 1960s and 1970s. Their aim was to define the stage and type of breast cancer in which local treatment alone would be highly effective. Using mammographic histologic correlation, they calculated that the probability of lymph node involvement would be 10% or less for all cases of lobular carcinoma in situ (LCIS) and DCIS, regardless of size, and for those cases of invasive ductal or invasive lobular carcinoma having a volume no greater than that of a sphere 0.5 cm in diameter. They predicted that treatment of such cases by local means would enable 10 or 20 years' survival rates of 95%. Subsequent studies by other investigators have shown that the predictions of Gallager and Martin [31] were, if anything, overly pessimistic because the no-evidence-of-disease rate of such cancers at follow-up periods of 1 to 26 years was 97%. Today the definition of minimal carcinoma has evolved further and includes all cases of DCIS and those invasive cancers measuring 1 cm or less. LCIS currently is regarded as a marker of high risk rather than a true cancer [32]. All cases of DCIS are stage 0. Invasive carcinoma 2 cm or less without nodal involvement is considered stage I.

Desirable goals for surrogate measures of screening outcomes

The desirable goals for screening outcome parameters chosen by the AHCPR and endorsed by ACR are shown in Table 2. These goals were selected by panels of breast-imaging experts based on results from relatively small but well-run community and academic screening programs and had been published in the peer-review literature. These numeric values were intended to be advisory rather than restrictive. Somewhat different values have been selected by screening programs in the United Kingdom and Europe and have been used there to enforce standards for performance outcomes (see Table 1) [33–35]. Within the United States, the Food and Drug Administration (FDA)–regulated Mammography Quality Standards Act (MQSA) requires auditing of clinical outcomes for all screening and diagnostic examinations assessed as either suspicious for malignancy (BI-RADS category 4) or highly suggestive of malignancy (BI-RADS category 5) [36]. These rules pertain to data collection but do not involve enforcement of any standards of interpretative performance outcome.

Breast Cancer Surveillance Consortium benchmarks

The recently published benchmarks for screening and diagnostic mammography from the Breast Cancer Surveillance Consortium (BCSC) derive their data from different types of sources than those used to select outcome measures for the AHCPR report. The BCSC is a research initiative funded by the National Cancer Institute–with a Statistical Coordinating Center and six population-based research sites [37]: the Carolina Mammography Registry (Chapel Hill, North Carolina), Group Health Cooperative (Seattle, Washington), New Hampshire Mammography Network (Lebanon, New Hampshire), New Mexico Mammography Project (Albuquerque, New Mexico), Vermont Breast Cancer Surveillance System (Burlington, Vermont), and San Francisco Mammography Registry (San Francisco, California).

Approximately 188 screening mammography facilities (151 diagnostic mammography facilities) contributed to the pooled data [38,39]. These represent about 2% of the approximately 10,000 FDA-certified mammographic facilities throughout the United States. Results from a total of 2,580,151 screening mammography studies from 1,117,390 women performed between 1996 and 2002 and 332,926 diagnostic mammography studies performed on 239,751 women between 1996 and 2001 were analyzed. Demographic data, including race and economic status, from all six registries combined differed by less than 5% from those for the entire United States population. This robust practice data from the BCSC may be considered representative of that for the entire country.

Benchmarks for screening mammography

In general, mean outcome values for the largely community-based radiologists in the BCSC registries fell within the "desirable" range of values suggested by AHCPR (see Table 2). Among screen-detected invasive cancers with known size detected at the BCSC sites, 37.1% were 1 cm or less, 41.7% were 1 to 2 cm, and 21.2% were larger than 2 cm. Among the invasive cancers, the median size was 1.3 cm, and the mean size was 1.6 cm [39]. These results are in accord with the recommendation of Tabar and colleagues [12] that at least 50% of screen-detected invasive cancers should be smaller than 1.5 cm. Thus, in terms of detection rates and stage of diagnosis, screening mammography in the United States seems to be functioning adequately.

Besides mean outcome values, BCSC outcome data also were presented as frequency plots, which provided the range of values for 50% (twenty-fifth to seventy-fifth percentile) and 80% (ninth to ninetieth percentile) of radiologists. It is unlikely that the performance of any given radiologist will approximate average values closely. Thus, frequency plots should be extremely helpful to radiologists who want to compare their own performance with that of their peers around the country.

Table 2: **Screening mammography: comparison of Breast Cancer Surveillance Consortium performance results with Agency for Health Care Policy and Research, European, and United Kingdom recommendations**

Parameter	BCSC Results (%)	AHCPR Goals (%)	European and United Kingdom Guidelines	
			Minimal (%)	*Desirable (%)*
Recall rate	9.7	≤ 10	–	–
Initial screen	12.3	–	< 7	≤ 5
Subsequent screen	8.8	–	< 5	≤ 3
Cancer detection rate[a]	4.4	2–10		
Initial screen	4.4	6–10	3	> 3
Subsequent screen	4.3	2–4	1.5	> 1.5
Interval cancer rate	–	–	–	–
0–11 months	–	–	30	< 30
12–23 months	–	–	50	< 50
PPV_1	4.5	5–10	–	–
PPV_2	25.0	25–40	–	–
PPV_3	33.8	–	–	–
Ductal carcinoma in situ	21.6	–	10	10–20
Minimal cancer	51.8	> 30	–	–
Stage 0 or I	76.0	> 50	–	–
Initial screening	–	–	75	> 75
Subsequent screening	–	–	80	> 80
Invasive cancers < 10 mm/total cancers detected	–	–	–	–
Initial screening	–	–	≥ 20	≥ 25
Subsequent screening	–	–	≥ 25	≥ 30
Node + cancer	18.8	< 25	–	–
Initial screening	–	–	30	< 30
Subsequent screening	–	–	25	< 25
Sensitivity (if measurable)	–	> 85	–	–
Specificity (if measurable)	–	> 90	–	–

[a] Cancers per 1000 women screened.

These types of data indicate moderate variability in interpretative performance among radiologists in the United States for both screening and diagnosis. Results for screening recall rates are of particular interest because, although the median recall rate of 9.7% was within the AHCPR recommendations, the spread was wide: about 50% of radiologists had recall rates that exceeded the upper limit of the recommended range, which is 10%. Some observers have suggested that this variability is of some concern because the medical literature suggests that wide variation in the processes of health care delivery may be associated with lower quality or worse outcomes [39,40]. Mammography interpretation, however, is highly challenging, is not totally objective, and depends on experience and skill; the variation in recall rates reflects this reality.

Setting goals for screening recall rates and positive biopsy rates

In a recent study, Smith-Bindman and colleagues [41] compared recall rates with cancer detection rates at three large-scale mammography registries or screening programs: the BCSC and the National Breast and Cervical Cancer Early Detection Program (NBCCEDP) in the United States and the National Health Services Breast Screening Program (NHSBSP) in the United Kingdom. Recall rates for the first screening mammogram in the two

American programs were about twice as high as those for the United Kingdom: 13.1 and 11.2, respectively, versus 7.4. On subsequent screens, recall rates in the United States still were about double those in the United Kingdom: 8.0 and 6.8, respectively, versus 3.6. Despite higher recall rates, cancer detection rates were not significantly higher among American women than among women in the United Kingdom. The authors suggested that radiologists in the United States are interpreting too many screening mammograms as abnormal. Additionally, Smith-Bindman and colleagues [41] found that negative open surgical biopsy rates per 100 screening mammograms were higher at the BCSC sites in the United States than at the NHSBSP sites in the United Kingdom: 0.82 versus 0.36 at first screenings and 0.22 versus 0.10 at subsequent screenings.

The purpose of breast cancer screening is to detect earlier cancers rather than just more cancers. Careful reading of the study by Smith-Bindman and colleagues [41] reveals that the BCSC and the NBCCEDP detection rates for DCIS were higher than those of the NHSBSP program. Detection rates for invasive cancers measuring less than 10 mm and 10 to 20 mm were higher at the BCSC in the United States than at the NHSBSP in the United Kingdom [41,42]. Higher detection rates for minimal cancers in the United States may be related in part to higher recall rates.

A study by Sant and colleagues [43] compared results from two population-based registries: the Survival, Epidemiology, and End Results Program in the United States and the European Concerted Action on Survival and Care of Cancer Patients Project that pooled data from 17 European countries. Early-stage breast cancers were more frequent (41% versus 24%) and overall 5-year breast cancer survival rates were higher (89% versus 79%) in the United States than in Europe. In the United Kingdom, only 26% of invasive breast cancers are detected at an early stage, versus 76% in the United States. In Europe, the excess relative risk of death from breast cancer was 37% higher than in the United States. The authors suggested that the higher breast cancer survival rates in the United States can be explained by earlier diagnosis. Comparison of the survival rate data of Sant and colleagues [43] and the recall rate data of Smith-Bindman [41,42] suggests that higher breast cancer survival rates in the United States may be related to higher recall rates at screening and lower PPVs at biopsy. Thus screening recall rates are two to three times higher in the United States than in Europe, the stage of cancer detected is lower, and breast cancer survival rates are higher [44]. Higher rates in the United States result in part from the more litigious medicolegal climate. Lower recall rates in Europe often are imposed by government policy.

A study from facilities throughout North Carolina found lower rates of cancer detection with recall rates below 4.9% but no significant benefit from recall rates above 10% [45]. PPV_1 began decreasing significantly at a recall rate of 5.9%. The authors concluded that a recall rate between 4.9% and 5.5% represents the best trade-off between detection sensitivity and PPV_1. A study by Gur and colleagues [46] from Pittsburgh found little or no gain in the detection rate beyond a 12% recall. The conclusions from the North Carolina study are supported by those from a more recent, larger study of 171,104 initial (prevalence) and 1,872,687 subsequent (incidence) screening mammograms from 172 and 139 facilities, respectively, in the six BCSC sites [47]. The number of additional women needed to be recalled at a given recall rate to detect one additional cancer was estimated as additional work-ups (AW) per additional cancer detected (ACD): AW/ACD. On this basis, the authors recommended a recall rate of 10% for first screenings and 6.7% for subsequent screenings. Recall rates above these values were associated with AW/ACD values of greater than 100.

The recall rate in the Dutch screening program (< 1% recall for subsequent screens) is the lowest worldwide. Otten and colleagues [48] estimated that increasing the recall rate to 4% would reduce substantially the number of late-detected interval cancers and cancers detected at later screenings. In my opinion, the European countries that have set recall rates of 5% or less need to recognize that this policy will result in a delayed diagnosis of too many cancers.

Elmore and colleagues [49] reviewed outcomes from community-based screening programs around the world. Wide variations were noted for the percentage of screening mammograms judged to be abnormal (1.2%–15.0%). This value was two to four percentage points higher for programs in the United States and Canada than for programs in other countries. The PPV_3 values for European programs were generally in the range of 40% to 80%, compared with 20% to 40% for North American programs and 33.8% at the BCSC sites.

Benchmarks for diagnostic mammography

Among the diagnostic cases, abnormal interpretation following work-up was defined as a recommendation for biopsy (fine-needle aspiration, core, or excisional), that is, BI-RADS category 4 or 5 [38]. Outcomes for diagnostic mammography, according to indications, are shown in Table 3. The likelihood of any specific clinical outcome for diagnostic

Table 3: **Abnormal interpretation rates, PPV_3, cancer detection rates, histology, and size according to indication for diagnostic mammography examination**

Parameter (%)	Screen-detected abnormality	Short-interval follow-up	Symptomatic but no Lump	Palpable Lump	Total
Abnormal interpretation rate	12.3	3.4	5.7	10.5	8.0
PPV_2	30.3	32.3	43.2	59.4	39.5
Cancer diagnosis rate per 1000 examinations[a]	30.8	8.4	18.1	49.0	25.3
Ductal carcinoma in situ	26.9	30.7	16.0	5.5	17.5
Invasive cancer	73.1	69.3	84.0	94.5	82.5
Minimal cancer	62.0	64.7	37.2	17.5	42.0

[a] Cancers per 1000 women screened.
Data from Sickles EA, Miglioretti DL, Ballard-Barbash R, et al. Performance benchmarks for diagnostic mammography. Radiology 2005;235:775-90.

mammography depends largely on the clinical indication for the examination. Abnormal interpretation rates (BI-RADS category 4 or 5) were, on average, 8.0%. These rates were highest for women having a screen-detected abnormality (12.3%) or a palpable mass (10.5%). They were lower for women having breast symptoms but no lump (5.7%) and were lowest for women having a short-interval follow-up for a probably benign (BI-RADS category 3) lesion (3.4%).

The likelihood of malignancy at biopsy (PPV_3) was 39.5% on average. It was highest for women presenting with a palpable mass (59.4%), next highest for those who had clinical symptoms other than a mass (43.2%), and lowest for those who had a screen-detected abnormality (30.3%) or a change in imaging appearance on short-interval follow-up (32.3%).

The overall cancer detection rate was 25.3 per 1000 diagnostic examinations. These rates were higher for women having a palpable mass (49.0/1000), lower for those with a screen-detected abnormality (30.8/1000), still lower among women with breast symptoms but no lump (18.1/1000), and lowest for women having short-interval follow-up (8.4/1000).

Among biopsy-proven malignancies, DCIS was more likely among women biopsied on the basis of a nonpalpable abnormality or a change on short-interval follow-up (26.9% and 30.7%, respectively) and was lower among those biopsied because of a palpable lesion (5.5%). A similar pattern was found for the relative likelihood of minimal carcinoma versus nonminimal carcinoma.

Because of these wide discrepancies, radiologists who want to compare their own interpretative performance of diagnostic mammography with the BCSC benchmarks would be well advised to make indication-specific rather than overall comparisons.

Comparison of screening outcomes among radiology practice groups

Finally, although radiologists may benefit from comparing screening performance data for themselves or their practice group with BCSC performance benchmarks, this comparison should be made with caution. Several caveats must be kept in mind. Outcome data are, of course, influenced by radiologists' skill, experience, and interpretive threshold [50]. They also are affected by the demographic characteristics and risk factors, including patient age, family history, diet, and environment, that affect the prior probability of disease [51].

Recall rates show only minimal variation with patient age. Cancer detection rates, however, are higher in older women, coincident with the increasing incidence of breast cancer with age. Compared with women in their forties, screening detection rates are twice as high among women ages 60 to 69 years and are almost three times higher for those ages 70 to 79 years. Positive predictive value at biopsy (PPV_3) at several screening programs in the United States generally has been 20% to 30%, 25% to 35%, 30% to 40%, and 40% to 60% for women ages 40 to 49, 50 to 59, 60 to 69, and 70 to 79 years, respectively [17]. DCIS generally has represented 40% to 50%, 30% to 40%, and 20% to 30% of all cancers detected at screening for women ages 40 to 49, 50 to 59, and 60 to 69 years, respectively [24].

The interval since the last screening examination, as well as the quality of the previous interpretation, also will affect results. Additionally, radiologists who interpret fewer mammograms and lower-volume screening facilities will be more subject to statistical variations in outcome. Robust data always provide more dependable conclusions. Low-volume readers and facilities may want to aggregate data from longer periods of time for their assessment.

Current and proposed audit requirements of the Mammography Quality Standards Act

Under current MQSA regulations, all BI-RADS category 4 and 5 recommendations must be recorded. All biopsy results must be collected, or an attempt to collect should be documented. Biopsy results from screening and diagnostic examinations may be combined. Annual analysis of biopsy outcome results for the facility and for each radiologist is required. Each facility must designate an audit-interpreting physician [36,52].

In its 2005 report "Improving Breast Imaging Quality Standards," the Institute of Medicine (IOM) recommended adding more outcome measures to those currently required by the MQSA [52]. Any such initiative cannot ignore the added cost and personnel required. Additional compensation must be provided for the substantial extra work in breast imaging, a field in which expenses and reimbursements are already narrowly separated.

The proposed new basic mammography audit would have additional data-collection requirements including

- **PPV_2, that is, results for all recommended biopsies**
- **Cancer detection rate per 1000 women screened**
- **Abnormal interpretation rate for additional imaging or biopsy**
- **Required tracking of BI-RADS category 4 and 5 and also BI-RADS category 0 images**
- **Separate audits for screening and diagnostic mammography**

The new rules would allow combined measurements for the same radiologist working at different facilities. Audit data collection and analysis would be verified at the annual FDA inspection but would not be collected by the FDA. Reimbursement rates would be increased to cover the costs of the new audit procedures.

The IOM also has proposed a voluntary advanced medical audit modeled on the BCSC. This audit would include collection of patient characteristics as well as tumor-staging information from the pathology report. There would be higher reimbursement rates for volunteer facilities in keeping with the "pay for performance" paradigm.

In addition, the IOM has proposed the establishment of "Breast Imaging Centers of Excellence." These facilities would participate in both basic and advanced audits. They would be used as clinical research sites to test the effects of initiatives such as high volume, double reading, and advanced audits on clinical outcomes from screening. These facilities could serve as test sites to develop and evaluate programs assessing interpretive skills. They could be training centers for breast imagers from other facilities. They also could assess a no-fault medical liability system.

Another IOM proposal is the establishment of a central data and statistics coordinating center that could release aggregate data that physicians could compare with their own performance. Using these data, the center could develop, implement, and evaluate self-improvement plans for radiologists. The center would be independent of regulatory authority, and all data would be protected from discoverability.

Summary

More than any other subspecialty of diagnostic radiology, breast imaging lends itself to the objective assessment of interpretive performance, which has been the subject of innumerable clinical research studies. Mammography outcome audits for individual radiologists and radiology groups allows comparison with recommended values and national benchmarks. Such initiatives allow each radiologist to determine how well he or she is doing in continuing to improve the prognosis for women with breast cancer. The substantial reduction of deaths from breast cancer has been one of the major medical accomplishments of this time.

References

[1] Humphrey LL, Helfand M, Chan BKS, et al. Breast cancer screening: a summary of the evidence for the U.S. Preventive Services Task Force. Ann Intern Med 2002;137:347–60.

[2] U.S. Preventive Services Task Force. Screening for breast cancer: recommendations and rationale. Ann Intern Med 2002;137:344–6.

[3] Smith RA, Saslow D, Sawyer KA, et al. American Cancer Society guidelines for breast cancer screening: update 2003. CA Cancer J Clin 2003; 53:141–69.

[4] Feig SA. Effect of service screening mammography on population mortality from breast cancer. Cancer 2002;95:451–7.

[5] Tabar L, Yen M-F, Vitak B, et al. Mammography service screening and mortality in breast cancer

patients: 20-year follow-up before and after the introduction of screening. Lancet 2003;361: 1405–10.
[6] Otto SJ, Fracheboud J, Looman CWN, et al. Initiation of population-based mammography screening in Dutch municipalities and effect on breast cancer mortality: a systematic review. Lancet 2003;361:1411–7.
[7] Olsen AH, Njor SH, Vejborg I, et al. Breast cancer mortality in Copenhagen after introduction of mammography screening: cohort study. BMJ 2005;330:220–4.
[8] Duffy SW, Tabar L, Chen TH-H, et al. Reduction in breast cancer mortality from organized service screening with mammography: 1. Further confirmation with extended data. Cancer Epidemiol Biomarkers Prev 2006;15:45–51.
[9] Parinven I, Helinius H, Anttila A, et al. Service screening mammography reduces breast cancer mortality among elderly women in Turku. J Med Screen 2006;13:34–40.
[10] Duffy SW, Tabar L, Chen TH-H. Effect of mammographic service screening on stage at presentation of breast cancers in Sweden. Cancer 2007; 109:2205–12.
[11] Day NE, Williams DRR, Khaw KT. Breast cancer screening programmes: the development of a monitoring and evaluation system. Br J Cancer 1989;59:954–8.
[12] Tabar L, Fagerberg G, Duffy SW, et al. Update of the Swedish two-county program of mammographic screening for breast cancer. Radiol Clin North Am 1992;30:187–219.
[13] Feig SA. Determination of mammographic screening intervals with surrogate measures for women age 40-49 years. Radiology 1994;193: 311–4.
[14] Tabar L, Gad A, Holmberg L, et al. Significant reduction in advanced cancer: results of the first seven years of mammography screening in Kopparberg, Sweden. Diagn Imaging Clin Med 1985; 54:158–64.
[15] Michaelson JS, Satija S, Kopans DB, et al. Gauging the impact of breast carcinoma screening in terms of tumor size and death rate. Cancer 2003;98:2114–24.
[16] Wilson JMG, Jungren G. Principles and practice of screening for disease. Public Health Paper (No. 34). Geneva: World Health Organization; 1968. p. 26.
[17] Feig SA. Adverse effects of screening mammography. Radiol Clin North Am 2004;42:807–20.
[18] D'Orsi CJ. Mammography: will adequate manpower exist? Radiol Clin North Am 2004;42: 975–8.
[19] Bassett LW, Hendrick RE, Bassford TL, et al. Clinical practice guideline number 13: quality determinants of mammography. AHCPR Publication 95–0632. Rockville (MD): U.S. Department of Health and Human Services, Agency for Health Care Policy and Research, Public Health Service; 1994. p. 83.
[20] D'Orsi CJ, Bassett LW, Feig SA, et al. Illustrated breast imaging reporting and data system (BI-RADS). 3rd edition. Reston (VA): American College of Radiology; 1998. p. 180–1.
[21] D'Orsi CJ, Bassett LW, Berg WA, et al. Breast imaging reporting and data system: ACR BI-RADS. In: . 4th edition. Reston (VA): American College of Radiology; 2003. p. 229–51.
[22] Hunt KA, Rosen EL, Sickles EA. Outcome analysis for women undergoing annual versus biennial screening mammography: a review of 24,211 examinations. AJR Am J Roentgenol 1999; 173:285–9.
[23] Morrison AS. Screening for chronic disease. 2nd edition. New York: Oxford University Press; 1992.
[24] Feig SA. Ductal carcinoma in situ: implications for screening mammography. Radiol Clin North Am 2000;38:653–8.
[25] Sanders ME, Schuyler PA, DuPont WD, et al. The natural history of low-grade ductal carcinoma in situ of the breast in women treated by biopsy only revealed over 30 years of long-term follow-up. Cancer 2005;103:2481–4.
[26] Collins LC, Tamini RM, Baer HJ, et al. Outcome of patients with ductal carcinoma in situ untreated after diagnostic biopsy: results from the Nurses' Health Study. Cancer 2005;103: 1778–84.
[27] Yen M-F, Tabar L, Smith RA, et al. Quantifying the potential problem of over diagnosis of ductal carcinoma in situ in breast cancer screenings. Eur J Cancer 2003;39:1746–54.
[28] McCann J, Treasure P, Duffy S. Modeling the impact of detecting and treating carcinoma in situ in a breast screening programme. J Med Screen 2004;11:117–25.
[29] Gallager HS, Martin JE. An orientation to the concept of minimal breast cancer. Cancer 1971; 28:1505–7.
[30] Gallager HS. Minimal breast cancer: origin of the concept and definition. In: Feig SA, McLelland R, editors. Breast carcinoma: current diagnosis and treatment. New York: Masson Publishing USA and American College of Radiology; 1983. p. 251–6.
[31] Gallager HS. Minimal breast cancer: results of treatment and long-term follow-up. In: Feig SA, McLelland R, editors. Breast carcinoma: current diagnosis and treatment. New York: Masson Publishing USA and American College of Radiology; 1983. p. 291–4.
[32] Sewell CW. Pathology of high-risk breast lesions and ductal carcinoma in situ. Radiol Clin North Am 2004;42:821–30.
[33] Liston J, Wilson R, editors. Quality assurance guidelines for breast cancer screening radiologists. NHS breast screening programmes publication no. 59. Sheffield (UK): NHS Cancer Screening Programmes; 2005.
[34] Advisory Committee on Cancer Prevention. Recommendation on cancer screening in the European Union. Eur J Cancer 2000;36:1473–8.

[35] Roselli del Turco M, Hendrik JH, Perry NM. Radiological guidelines. In: Perry N, Broeders M, de Wolf CJM, et al, editors. European guidelines for quality assurance in mammography screening. 3rd edition. Luxembourg: Office for Official Publications of the European Commission; 2001. p. 366–75.
[36] Monsees BS. The Mammography Quality Standards Act: an overview of the regulations and guidance. Radiol Clin North Am 2000;38: 759–72.
[37] Ballard-Barbash R, Taplin SH, Yankaskas BC, et al. Breast cancer surveillance consortium: a national mammography screening and outcomes database. AJR Am J Roentgenol 1997;169:1001–8.
[38] Sickles EA, Miglioretti DL, Ballard-Barbash R, et al. Performance benchmarks for diagnostic mammography. Radiology 2005;235:775–90.
[39] Rosenberg RD, Yankaskas BC, Abraham LA, et al. Performance benchmarks for screening mammography. Radiology 2006;241:55–66.
[40] Hewitt M, Simone JV, editors. Ensuring the quality of cancer care. National Cancer Policy Board, Institute of Medicine and National Research Council. Washington DC: National Academies Press; 1999.
[41] Smith-Bindman R, Chu PW, Miglioretti DL, et al. Comparison of screening mammography in the United States and the United Kingdom. JAMA 2003;290:2129–37.
[42] Smith-Bindman R, Kerlikowske K. Optimal recall rates following mammography. [letter to the editor]. JAMA 2004;291:821–2.
[43] Sant M, Allemani C, Berrino F, et al. Breast carcinoma survival in Europe and the United States: a population-based study. Cancer 2004;291: 715–22.
[44] Feig SA. Should there be prescribed standards for screening mammography recall rates? Breast Diseases, A Year Book Quarterly 2005;15:336–59.
[45] Yankaskas BC, Cleveland RJ, Schell MJ, et al. Association of recall rates with sensitivity and positive predictive value of screening mammography. AJR Am J Roentgenol 2001;177:543–9.
[46] Gur O, Sumkin JH, Hardesty LA, et al. Recall and detection rates in screening mammography: a review of clinical experience—implications for practice guidelines. Cancer 2004;100:1590–4.
[47] Schell MJ, Yankaskas BC, Ballard-Barbash R, et al. Evidence-based target recall rates for screening mammography. Radiology 2007;243:681–9.
[48] Otten JDM, Karssemeijer N, Hendriks JHCL, et al. Effect of recall rate on earlier screen detection of breast cancers based on the Dutch performance indicators. J Natl Cancer Inst 2005;97: 748–54.
[49] Elmore JG, Nakano CY, Koepsell TD, et al. International variation in screening mammography interpretation in community-based programs. J Natl Cancer Inst 2003;95:1384–93.
[50] Warren-Burhenne LJ. Proficiency in mammography interpretive skills, computer-aided detection and double reading. In: Feig SA, editor. Categorical course in diagnostic radiology: breast imaging, 2005 syllabus. Oak Brook (IL): Radiological Society of North America; 2005. p. 93–106.
[51] Kopans DB. The positive predictive value of mammography. AJR Am J Roentgenol 2002;158: 521–6.
[52] Nass S, Ball J, editors. Improving breast imaging quality standards. Committee on Improving Mammography Quality Standards, National Research Council. Washington DC: National Academics Press; 2005.

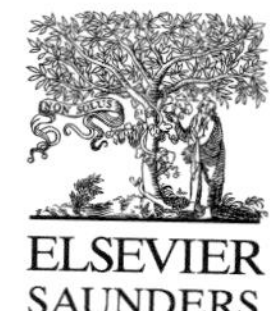

ELSEVIER
SAUNDERS

RADIOLOGIC
CLINICS
OF NORTH AMERICA

Radiol Clin N Am 45 (2007) 801–811

Improving Mammographic Interpretation: Double Reading and Computer-Aided Diagnosis

Mark Helvie, MD

Mammographic assessment is a difficult and complex task. It involves image interpretation and a clinical decision threshold regarding the need for tissue biopsy or follow-up. This process is different than other aspects of radiology interpretation that concentrate on differential diagnosis or diagnosis and not biopsy decisions. The radiologist interpreting mammography acts as a clinician. For these reasons, a myriad of factors influence a breast-imaging final assessment category.

This article discusses two commonly used techniques advocated to improve screening mammography performance: double reading (DR) and computer-aided detection (CAD). Analysis of these methods is incomplete because no randomized controlled trials have been performed to assess changes in survival. Although DR and CAD have shown improvement in sensitivity, specificity has often decreased. Balancing which parameter is more important involves health care policy, costs, cultural factors, legal risk, and patient preference. Similar to other areas of human endeavor, one must decide whether "two heads are better than one" or if "too many cooks spoil the broth."

Mammographic interpretation involves different processes. These can be dichotomized into detection (perception) of an area of possible abnormality and characterization (analysis, classification, "diagnosis") of a found abnormality. A practicing radiologist may perform both of these functions rapidly in a clinical setting. Coarse calcifications may be detected and characterized immediately as a benign calcified fibroadenoma. For more subtle lesions, an area is detected as possibly abnormal and much effort is spent deciding whether the detected area is a true lesion. Achieving high cancer sensitivity involves the ability to detect the myriad of appearances known to possibly represent cancer. High specificity requires the ability to characterize these found lesions as possible cancer requiring biopsy or not cancer with follow-up imaging recommended. As currently practiced in the United States, achievement of high sensitivity at the expense of lower specificity is an accepted philosophical goal. Other health systems may emphasize specificity more than the United States. As cost constraints increase for the United States medical system, documented improvement in test accuracy will become more important before clinical use.

Department of Radiology, University of Michigan Health System, 1500 East Medical Center Drive, TC 2910N, Ann Arbor, MI 48109-0326, USA
E-mail address: mahelvie@umich.edu

0033-8389/07/$ – see front matter
radiologic.theclinics.com
doi:10.1016/j.rcl.2007.06.004

Efforts to improve mammographic interpretative performance with DR and CAD have been driven by two persistent observations: (1) performance variability exists among radiologists and (2) retrospective review of screening mammograms of women eventually diagnosed with breast cancer often shows abnormalities that can be perceived on older studies.

DR and CAD have been proposed and implemented to overcome potential deficiencies of the human reader of mammograms for detection and characterization.

Before discussion of DR and CAD, a basic understanding of several factors known to influence radiologist performance are reviewed because these affect reader performance independent of DR and CAD. These include the nature of "expertise," the relationship between sensitivity and recall rate, and observation time and sensitivity.

Radiologist interpretive variability may represent "the weakest link" in the imaging chain [1]. Elmore and colleagues [2] noted moderate variation (agreement 78%) among radiologists interpreting mammograms in an enriched experimental population. Using an enriched experimental population, Beam and colleagues [3,4] found marked variation among United States' practicing breast-imaging radiologists. Sensitivity varied from 59% to 100% overall, but 10% to 80% at the 1% false positive (FP) level (Fig. 1). Specificity ranged from 35% to 98%. The reasons for the difference in interpretation skill are complex but involve overlooked findings (detection errors) and incorrect characterization. In an effort to define mammographic expertise, Sickles and colleagues [5] noted significant interpretation differences among specialists and generalists in a single academic center. A cancer detection rate of 6/1000 was noted for specialists, whereas the rate was 3.4/1000 for generalists. Parameters associated with higher performance were higher volume, fellowship training, continuing medical education, and regular participation in radiologic-pathologic correlation conference (which provided case-specific outcomes feedback). Esserman and colleagues [6] noted improved sensitivity among American radiologists practicing at higher volumes. Using receiver operating characteristic (ROC) curve analysis at a 90% specificity cutoff, high-volume readers scored 0.76, mid-volume readers scored 0.70, and low-volume readers scored 0.65. Beam and colleagues [7], however, did not find reading volume to be associated strongly with improved sensitivity. They reported expertise to be complex and multifactorial. To increase mammographic accuracy by 10% would require the unacceptable prohibition of 57% of radiologists from practicing, which would severely limit access to mammographic services.

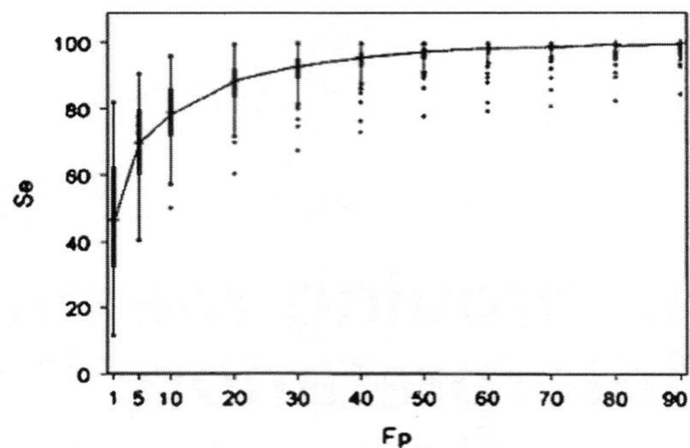

Fig. 1. Mammographic interpretive variability among radiologists. Sensitivity at any false positive (Fp) rate shows a range of values among 110 radiologists in the experimental Variability in Diagnostic Interpretation (VIDI) study. Box plots are radiologist sensitivity (Se) at different Fp probabilities. Box plots show the minimum, first quartile, median, third quartile, and maximum sensitivity at any Fp level. For example, at a 1% Fp ratio, radiologists' sensitivity ranged from 10% to 80%. Statistical outliers are identified by black dots. (*From* Beam CA. Reader strategies: variability and error-methodology, findings, and health policy implications from a study of the U.S. population of mammographers. In: Chakraborty DP, Krupinski EA, editors. Medical imaging 2002: Image perception, observer performance, and technology assessment. San Diego (CA): SPIE; 2002. p. 164; with permission.)

Detection is a skill, not an inherent ability, which can be improved with effective training. Expert readers likely follow similar ROC curves, and performance differences reflect the threshold point used for clinical decisions. Achieving high sensitivity requires recalling a sufficient number of cases from screening for diagnostic evaluation. Within ranges, increasing the recall rate will improve sensitivity and decrease specificity independent of DR or CAD. Yankaskas and colleagues [8] reported improved sensitivity for practicing North Carolina radiologists as the recall rate increased. Sensitivity of 65% at a callback rate of 1.9% to 4.4% improved to 80% at callback rate of 5.8% to 8.7%, an increase of 23%. Otten and colleagues [9] showed sensitivity changes in an experimental study of 15 high-volume breast radiologists. Increasing the FP rate from 1% to 4% resulted in an increase in the sensitivity rate from 14.6% to 21.5%—an improvement of 47% (Fig. 2). Gur and colleagues [10] studied 10 experienced high-volume readers in a large United States academic practice. They found a direct relationship between the recall rate and sensitivity over a wide recall range (7.7%–17.2%; $P<.05$). On average, a 0.22/1000 cancer detection rate improvement occurred for every 1% absolute increase in recall rate. For example, a 14.7% increase in

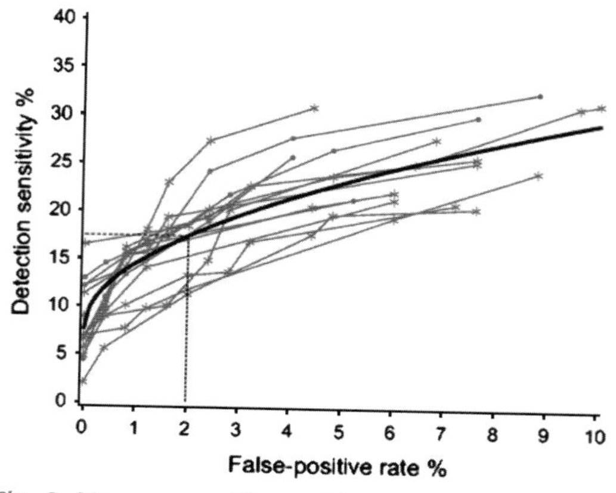

Fig. 2. Mammographic sensitivity compared with FP rates. Fifteen radiologists' (gray lines) performance in an experimental enriched population using localization-response ROC curve. The black line represents the average curve for all 15 radiologists. The dotted lines represent the average sensitivity (17.4%) at a 2% FP rate. The asterisks represent Dutch radiologists, and the circles represent non-Dutch radiologists. (*From* Otten JDM, Karssemeijer N, Hendriks JHCL, et al. Effect of recall rate on earlier screen detection of breast cancers based on the Dutch performance indicators. J Natl Cancer Inst 2005;97: 750; with permission.)

sensitivity would occur if recall increased from 8% to 10% (3.0/1000 to 3.4/1000). Hardesty and colleagues [11] explored the positive relationship between recall rate and sensitivity in experimental models.

Radiologic detection sensitivity is increased with observation time. Christensen and colleagues [12] found that even experienced readers stop searching chest radiographs while true positive (TP) detections are still being made. They noted a biphasic detection pattern, with a rapid detection of most abnormalities and then a slower detection of other abnormalities. Nodine and colleagues [13] assessed time of unilateral mammographic interpretation in an enriched experimental study. Experienced mammographers made 71% of detections in the first 25 seconds, and trainees made 46% of detections in the first 40 seconds. Continued detection of TP cases continued for about 80 seconds but at a much slower rate. Stated differently, 29% of decisions occurred after 26 to 80 seconds of reviewing a unilateral mammogram. Krupinski [14] studied mammographic lesions deemed to be subtle. Detection of subtle abnormalities occurred later than obvious abnormalities and required longer visual dwell time for correct assessment. Mello Thoms and colleagues [15] reported the median time for experienced academic radiologists to assess experimental unilateral mammographic mass cases to be 29 to 32 seconds. This body of work suggests that although quick reading of a mammographic image by experienced radiologists detects most malignancies, a minority of cases may be overlooked. Application of DR and CAD after a quick mammographic visual assessment would be expected to improve sensitivity more than after a thorough review. Unfortunately, reading speed is measured infrequently in DR and CAD studies.

The process of characterization leads to a decision to biopsy or not to biopsy a potential abnormality. Practices achieving extremely high positive predictive values (PPVs) for biopsy may be associated with a higher false negative (FN) rate. The US Department of Health and Human Services has suggested a 25% to 40% goal for biopsy PPV [16]. The annual incident cancer detection rate should be 2 to 4/1000, and the prevalent detection rate (6–10/1000) will be 1.5 to 5 times higher.

The implications of these factors for DR and CAD are significant. Increasing the recall rate, observation time, and level of expertise and decreasing the PPV often will, by themselves, result in sensitivity improvements. Because DR and CAD studies may have important variations in these parameters, isolating DR or CAD as the key variable is difficult. Applying DR and CAD as prevalent technology (first year) may inflate performance compared with incident (second and later years) application.

Assessment of double reading and computer-aided diagnosis

Because no randomized controlled trials (RCTs) have been performed to document changes in survival from use of DR or CAD, surrogate end points, such as cancer detection rate, stage of cancer, frequency of interval cancers, change in recall rate, and change in biopsy PPV are used. Lacking RCTs, ROC methodology can be assessed to compare test accuracy. ROC analysis rewards improvements in sensitivity but penalizes loss of specificity. But ROC analysis is imperfect because clinical decisions are binary – biopsy or follow. If DR and CAD provide true test improvements, ROC values should increase, especially at clinically relevant FP levels. If sensitivity increases yet ROC values are unchanged, a change in threshold toward higher sensitivity has occurred although test accuracy may not change. Individual patients, physicians, and communities usually opt for higher sensitivity at the expense of lower specificity and view this as a favorable tradeoff because the goal of screening is early cancer detection. One can debate philosophically whether improvement in sensitivity is worth decline in specificity from complex medical, legal, heath system, costs, and cultural perspectives; however, the academic question for DR and CAD is whether overall test accuracy is improved or whether one is changing the decision threshold point toward sensitivity while operating on the same ROC curve. Clinically, most United States patients may care less how sensitivity is improved and when asked, often choose sensitivity over lower recall rate [17], especially when the cost is not paid directly by patients.

Double reading

DR has been advocated as a method to improve detection of overlooked findings by a single reader. DR may be practiced in various ways, including independent reading by two readers, one reader providing the primary interpretation and the second an overview, "expert" review by a second reviewer, consensus review by a team, and other variations. Handling discordant recalls may involve recall of all for independent DR, recall of some, consultation among two readers, or deferral to expert physician, consensus, or panel. A summary of DR studies is presented in Table 1. Because each study was performed and reported differently, changes in detection and recall rates listed may reflect different methods and may not be exactly comparable. When possible, calculated detection rate change is incremental new cancers found by the second reader/cancers detected by the first reader. For example, if 100 cancers are found by reader one and 10 incremental cancers are found by reader two, the change is 10/100 = 10%. Recall rate change is defined as the number of incremental recalls by second reader/total recalls of first reader.

Anttinen and colleagues [18] reported on 15,457 Finish screening mammograms with 67 cancers interpreted by then consensus between the two readers. Sensitivity increased by 6.3% for reader 1 and 11.5% for reader 2 (mean 9%), showing differences between readers. Consensus discussion decreased the recall rate to 2.5% from 5.5% if independent recall had been used. One reader decreased the recall number from 412 to 104. The recall rate would increase by 120% if an independent DR system was used compared with consensus review; however, two (3%) cancers found at subsequent screens would have been recalled if independent recall had been used. A biopsy PPV of 63% was observed.

Anderson and colleagues [19] reported on a Scottish screening program using an independent DR program. Twelve percent of cases were missed by one of the readers but were picked up by DR. Recalled patients increased by 45%. Findings that may limit application to North American radiologists include the single mediolateral oblique view obtained during screening and radiologists' reading speed of 200 cases per hour (18 seconds per bilateral mammogram), a speed faster than typical in the United States.

Table 1: Double reading of screening mammograms

Study	Country	N	Method	Final recall rate (%)	Bx PPV (%)	Detection rate/1000	Detection rate change (%)	Recall rate change (%)
Anttinen et al, 1993 [18]	Finland	15,457	Consensus	2.5	63	4.3	+9	−45
Anderson et al, 1994 [19]	Scotland	31,146	Independent	5.9	73	6.1	+12	+45
Thurfjell et al, 1994 [20]	Sweden	11,343	Independent, discussion	4.8	58	6.7	+15	NR
Ciatto et al, 1995 [21]	Italy	18,817	Independent	4.0	80	6.6	+4.6	+15.1
Warren & Duffy, 1995 [22]	United Kingdom	33,734	Consensus, expert review	4.4	78	8.0	+14	−39
Seradour et al, 1996 [23]	France	77,236	Independent, expert	4.4	54	5.5	+17	+23
Harvey et al, 2003 [24]	USA	25,369	Independent	14	21	5.6	+6.7	+11.5
Beam et al, 1996 [25]	USA	131 MD pairs	Experimental	NA	NA	NA	+11	+7
Taplin et al, 2000 [26]	USA	31 MDs	Experimental	NA	NA	NA	+8.9	+13.6

Because each study was performed and reported differently, changes in the detection and recall rate reflect different methodologies and may not be exactly comparable.
Abbreviations: Bx, biopsy; NA, non applicable; NR, not recorded.

Thurfjell and colleagues [20] reported a Swedish experience of DR that involved independent reading and discussion of potential recalls by screen readers on duty. Sixty-four percent of cases involved a two-view study. In this trial of 11,343 cases, the addition of a second reader resulted in 8.6% improvement in sensitivity for reader one and 23% for reader two. This study showed variability of DR effect by reader. The average improvement in detection for both readers was 15% with no change in biopsy PPV of 58%. Tumors found by a second reader tended to be smaller than found by both readers.

In Italy, Ciatto and colleagues [21] found a modest improvement in sensitivity in a study of independent DR involving 18,817 women. On average, a 4.6% increase in sensitivity was attributed to DR. This effect varied from 7.8% to 1.9% for reader 1 and reader 2. This was balanced by a 15.1% average increase in recall rate. Sensitivity improvement for first screen (4.8%) was greater than for second incident screen (3.4%). Because the recall rate increased for second screen (16.4%) more than first screen (15%), it suggested a decline in reading performance on incident cases compared with first screens. Second reader detected cancers were lower stage than other cancers. An 8.5% cost increase was attributed to DR. The investigators concluded that it would be preferable to use the extra money to extend screening to unscreened women rather than to fund DR.

In the United Kingdom, Warren and Duffy [22] reported 33,734 cases using consensus reading and review by a senior radiologist after independent DR. An improvement in sensitivity of 14% was observed at a PPV of 78%. The recall rate decreased by 39% for reader 1 using consensus/expert reading. If independent reading had occurred without consensus, the recall rate would have increased 44%. Three cancers (1.1%) were detected by independent DR but were considered negative at consensus expert review and only diagnosed at subsequent screening.

Seradour and colleagues [23] reported a French experience. In their screening program, a field radiologist interpreted the mammogram initially, which was read independently by a high-volume expert. In reporting 77,236 cases, DR by the expert resulted in a 17% increase in cancer detection. If the expert radiologist had read the case first and the field radiologist had acted as the second reader, it would have resulted in a 10% increase in detection; therefore, the impact of DR depended upon the level of expertise of the second reader compared with the first. The recall rate was noted to increase by 23%. High-volume throughput (120–200 cases per 1.5–2 hours) by the expert reader was noted.

In the United States, Harvey and colleagues [24] reported independent DR of 25,369 cases in an academic practice. They observed a sensitivity improvement of 6.7% balanced by a recall rate increase of 11.5%. The PPV was 21%, and the final recall rate was 14%. These parameters, although reflective of United States practices, contrast markedly with European examples regarding recall rate and PPV. The 6.7% sensitivity change is at the lower range of European values.

Experimental studies also have evaluated DR. Beam and colleagues [25] found the DR effect to be dependent upon the types of reading pairs. Overall TP rate increased by 11%, and the FP rate increased by 7%. Some reading pairs resulted in improvement and others did not. Physicians with lower reading performance improved when paired with a skilled second reader. Conversely, a skilled reader could decrease the performance because of increased FP cases when paired with an unskilled reader.

Taplin and colleagues [26] attempted to answer the fundamental question of whether independent DR improves accuracy or merely shifts decision threshold toward higher sensitivity. They tested 31 community radiologists using an enriched test set of 113 cases and compared 465 potential DR pairs using ROC methods. They found that test accuracy did not change as measured by ROC. Although the readers' average sensitivity increased from 79% to 86% (8.9%), a decrease in specificity from 81% to 70% (13.6%) balanced the sensitivity improvements. The investigators suggested that DR moves the threshold point on the ROC curve toward higher sensitivity without changing the accuracy. Higher sensitivity from DR would benefit women who have cancer, but it would harm women who do not have cancer because of the higher recall rate and associated costs.

In summary, DR studies from most centers have resulted in higher cancer detection rates that vary by reader and study. Independent DR is associated with a loss of specificity as evidenced by higher recall rates. Consensus reading or expert reading after DR seems to maintain most, but not all, of the improvement in sensitivity without sacrificing specificity. Some of this improvement likely relates to the expertise of the consensus reader. There is experimental evidence to suggest that independent DR does not change accuracy although sensitivity improvement occurs. There will be associated increased costs of radiologist time, increased diagnostic imaging, and incremental biopsies with independent DR.

An example of how DR may impact a typical North American clinical practice can be illustrated. Assume that a DR program of 7% increased sensitivity and 12% increased recall is applied to an annual screening population (3/1000 cancer incidence) with a 10% callback rate. Screening 10,000 women will cause 1000 recalls and detect 30 cancers. DR would cause 120 extra recalls and detect 2 incremental cancers. The ratio of DR recalls/cancer detections is 120:2 or 60:1. Two of 10,000 patients (0.02%) patients may benefit from DR. For an American radiologist reading the Mammography Quality Standards Act minimum of 480 cases per year, DR would be expected to detect a single incremental cancer once in every 10 years of practice.

There is a paucity of literature and experience testing independent triple reading or the application of DR to diagnostic cases, logical extensions for clinical advocates of DR. Because a 10 to 20 fold higher disease prevalence exists in diagnostic breast imaging compared with annual screening, more patients with disease per 1000 tested may benefit from a diagnostic DR if other factors remain the same. Within nonbreast diagnostic radiology, DR is rarely practiced, although reader variability and oversight are not unique to breast imaging. Outside of radiology, our clinical colleagues rarely practice double office visits and double clinical examinations, except in training situations, even though physician variability and discordant opinions exist among clinicians. The economic implication of health system–wide double examinations is untenable.

Computer-aided detection

CAD has shown promise in improving reader sensitivity performance. CAD was developed to act as a second reader, similar to DR, with the goal of gaining sensitivity without the human costs of DR. Current CAD methods will advance with the explosive improvements in computer technology, so any discussion of CAD is immediately dated. CAD systems analyze digitized or digital mammography images using software programs to find features that are associated with breast cancer. A "mark" is placed at the site of these findings for the radiologist to review, similar to DR. Independent radiologist reading should occur before knowledge of the CAD result. If the proper sequence is followed, CAD acts as a second reader with consensus expert opinion by the radiologist. If the radiologist reviews the CAD results before review of the mammogram, CAD acts as the first reader and the radiologist acts as a second, expert reader. There are several manufacturers of CAD systems, both commercial and noncommercial, which use their own software systems. Some of these systems have achieved FDA approval for clinical use. Because CAD acts as a second reader, many of the DR issues are mirrored in the CAD literature.

Current CAD systems are programmed to balance sensitivity and specificity, with a strong emphasis on sensitivity. These programs can be adjusted, depending upon the desires of the customer, toward sensitivity or specificity. A typical four-view bilateral screening mammogram will have several CAD marks per case, most of which will prove to be FPs. The radiologist determines (characterizes) which CAD marks warrant further investigation with diagnostic imaging or intervention. The radiologist may choose to actually overrule his/her own detection if CAD is negative, thereby using CAD as the expert. Although CAD is believed to be for "detection," all CAD systems characterize findings to determine thresholds for placing marks. A characterization score proportional to the probability of malignancy can be provided. The primary purpose of current CAD systems is to identify areas overlooked by the radiologist during routine care. Although much research is ongoing regarding characterization by CAD [27], this discussion is limited to detection issues. Currently, no CAD system approaches reader performance, and these systems are not to be used as stand-alone readers.

To understand the potential magnitude of CAD performance in clinical practice, it is illustrative to review what may occur in a typical annual incident screening practice, similar to the DR example of 10,000 cases with a cancer incidence of 3/1000 and CAD sensitivity of 80% at three marks per case allowed. Assume CAD will detect 10% incremental cancer cases not detected by the radiologist. Of the 30 cancers, 24 cases (0.80×30) will be marked correctly by CAD, 27 will be identified without CAD, and 3 cases will be incremental CAD detections. Of the 10,000 cases, there will be 30,000 total CAD marks; all will be FPs except 48 (24 cancer cases $\times$ two views). Of these 48 correct TP marks, only 3 cancers (six marks) will be true incremental TP CAD detections. The radiologist faces 29,952 FP marks and 48 TP marks or 624 FP marks for every TP mark. For the 3 cancers detected exclusively by CAD, the ratio of redundant and FP CAD marks to unique TP CAD marks is 29,994/6 or 4999 nonhelpful marks for a single unique TP. The actual ratios will be higher because CAD may not mark a cancer on both views. Most studies showed that many of these incremental detections are ductal carcinoma in situ (DCIS) and not invasive cancers. Similar to DR, these incremental detections may or may not impact survival or morbidity.

Although this exercise shows the drawbacks of CAD, the actual radiologist "burden" may be much less in practice. The mammographic surface area to be reviewed visually based upon CAD marks is small. If a CAD mark is about 1 cm^2 and a typical mammogram view (our data) is approximately 110 cm^2, each CAD mark is less than 1% of the visual mammographic area to review. The three typical CAD marks require review of 0.75% of the total surface area of a bilateral mammogram. This suggests that the post-CAD review can occur quickly when CAD functions as a second reader because only a limited area requires radiologist visual attention.

The clinical impact of these systems requires careful analysis because human behavior, psychology, visual cognitive processes, and decision processes change when reading with CAD systems. Although it is intuitive that CAD can help performance only by detecting overlooked findings, actual results may be much more complex. For example, the safety advantage conferred by antilock brake systems (ABS) can be lost when driving speeds on icy roads are increased because one is driving a car with ABS. Conversely, ABS should usually benefit if stable speeds are maintained. Therefore, the radiologist who does less than a full image evaluation knowing that CAD support will follow effectively may be diminishing the magnitude of the support that CAD provides.

Retrospective computer-aided diagnosis studies

CAD systems have been applied to retrospective review of problematic mammograms, especially prior mammograms of patients who later developed cancer. These studies assume that the radiologist will act on the placed marks, an assumption requiring clinical verification in a realistic prospective testing. These studies assume that there will be no negative impact of CAD on the reader's own detections if CAD is FN.

Warren Burhenne and colleagues [28] applied CAD to a set of 115 prior mammograms of women who eventually developed cancer. CAD correctly marked many of these cases and was estimated to have the potential to decrease the radiologists 21% FN rate by 77%. Ikeda and colleagues [29] applied CAD to 172 prior mammograms, which had subtle findings, of patients later found to have cancer. The CAD program marked 42% of areas that subsequently developed cancer. As findings became more obvious to the radiologists, CAD had similar higher detection performance. Brem and colleagues [30] applied CAD to 377 mammograms initially interpreted as negative in women who eventually developed cancer. Retrospective review identified 177 possible abnormalities. CAD marked 63% of these cases. The investigators estimated the potential detection improvement by using CAD to be 21.2%.

In 1998, Thurfjell and colleagues [31] reviewed the effect of CAD on an enriched set of 120 (74 cancer cases) mammograms presented to 3 radiologists defined as an expert, a screening radiologist, and a clinical radiologist. The sensitivity for CAD was 50% compared with 59% for the expert. CAD resulted in no incremental detections for the expert, but did result in a 9% detection improvement for the least experienced reader. Ciatto and colleagues [32] used CAD in an enriched data set of 150 cases, including 17 cancers. When used by 10 radiologists of variable experience, a nonsignificant 4.2% increase in sensitivity was noted. There was a significant 44% ($P = .003$) increase in the recall rate from 7.9 to 11.4%. Overall CAD sensitivity was 94%, and 5.1 marks per case were allowed. Most improvement occurred for less experienced radiologists.

Taylor and colleagues [33] applied a commercial CAD system to a test set of 180 cases, which included 60 cancers to 50 high-volume (5000 cases/y) study readers. CAD sensitivity was 73% with about two marks per case. Cases were read without CAD or with CAD in a randomized manner. There was no significant difference in reader performance with CAD for sensitivity or specificity. The investigators postulated that the large number of CAD FPs limited CAD's effectiveness in screening. Of 10,000 CAD prompts per year that a reader would experience, they estimated that only 5 CAD prompts would represent TPs that were not recognized by the readers.

Alberdi and colleagues [34,35] attempted to determine the effect of FN CAD assessments. An experimental data set of 60 enriched cases (30 cancers) was assessed by 39 physicians. The researchers decreased the performance of a CAD system and then presented the cases to radiologists with CAD annotations or without CAD in a test situation. Average reader sensitivity with CAD decreased significantly compared with reading without CAD (61% versus 73%). Specificity was without significant change (90% with CAD and 86% without CAD). Most of the decline in sensitivity was for cases that were FN by CAD. The investigators noted that incorrect CAD output could have a detrimental effect on human decision making. They offered several explanations for these phenomena, including "automation bias," in which physicians faced with a negative CAD decreased their interpretation vigilance. Another possibility was characterization bias: physicians defer to CAD and ignore their own opinions. The study has important implications for clinical radiologists, especially those who choose off-label use of CAD as the first reader.

Destounis and colleagues [36] attempted to determine whether CAD provides incremental information for cases that have already undergone DR.

In this situation, CAD is acting as a "triple" reader. CAD was applied retrospectively to 52 screening cancer cases not originally detected by clinical DR. In this experiment, 71% of these screening mammograms were retrospectively marked correctly by CAD, suggesting the potential for CAD to reduce FN cases, even when assessed by DR.

Clinical computer-aided diagnosis trials

There have been two methods used to test CAD in clinical trials. One method (sequential) presents the radiologist with an image without CAD information, requires interpretation, and then presents the same image with CAD markings and allows the radiologist to modify one's assessment. Changes in sensitivity, specificity, recall rate, biopsy rate, and cancer detection are calculated. The second method uses historical control periods without CAD followed by the time period after CAD introduction. Both experimental methods are subject to potential bias. In the sequential method, radiologists may decrease their vigilance in interpretation of the examination without CAD, knowing that CAD has high sensitivity, especially for microcalcifications. This would tend to decrease sensitivity without CAD. Conversely, radiologists may "compete" versus CAD and be more sensitive than usual care. Because sequential studies are designed like independent DR, the effect of an FN CAD is not assessed. In practice, radiologists may choose to ignore an MD-detected region if CAD is FN at that site. Historical controls may exaggerate the benefit of CAD, because technology, quality, and image interpretation ability may improve with time, and this improvement may be caused by factors unrelated to CAD. CAD also may act as a "teacher" with diminishing return on subsequent screens. CAD effect on the first prevalent screen may be greater than on subsequent incident screens because the CAD positive cases are removed from the population by biopsy. Conversely, CAD may be at a disadvantage because more latter cases are incident screens, which decreases the cancer rate. DCIS detection has been considered an improvement in sensitivity for CAD. Controversy exists regarding the biologic significance of DCIS detection and impact on survival of earlier DCIS detection.

Table 2 summarizes United States clinical trials of CAD. In 2001, Freer and Ulissey [37] reported the first sequential clinical CAD study of a community practice. They noted a 19.5% improvement in mammographic cancer detection in a study of 12,860 patients. Of the incremental cancers detected by CAD, 87% were microcalcifications; 75% of incremental detections (six of eight) were

Table 2: **United States clinical trials of screening mammography with computer-aided diagnosis**

Study	N	Method	Final recall rate (%)	Bx PPV (%)	Detection rate/1000	CAD sensitivity (%)	Detection rate change (%)	Recall rate change (%)
Freer et al, 2001 [37]	12,860	S	7.7	38	3.8	82	+19.5	+18.5
Gur et al, 2004 [10,38]	115,571	H	11.4	NR	3.5	NR	+1.7	+0.1
Helvie et al, 2004 [40]	2389	S	15.8	NR	4.6	91	+9.1	+9.7
Birdwell et al, 2005 [41]	8682	S	9.9	18	3.3	79	+7.4	+8.3
Cupples et al, 2005 [42]	27,274	H	8.3	29	4.3	NR	+16	+8.1
Morton et al, 2006 [43]	21,349	S	10.8	41	5.3	76	+7.6	+9.5
Dean & Ilvento, 2006 [44]	5631	S	7.8	26.3	6.2	89	+13.3	+26
Ko et al, 2006 [45]	5016	S	13.9	36	9.0	79	+4.7	+14.7

Abbreviations: Bx, biopsy; H, historical control without CAD; NR, not recorded; S, sequential reads with CAD.

DCIS. There was a 5% invasive cancer detection improvement. Specificity was noted to decline. Recall rates increased by 18.5%, and short-term follow-up for Category 3 probably benign cases increased by 38%. CAD was an imperfect test, missing 33% of invasive cancers manifest as masses but found by the radiologist. Overall, CAD detected 82% of cancers.

Gur and colleagues [38] reported the largest clinical trial involving 24 radiologists and 115,571 examinations. They found no significant difference in the malignancy detection rate or recall rate in a study using a historical control model following institution of a commercial CAD program at a large academic practice. A 1.7% increase in cancer detection rate was observed (3.49/1000 without CAD versus 3.55/1000 with CAD; $P = .68$). The recall rate (11.4%) increased by 0.1%. Although subset analyses noted sensitivity improvement for low-volume radiologists, high-volume readers had a nonsignificant decrease in their sensitivity with CAD [38,39]. Similar to DR, the effect of CAD may depend upon radiologist expertise.

The author and colleagues [40] reported a sequential multi-institutional trial using a noncommercial system at academic centers. A 9% increase in sensitivity was matched by a 10% increase in recall rate. Incremental detection was solely for DCIS manifest as calcifications. CAD sensitivity was 91%. Of interest, the study baseline recall rate increased 31% compared with nonstudy cases, suggesting study radiologists were more sensitive in the CAD experiment compared with usual care by attempting to outperform CAD.

In 2005, Birdwell and colleagues [41] reported on 8682 consecutive cases using the sequential methodology during a 19-month period at StanfordUniversity. The investigators found a 7% increase in cancer detection and an associated 8% increase in recall rate. The overall cancer detection rate was 3.3/1000. CAD detected 79.3% of cancers. Both incremental cancers prompted by CAD were invasive tumors.

Cupples and colleagues [42] reported a historical control study involving 7872 patients examined before institution of a CAD program and 19,402 patients following the introduction of a commercial CAD program in a community practice. An increase in the detection rate from 3.7/1000 to 4.3/1000 with CAD (16%) was found. This increased detection rate was accompanied by an 8.1% increase in the recall rate (from 7.7% to 8.3%) and a 6.7% increase in the biopsy rate. Forty-seven percent of the CAD cases were examined by a reader not present in the pre-CAD arm of the study, although the readers present during both study periods had sensitivity improvement.

In 2006, Morton and colleagues [43] reported a sequential Mayo Clinic experience using a commercial CAD system; they found a nonsignificant 7.6% increase in cancer detection (from 4.92/1000 to 5.29/1000). The recall rated increased 9.5%, from 9.84% to 10.77% with CAD. PPV remained stable at 41%. In this trial, the commercial CAD system marked 76% of cancers, which included 65% of masses and 100% of calcification cases. Five of eight (63%) cancers not detected by routine care but detected by CAD were microcalcifications, and all were low- to intermediate-grade DCIS. There was a 2.8% increase in the detection of invasive cancers (3/105).

Dean and Ilvento [44] reported a single institution experience for CAD in screening and diagnostic cases in a private practice setting. A 13% improvement in cancer detection was noted for 5631 screening cases using a sequential clinical model. The recall rate increased 26%, from 6.2% to 7.8%. CAD marked 89% of all screening cancer cases and 83% of combined screening and diagnostic cases. CAD detected 64% of invasive lobular cancers and 83% of invasive ductal cancers. Overall, 30% of CAD incremental detections were for DCIS.

Ko and colleagues [45] reported a sequential CAD experience involving 5016 screening cases (45 cancers). A 4.7% increase in cancer detection was matched by a 14.7% increase in the recall rate. CAD resulted in a 2% increase in incremental invasive cancer clinical detection (50% of CAD incremental cases were DCIS). Like other studies, CAD performance for malignant calcification cases was greater than for masses (100% versus 67%). A single-interval cancer that had been marked by CAD was dismissed by the radiologist, showing that CAD marks may not always be acted upon because of the large number of FP marks. In this study, CAD produced one mark per image. PPV declined from 37% to 36%.

Overall, CAD trials have generally, but not always, shown detection improvement and loss of specificity. In clinical practice, CAD may have positive and negative attributes, and the clinical situation may explain some of the differences. The three community-practice CAD studies (see Table 2) showed a 16.6% weighted average sensitivity improvement (16.2% nonweighted average). This contrasts with the 3.1% weighted average improvement from five academic or affiliated medical centers (6.1% nonweighted average). Changes in CAD performance used as prevalent test compared with use as an incident test are insufficiently reported.

If a reader does not become immune to CAD marks, oversight errors should be corrected by CAD prompts. Associated increases in recall rates with CAD would be expected to follow an ROC curve, leading to higher sensitivity and a higher cancer detection rate based on experimental and clinical models of recall. Although proponents of CAD argue that even this is a true incremental detection, critics argue that increasing the recall rate may result in a similar result, even without the introduction of CAD; however, a blanket recommendation to increase the recall rate cannot guarantee a specific increase in detection in practice. Clinically, appropriate prompts for overlooked cancers should remain a valuable tool, even if associated with recall rate increases for United States readers, who value sensitivity.

With any new technology, human interaction with the technology will prove to be critical until the technology is perfected. This complex interaction has just begun to be studied. CAD is in its infancy, and progress will continue to be made; however, overdependence on CAD is to be avoided. CAD programs should not be applied until image interpretation without CAD has been performed. Given the time constraints in current North American practice, it is likely that this sequential procedure will not be followed uniformly. For example, if radiologists depend upon CAD for calcification detection, there may be less interest in careful review of a mammogram to detect calcifications because calcification performance by CAD is already good. This may be problematic. Soo and colleagues [46], in an assessment of amorphous calcifications in 85 cases, noted a CAD detection rate of only 51%. Only 57% of malignant cases and 29% of high-risk lesions were identified by CAD.

Summary

CAD is in its infancy. Exciting progress is being made for detection and characterization of found abnormalities, and this should lead to marked improvements of future systems. Much more work is necessary to understand aspects of human interaction with CAD systems. Current clinical trial literature suggests modest improvements in invasive cancer detection associated with decreased specificity. CAD should only be applied after prospective radiologist reading without CAD, and it should not be used to discount radiologist detections if sensitivity improvement is the desired goal. Misapplication of CAD may defeat CAD strengths and may decrease radiologist performance.

References

[1] Robinson PJ. Radiology's Achilles' heel: error and variation in the interpretation of the roentgen image. Br J Radiol 1997;70:1085–98.

[2] Elmore JG, Wells CK, Lee CH, et al. Variability in radiologists' interpretations of mammograms. N Engl J Med 1994;331:1493–9.

[3] Beam CA. Reader strategies: variability and error-methodology, findings, and health policy implications from a study of the U.S. population of mammographers. In: Chakraborty DP, Krupinski EA, editors. Medical imaging 2002: image perception, observer performance, and technology assessment. San Diego (CA): SPIE; 2002. p. 157–68.

[4] Beam CA, Conant EF, Sickles EA. Association of volume and volume-independent factors with accuracy in screening mammogram interpretation. J Natl Cancer Inst 2003;95:282–90.

[5] Sickles E, Wolverton D, Dee K. Performance parameters for screening and diagnostic mammography: specialist and general radiologists. Radiology 2002;224:861–9.

[6] Esserman L, Cowley H, Eberle C, et al. Improving the accuracy of mammography: volume and outcome relationships. J Natl Cancer Inst 2002;94:369–76.

[7] Beam CA, Conant EF, Sickles EA, et al. Evaluation of proscriptive health care policy implementation in screening mammography. Radiology 2003;229:534–40.

[8] Yankaskas BC, Cleveland RJ, Schell MJ, et al. Association of recall rates with sensitivity and positive predictive values of screening mammography. Am J Roentgenol 2001;177:543–9.

[9] Otten JDM, Karssemeijer N, Hendriks JHCL, et al. Effect of recall rate on earlier screen detection of breast cancers based on the Dutch performance indicators. J Natl Cancer Inst 2005;97:748–54.

[10] Gur D, Sumkin J, Hardesty L, et al. Recall and detection rates in screening mammography. Cancer 2004;100:1590–4.

[11] Hardesty LA, Klym AH, Shindel BE, et al. Is maximum positive predictive value a good indicator of an optimal screening mammography practice? Am J Roentgenol 2005;184:1505–7.

[12] Christensen EE, Murry RC, Holland K, et al. The effect of search time on perception. Radiology 1981;138:361–5.

[13] Nodine CF, Mello-Thoms C, Kundel HL, et al. Time course of perception and decision making during mammographic interpretation. Am J Roentgenol 2002;179:917–23.

[14] Krupinski EA. Visual search of mammographic images: influence of lesion subtlety. Acad Radiol 2005;12:965–9.

[15] Mello-Thoms C, Hardesty L, Sumkin J, et al. Effects of lesion conspicuity on visual search in mammogram reading. Acad Radiol 2005;12:830–40.

[16] U.S. Dept. of Health & Human Services. Quality determinants of mammography. Clin Pract Guidel 1994;13:83.

[17] Ganott MA, Sumkin JH, King JL, et al. Screening mammography: do women prefer a higher recall

rate given the possibility of earlier detection of cancer? Radiology 2006;238:793–800.

[18] Anttinen I, Pamilo M, Soiva M, et al. Double reading of mammography screening films-one radiologist or two? Clin Radiol 1993;48:414–21.

[19] Anderson EDC, Muir BB, Walsh JS, et al. The efficacy of double reading mammograms in breast screening. Clin Radiol 1994;49:248–51.

[20] Thurfjell E, Lernevall K, Taube A. Benefit of independent double reading in a population-based mammography screening program. Radiology 1994;191:241–4.

[21] Ciatto S, Del Turco MR, Morrone D, et al. Independent double reading of screening mammograms. J Med Screen 1995;2:99–101.

[22] Warren RM, Duffy SW. Comparison of single reading with double reading of mammograms, and change in effectiveness with experience. Br J Radiol 1995;68:958–62.

[23] Seradour B, Wait S, Jacquemier J, et al. Dual reading in a non-specialized breast cancer screening programme. The Breast 1996;5:398–403.

[24] Harvey SC, Geller B, Oppenheimer RG, et al. Increase in cancer detection and recall rates with independent double interpretation of screening mammography. Am J Roentgenol 2003;180: 1461–7.

[25] Beam C, Sullivan D, Layde P. Effect of human variability on independent double reading in screening mammography. Acad Radiol 1996;3: 891–7.

[26] Taplin SH, Rutter CM, Elmore JG, et al. Accuracy of screening mammography using single versus independent double interpretation. Am J Roentgenol 2000;174:1257–62.

[27] Hadjiiski L, Chan H-P, Sahiner B, et al. Improvement in radiologists' characterization of malignant and benign breast masses on serial mammograms with computer-aided diagnosis: an ROC study. Radiology 2004;233:255–65.

[28] Warren Burhenne LJ, Wood SA, D'Orsi CJ, et al. Potential contribution of computer-aided detection to the sensitivity of screening mammography. Radiology 2000;215:554–62.

[29] Ikeda DM, Birdwell RL, O'Shaughnessy KF, et al. Computer-aided detection output on 172 subtle findings on normal mammograms previously obtained in women with breast cancer detected at follow-up screening mammography. Radiology 2004;230:811–9.

[30] Brem RF, Baum J, Lechner M, et al. Improvement in sensitivity of screening mammography with computer-aided detection: a multi-institutional trial. Am J Roentgenol 2003;181:687–93.

[31] Thurfjell E, Thurfjell MG, Egge E, et al. Sensitivity and specificity of computer-assisted breast cancer detection in mammography screening. Acta Radiologica 1998;39:384–8.

[32] Ciatto S, Del Turco MR, Risso G, et al. Comparison of standard reading and computer-aided detection (CAD) on a national proficiency test of screening mammography. Eur J Radiol 2003; 45:135–8.

[33] Taylor PM, Champness J, Given-Wilson RM, et al. An evaluation of the impact of computer-based prompts on screen readers' interpretation of mammograms. Br J Radiol 2004;77:21–7.

[34] Alberdi E, Povyakalo A, Strigini L, et al. Effects of incorrect computer-aided detection (CAD) output on human decision-making in mammography. Acad Radiol 2004;11:909–18.

[35] Alberdi E, Povyakalo AA, Strigini L, et al. Use of computer-aided detection (CAD) tools in screening mammography: a multidisciplinary investigation. Br J Radiol 2005;78:S31–40.

[36] Destounis SV, DiNitto P, Logan-Young W, et al. Can computer-aided detection with double reading of screening mammograms help decrease the false-negative rate? Initial experience. Radiology 2004;232:578–84.

[37] Freer TW, Ulissey MJ. Screening mammography with computer-aided detection: prospective study of 12,860 patients in a community breast center. Radiology 2001;220:781–6.

[38] Gur D, Sumkin JH, Rockette HE, et al. Changes in breast cancer detection and mammography recall rates after the introduction of a computer-aided detection system. J Natl Cancer Inst 2004;96:185–90.

[39] Feig SA, Sickles EA, Evans WP, et al. Re: changes in breast cancer detection and mammography recall rates after the introduction of a computer-aided detection system. J Natl Cancer Inst 2004;96:1260–1.

[40] Helvie MA, Hadjiiski L, Makariou E, et al. Sensitivity of noncommercial computer-aided detection system for mammographic breast cancer detection: pilot clinical trial. Radiology 2004; 231:208–14.

[41] Birdwell RL, Bandodkar P, Ikeda DM. Computer-aided detection with screening mammography in a university hospital setting. Radiology 2005; 236:451–7.

[42] Cupples TE, Cunningham JE, Reynolds JC. Impact of computer-aided detection in a regional screening mammography program. Am J Roentgenol 2005;185:944–50.

[43] Morton MJ, Whaley DH, Brandt KR, et al. Screening mammograms: interpretation with computer-aided detection–prospective evaluation. Radiology 2006;239:375–83.

[44] Dean JC, Ilvento CC. Improved cancer detection using computer-aided detection with diagnostic and screening mammography: prospective study of 104 cancers. Am J Roentgenol 2006;187:20–8.

[45] Ko JM, Nicholas MJ, Mendel JB, et al. Prospective assessment of computer-aided detection in interpretation of screening mammography. Am J Roentgenol 2006;187:1483–91.

[46] Soo MS, Rosen EL, Xia JQ, et al. Computer-aided detection of amorphous calcifications. Am J Roentgenol 2005;184:887–92.

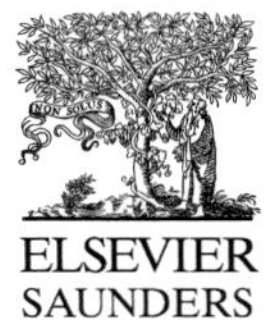

ELSEVIER
SAUNDERS

RADIOLOGIC
CLINICS
OF NORTH AMERICA

Radiol Clin N Am 45 (2007) 813–830

Issues to Consider in Converting to Digital Mammography

Etta D. Pisano, MD[a,b,c,d,*], Margarita Zuley, MD[e], Janet K. Baum, MD[f,g], Helga S. Marques, MS[h]

This article outlines the reasons that many radiology practices are converting to digital mammography. In addition, it provides basic information about the issues that must be considered in making the transformation. These issues include technical matters regarding image display, storage, and retrieval as well as clinical and ergonomic considerations.

Why should a radiology practice convert to digital mammography?

Digital mammography has been on the horizon as a tool for breast cancer detection and diagnosis since the early 1990s when the National Cancer Institute funded the International Digital Mammography Development Group [1]. The first clinical digital mammography system received Food and Drug Administration (FDA) approval in early 2000. Despite high hopes, adoption of this new technology has been slower than anticipated. Besides its high cost and the unwillingness of insurers to provide higher reimbursement for the more expensive technology, the dissemination of this promising tool undoubtedly was slowed by a lack of data supporting improved diagnostic accuracy. Early studies comparing digital and film mammography [2–5] showed no significant difference between digital and film mammography, with digital in fact

[a] Department of Radiology, University of North Carolina School of Medicine, CB 7000, Room 4030 Bondurant Hall, Chapel Hill, NC 27599-7510, USA
[b] Department of Biomedical Engineering, University of North Carolina School of Medicine, CB 7000, Room 4030 Bondurant Hall, Chapel Hill, NC, USA
[c] University of North Carolina Biomedical Research Imaging Center, CB 7000, Room 4030 Bondurant Hall, Chapel Hill, NC 27599-7510, USA
[d] University of North Carolina -Lineberger Comprehensive Cancer Center, UNC School of Medicine, CB 7000, Room 4030 Bondurant Hall, Chapel Hill, NC 27599-7510, USA
[e] University of Pittsburgh Medical Center, Magee Women's Hospital, 300 Halkett Street, Department of Radiology, Pittsburgh, PA 15213, USA
[f] Department of Radiology, Cambridge Health Alliance, Cambridge, MA, USA
[g] Harvard Medical School, 1493 Cambridge St., Boston, MA 02139, USA
[h] Center for Statistical Sciences, Brown University, Box G-S121-7, 121 South Main Street, Providence, RI 02912, USA
* Corresponding author. CB 7000, Room 4030 Bondurant Hall, Chapel Hill, NC 27599-7510.
E-mail address: Etta_Pisano@med.unc.edu (E.D. Pisano).

doi:10.1016/j.rcl.2007.06.007
radiologic.theclinics.com

performing nonsignificantly slightly worse than film mammography when the area under the receiver operator curve (AUC) or cancer detection rate was measured. These early studies were limited by comparing only one digital system versus film, and their sample size was relatively small.

Two larger recently published studies have added impetus to the more widespread adoption of digital mammography. These studies are the Oslo II Trial and the Digital Mammographic Imaging Screening Trial (DMIST) [6,7].

The Oslo II study enrolled 25,263 women who were assigned randomly to either film or digital mammography for breast cancer screening. The rate of cancer detection across the entire population and for the group of women ages 50 to 69 years was greater for digital mammography than for film mammography. The overall detection rates were 0.41% for film and 0.59% for digital mammography (P = .06). For the group aged 50 to 69 years, the detection rates were 0.54% for film and 0.83% for digital mammography (P = .053). These results approached statistical significance. The trend in cancer detection rate for women under 50 years favored digital mammography (0.22% for film and 0.27% for digital). Recall rates in all population subgroups were statistically significantly higher for digital than for film mammography without a significant difference in positive predictive value [6]. The results of the Oslo II study may not be immediately generalizable to the practice of mammography in the United States because the number of readers was quite small, only one digital mammography system was compared with film, and the study was performed in Norway where the screening paradigm for breast cancer is different from that used in the United States. This last point is evidenced by recall rates in the study, which ranged from 2.5% to 3.8% [6], whereas one recent large consortium study found the mean recall rate for the middle two quartiles of United States radiologists to be 9.8% [8].

The DMIST, funded by the National Cancer Institute under the auspices of the American College of Radiology Imaging Network, enrolled 49,528 women at 33 institutions in the United States and Canada, with 42,760 evaluable cases. Women underwent both digital and film mammography. A detailed description of the study methodology is provided elsewhere [9]. Five different types of digital machine were used by 164 radiologists, with each patient's digital and film mammograms read independently by two readers. The digital systems that were included in the study were the Fischer SenoScan (Fischer Medical Corporation, Denver, Colorado), the Fuji 5000 Computed Radiography (CR) System for Mammography (Fujifilm Medical Systems USA, Stamford, CT), the General Electric Senographe 2000D (GE Health care, Milwaukee, Wisconsin), the LORAD/Trex Digital Mammography System (Hologic Inc, Bedford, Massachusetts), and the LORAD/Hologic Selenia Full Field Digital Mammography System (Hologic Inc, Bedford, Massachusetts).

The DMIST showed that, for the entire population of women, there was no significant difference in diagnostic accuracy, as measured by the AUC, between digital and film mammography for breast cancer screening. The difference in the AUC was 0.03 (P = .182). For women who had dense breasts, women under age 50 years, and pre- and perimenopausal women, however, digital mammography was statistically significantly better, even after accounting for multiple comparisons. The difference in the AUC for these three groups was 0.106 for women who had dense breasts (P = .0033), 0.151 for women under age 50 years (P = .0023), and 0.149 for pre- and perimenopausal women (P = .0022). The corresponding differences for women who had fatty breasts, women aged 50 years and over, and postmenopausal women were −0.03 (P = .32), 0.004 (P = .87), and −0.02 (P = .55), respectively. (Negative numbers indicate that the AUC was higher for film than for digital.) (Table 1) [7].

Measurement of sensitivity, specificity, and positive predictive value 1 (PPV1) across the entire study population also showed no differences between digital and film mammography. For women under age 50 years, the sensitivity of digital mammography was superior to that of film, 0.78 versus 0.51. Similar trends were evident in the sensitivity comparisons in the other population subsets in which the AUC was better for digital than for film. There were no differences in specificity or PPV1 measured in the DMIST, either across the entire population or in the subpopulations in which the AUC for digital significantly exceeded film. These values are shown in Table 1 [7].

There has been great interest in the reasons behind the DMIST results, including understandable concern about the performance of digital mammography in other population subsets. Those interested in breast cancer screening worry that there must be a population subset for which film outperformed digital because, although digital outperformed film in some population subsets, the results were similar in the entire population [10]. In addition, the cost effectiveness of this technology, given its relative performance in the overall population, is of great concern. These topics and a careful review of the DMIST cancer cases by experts to ascertain the causes for these results are ongoing and will be published shortly.

One factor not previously published but of great interest to radiologists is the performance of the

Table 1: **Difference in area under the curve, sensitivity, specificity, and positive predictive values-1 in the Digital Mammographic Imaging Screening Trial for different population subsets**

Population	AUC digital	AUC film	AUC difference	Sensitivity digital	Sensitivity film	Specificity digital	Specificity film	PPV1 digital	PPV1 film
All	0.775 (0.020)[a]	0.744 (0.022)	0.032 (0.024)	0.697 (0.029)	0.657 (0.030)	0.918 (0.001)	0.917 (0.001)	0.048 (0.004)	0.045 (0.003)
Age < 50 years	0.843 (0.030)	0.692 (0.050)	0.151[b] (0.050)	0.780[b] (0.054)	0.508[b] (0.065)	0.901 (0.003)	0.901 (0.003)	0.032 (0.005)	0.021 (0.004)
Age ≥ 50 years	0.755 (0.024)	0.751 (0.025)	0.004 (0.027)	0.672 (0.034)	0.703 (0.033)	0.926 (0.002)	0.926 (0.002)	0.059 (0.005)	0.061 (0.005)
Pre or perimenopausal	0.815 (0.030)	0.666 (0.046)	0.149[b] (0.049)	0.716 (0.050)	0.506 (0.056)	0.904 (0.002)	0.902 (0.002)	0.037 (0.005)	0.026 (0.004)
Post-menopausal	0.758 (0.025)	0.775 (0.024)	−0.016[c] (0.027)	0.695 (0.036)	0.737 (0.034)	0.926 (0.002)	0.927 (0.002)	0.057 (0.005)	0.061 (0.005)
Dense breasts	0.785 (0.025)	0.679 (0.033)	0.106[b] (0.036)	0.696 (0.041)	0.552 (0.044)	0.906 (0.002)	0.902 (0.002)	0.045 (0.005)	0.034 (0.004)
Nondense breasts	0.762 (0.030)	0.793 (0.028)	−0.031 (0.031)	0.698 (0.040)	0.760 (0.038)	0.928 (0.002)	0.931 (0.002)	0.052 (0.005)	0.059 (0.006)

[a] Numbers in parentheses are standard errors.
[b] *P* is significant at < .0033 to allow for multiple comparisons.
[c] Negative numbers indicate film AUC is greater than digital AUC.
Data from Pisano ED, Gatsonis C, Hendrick E, et al., DMIST Investigators Group. Diagnostic performance of digital versus film mammography for breast-cancer screening. N Engl J Med 2005;353(17):1773–83.

individual types of machine in the DMIST. Because machine types were not represented in equal numbers in the trial, and all of the Trex/Hologic units were replaced midtrial by the Selenia Hologic machines (both from Hologic Corporation, Danbury, CT), patient accrual using the various machines was quite variable. Table 2 gives the number of patients and cancers detected per machine type in the DMIST. Although no significant differences between digital and film mammography in the AUC, sensitivity, specificity, and PPV1 were measured by machine type, the ability to measure such differences varied substantially across the various manufacturers. Because of the very small number of cancers included in the study that were imaged using both of the Hologic systems (only 22 cases were imaged by both systems), estimates of the AUC and sensitivity had extremely wide confidence intervals and may not be reliable. The receiver operating characteristic curves for the other three manufacturers are shown in Fig. 1A–C.

Table 3 shows the AUC, sensitivity, specificity, and PPV1 for the three manufacturers that imaged 60 or more cancers in the study. Because patients and readers varied across the manufacturers, it is not readily evident how to compare the performance of digital mammography across the manufacturers in Table 3. That is, differences in the authors' estimates of performance of the various machine types may result from differences in patient and reader populations, not from differences in the characteristics of the machines themselves. This possibility is confirmed by the comparison of film mammography across the three populations of readers and patients: the AUC for film varied from 0.695 to 0.775.

Based on the results of the DMIST, the authors of this article believe that there is ample reason to consider converting to digital mammography, at least for the patient populations for which the

Table 2: **Evaluable cases and cancers per machine type in the Digital Mammographic Imaging Screening Trial**

Machine type	Evaluable cases	# Cancers (%)
Fischer	10,103	84 (25.1)
Fuji	8957	60 (17.9)
General Electric	19,250	169 (50.4)
Hologic Trex	1483	6 (1.8)
Hologic Selenia	2967	16 (4.8)
Totals	42,760	335

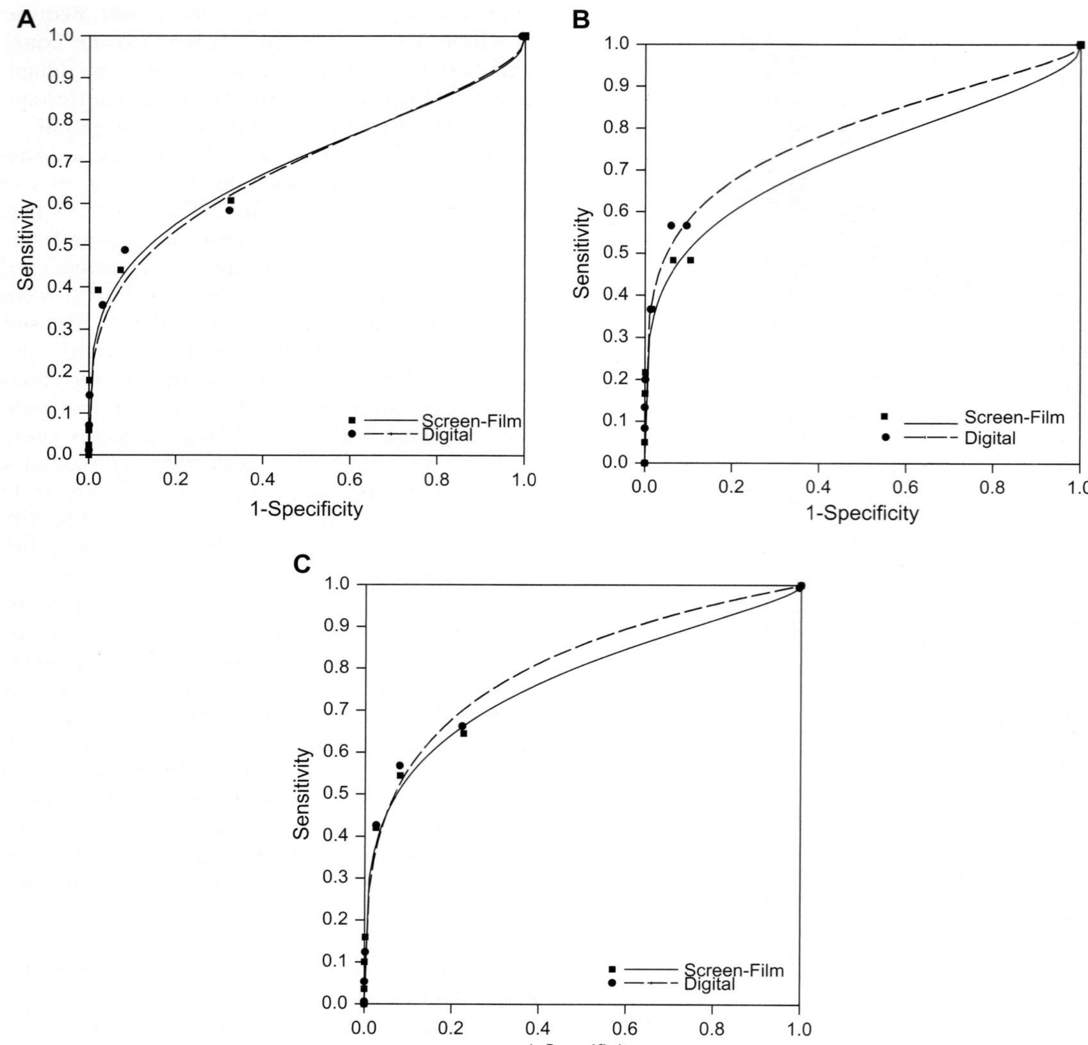

Fig. 1. Receiver operating characteristic analysis. (*A*) Fischer digital versus film. (*B*) Fuji digital versus film. (*C*) General Electric digital versus film.

DMIST showed digital mammography to have better diagnostic accuracy than film. Other reasons to consider the conversion are discussed in more detail in the sections that follow. These advantages include the ease of image storage, retrieval, and transmission, including the ability to get second opinions from other radiologists at remote sites. In addition, if breast imaging is the only nondigital part of the entire radiology department, the savings in costs in eliminating film processing, storage, and display for the department may be substantial, although the authors are not aware of any formal studies documenting those reductions in cost, and the DMIST cost-effectiveness analysis will take the payer's rather than the provider's perspective.

Technical issues to consider in converting to digital mammography

Because the DMIST demonstrated enhanced performance in some population subsets, there has been increased impetus to convert to digital mammography. There are many technical issues to consider before a transition occurs. This section describes those technical issues in detail.

Image display issues

For technologists and radiologists to perform and interpret digital mammography images correctly and expeditiously, they must understand the issues that surround image display. The first aspect of understanding display of an image is to understand

Table 3: **Area under the curve, difference in AUC, sensitivity, specificity, and positive predictive values 1 (PPV1) in the Digital Mammographic Imaging Screening Trial by machine type[a]**

Machine type	AUC digital	AUC film	AUC difference	Sensitivity digital	Sensitivity film	Specificity digital	Specificity film	PPV1 digital	PPV1 film
All	0.775 (0.020)[b]	0.744 (0.022)	0.032 (0.024)	0.697 (0.029)	0.657 (0.030)	0.918 (0.001)	0.917 (0.001)	0.048 (0.004)	0.045 (0.003)
Fischer	0.688 (0.045)	0.695 (0.045)	−0.007[c] (0.049)	0.619 (0.061)	0.651 (0.060)	0.908 (0.003)	0.916 (0.003)	0.041 (0.006)	0.046 (0.007)
Fuji	0.788 (0.054)	0.730 (0.063)	0.058 (0.068)	0.727 (0.067)	0.591 (0.074)	0.934 (0.003)	0.930 (0.003)	0.052 (0.009)	0.040 (0.008)
General Electric	0.809 (0.024)	0.775 (0.028)	0.034 (0.031)	0.709 (0.040)	0.685 (0.041)	0.917 (0.002)	0.917 (0.002)	0.054 (0.006)	0.052 (0.005)

[a] There were no comparisons where P is significant at < .0033.
[b] Numbers in parentheses are standard errors.
[c] Negative numbers indicate film AUC is greater than digital AUC.

the image itself. Digital mammograms start as a pixel map, with a numeric value in each pixel. These numeric values are called analog-to-digital units (ADU). They basically represent the amount of X-ray exposure to the digital detector in that pixel location. As one would expect, the highest ADU counts are in pixels where only air is between the tube and the detector surface, and the lowest counts are where dense structures such as bone or metal are present. The number and size of pixels available in the detector vary between vendors. Currently, in full-field digital mammography units, pixel sizes are 50, 70, or 100 microns in diameter. As in other modalities, spatial resolution improves as pixel size diminishes, but noise increases. Therefore the quality of the end image cannot be surmised from pixel size alone.

After the ADU map is created, the unit performs multiple processing algorithms to produce a readable image [11,12]. Some of the algorithms are intended to correct for detector inhomogeneities, and others are meant to manipulate the acquired data to render an interpretable image. One common algorithm is called "thickness equalization." This algorithm enhances the signal in the fatty subcutaneous region so that it is readily visible without the user having to adjust the window width and window level settings manually during interpretation. Other imaging processing algorithms are used in an effort to make lesions like mass borders and calcifications more obvious [11,13]. All these algorithms are currently proprietary to each manufacturer. The final resultant images that are produced are called the "for-presentation" images. These are the images that radiologists interpret. Every digital mammography unit also produces partially processed images. These images commonly are called "raw images," but they in fact are not raw images; they are images that have had some but not all of the processing applied to them. They are more correctly called "for-processing" images. The vendors of computer-assisted diagnosis (CAD) equipment use these for-processing images to apply their algorithm.

Digital Imaging and Communications in Medicine and Integrating the Health care Enterprise

Each digital image that is produced also has a Digital Imaging and Communications in Medicine (DICOM) header attached to it. The header carries all information necessary for accurate display, storage, and retrieval of the image such as patient demographics, acquisition parameters, and display requirements (Fig. 2). The DICOM standard assigns a specifice location to each piece of information

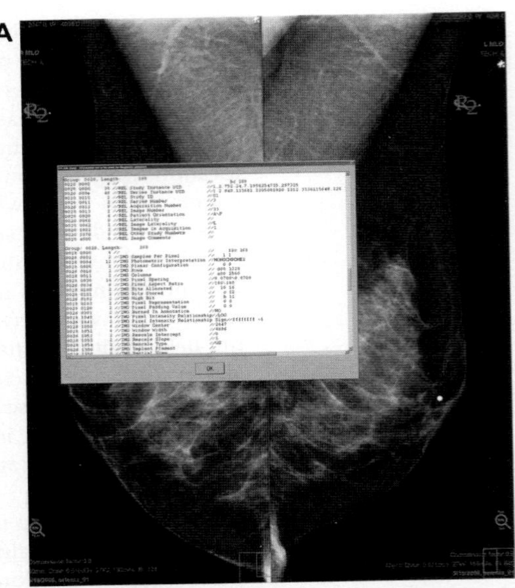

B

DICOM dump - Information not to be used for diagnostic purposes

```
Group: 0020, Length:         188
0020 0000        4 //                              //       bc 188
0020 000d       30 //REL Study Instance UID        //1.2.752.24.7.1956254735.297325
0020 000e       48 //REL Series Instance UID       //1.2.840.113681.2205081920.1212.3336115648.126.
0020 0010        2 //REL Study ID                  //01
0020 0011        2 //REL Series Number             //3
0020 0012        0 //REL Acquisition Number        //
0020 0013        2 //REL Image Number              //33
0020 0020        4 //REL Patient Orientation       //A\F
0020 0060        0 //REL Laterality                //
0020 0062        2 //REL Image Laterality          //L
0020 1002        2 //REL Images in Acquisition     //1
0020 1070        0 //REL Other Study Numbers       //
0020 4000        0 //REL Image Comments            //

Group: 0028, Length:         268
0028 0000        4 //                              //      10c 268
0028 0002        2 //IMG Samples Per Pixel         //    1 1
0028 0004       12 //IMG Photometric Interpretation //MONOCHROME2
0028 0006        2 //IMG Planar Configuration      //    0 0
0028 0010        2 //IMG Rows                      // d00 3328
0028 0011        2 //IMG Columns                   // a00 2560
0028 0030       14 //IMG Pixel Spacing             //0.0700\0.0700
0028 0034        8 //IMG Pixel Aspect Ratio        //180\180
0028 0100        2 //IMG Bits Allocated            //  10 16
0028 0101        2 //IMG Bits Stored               //   c 12
0028 0102        2 //IMG High Bit                  //   b 11
0028 0103        2 //IMG Pixel Representation      //   0 0
0028 0120        2 //IMG Pixel Padding Value       //   0 0
0028 0301        2 //IMG Burned In Annotation      //NO
0028 1040        4 //IMG Pixel Intensity Relationship//LOG
0028 1041        2 //IMG Pixel Intensity Relationship Sign//ffffffff -1
0028 1050        4 //IMG Window Center             //2047
0028 1051        4 //IMG Window Width              //4096
0028 1052        2 //IMG Rescale Intercept         //0
0028 1053        2 //IMG Rescale Slope             //1
0028 1054        2 //IMG Rescale Type              //US
0028 1300        0 //IMG Implant Present           //
0028 1350        0 //IMG Partial View              //
```

OK

Fig. 2. (*A, B*) Examples of a DICOM header.

recorded in the header . If each manufacturer uses the DICOM standard and interprets the meaning of the standard in the same way, information can be shared. If, however, two vendors interpret the standard differently, and any piece of information is stored in a different location in the header, the pieces of equipment cannot communicate that information; that is, there is a DICOM incompatibility. One of the main reasons that digital transitions are complicated is that these DICOM incompatibilities are common, between vendors and between different generations of equipment from the same vendor. Like all else in medicine, the standard has evolved and changed with advances in technology and experience. Multiple DICOM committees exist to keep the standards up to date. Frequently, the committees accept proposals for changing the standard. Vendors then must implement the new standard and make changes in their equipment to be compliant. It sometimes is not cost beneficial for vendors to make the necessary DICOM updates to equipment that is already deployed in the market. As a result, when a facility tries to add a new piece of equipment to an older system, there are often DICOM incompatibility problems. These problems may be corrected with software patches or site-specific workarounds. In some cases, however, these differences are so significant that old equipment must be replaced or choices for new equipment are limited.

Unfortunately, even when vendors comply with the same version of the DICOM standard, incompatibilities still exist between products because of variable interpretations of the standard. In 1998, a joint effort by the Radiological Society of North America and the Health care Information and Management Systems Society was created to address this problem. The effort is called "Integrating the Health care Enterprise" (IHE). IHE defines how standards such as DICOM and Health Level 7 should be used by defining the transactions that must occur between pieces of equipment to solve clinical problems [14,15]. These precise scenarios, called "profiles," allow integration of heterogeneous information systems. Each profile is meant to solve a related group of clinical problems. IHE also uses a specific vocabulary to avoid confusion. The profiles and the vocabulary make up the technical framework [16]. When vendors follow the IHE profiles and DICOM standards, their equipment can be integrated into a facility far more easily.

Food and Drug Administration classification

In 1999, the FDA classified full-field digital mammography as a class III device. Part of the FDA requirement for product approval has been that vendors ensure the integrity of the image from acquisition to display, storage, and printing. As a result, products have evolved as insular, proprietary systems that function well internally but have little ability to communicate with other equipment. For users, that configuration meant that the only choice to be made was which acquisition unit to purchase; the workstation, monitors, and printer that were developed to function with the acquisition unit had to be used for any images produced by that gantry. In 2001, the FDA allowed printers to be removed from this chain and have separate clearance as class II devices. Shortly thereafter, in 2002, the FDA chose to allow other third-party monitors and then diagnostic workstations to apply for approval for digital mammography display. Users now are free to use any FDA-approved workstation for interpretation, but, unfortunately, FDA approval for display does not mean that the images actually are displayed correctly. The user must be careful.

Compatibility

The problems with the display of images on foreign workstations stem from the different pixel sizes at acquisition, variable interpretations of the DICOM standard, and the proprietary development of products. The most obvious discrepancy between the systems is pixel size at acquisition. There are four ways to display a digital image on soft copy: fit to viewport, true size, full resolution, and magnification. In the fit-to-viewport mode, the image is scaled to fit on the portion of the monitor to which it is allocated. This scaling is accomplished by displaying an average ADU for a group of adjacent pixels. For instance, an image acquired at 70 microns might be displayed at 120-micron resolution. The smaller the pixel size of acquisition, the more the image must be down-sampled for display, so a breast imaged at 50 microns will look smaller to the radiologist than the same breast imaged at 100 microns (Fig. 3). To complicate matters more, some smart applications can identify skin line and display only the breast area while ignoring the air around the breast. Others do not have this ability and display the entire detector surface in the display. Mammograms displayed on workstations that do not have skin-line detection capability therefore look smaller than the same images displayed on smart workstations where skin line is known. As a result, if a patient has mammograms done on units of differing pixel size from year to year, and the workstation cannot adjust the display to compensate, evaluating the images for lesion growth and developing asymmetries is very difficult. Some smart workstations now can make the images look the same size by scaling the display in the fit-to-viewport mode, based on acquired pixel size (Fig. 4).

The second way to display images is true size. True size means that the display matches the actual physical size of the breast. This display is important for procedures such as stereotactic core biopsy and surgery, so that a lesion's size and location relative to skin, nipple, and chest wall can be ascertained easily. Some workstations currently are incapable of displaying true size.

The third display is full resolution. In this mode, each acquired pixel from the acquisition detector is displayed by one pixel on the monitor at the diagnostic workstation. Therefore, by definition, this is the mode in which all of the information in the acquisition is presented. Full resolution is important for evaluation of subtle lesions such as faint calcifications or mass margins. Because

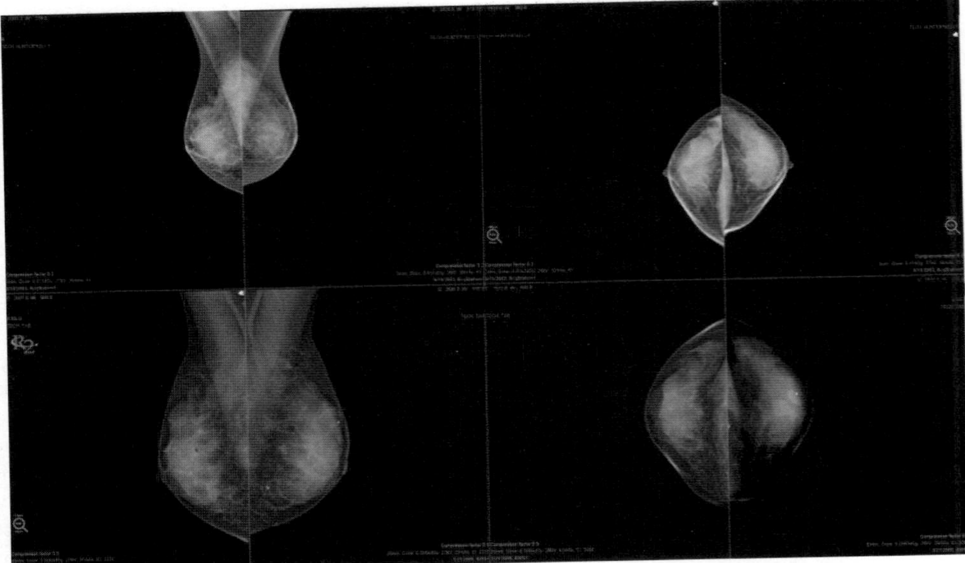

Fig. 3. The same patient imaged in 2 consecutive years on systems with different pixel pitch. In this fit to viewport mode,the four view mammogram in the upper right and upper left panels, which were acquired at 50 microns, look smaller than the four view mammogram in the lower right and lower left panels, which were acquired at 100 microns.

acquisition matrices are all larger than display matrices, unless the breast is small and the workstation is smart enough to detect skin line and exclude the area around the breast, this mode requires that the user be able to move around the displayed breast to see it all (with the pan function) or magnify subsets of the breast (with the zoom function).

The fourth mode of display is magnification. In this mode, an acquired pixel is displayed by more than one pixel on the workstation. Display can be achieved by use of a segmental magnification such as quadrant zoom (in which the radiologist steps through tiles of the image), a magnification glass that is moved around the image, or magnification

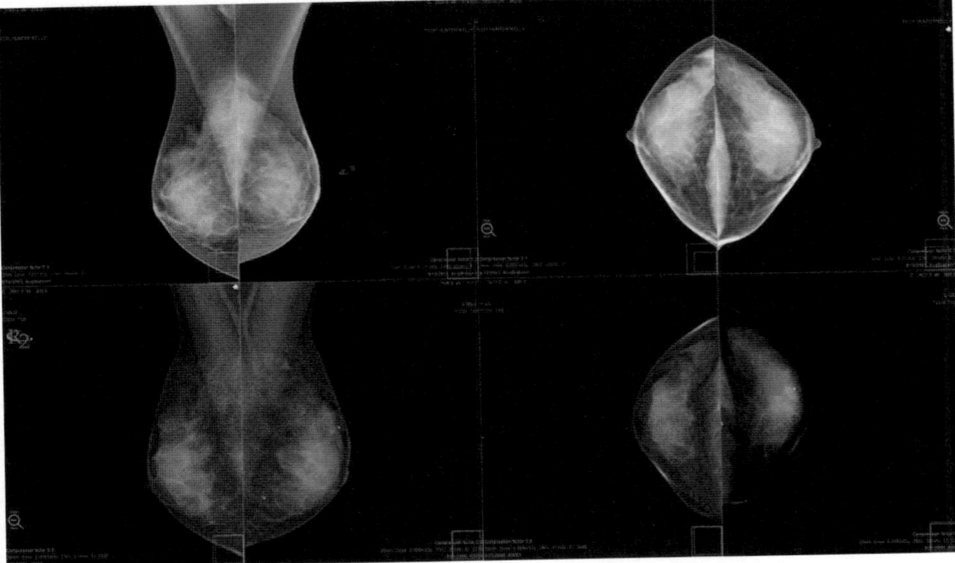

Fig. 4. In the fit-to-viewport mode, the images shown in Fig. 3 are all scaled to be displayed at the same size. This scaling allows the radiologist to compare the images for developing densities and lesion size changes.

of the entire image and use of the pan function. Inspecting images at resolutions greater than acquisition is performed by a variety of interpolation algorithms and may make review of mammograms easier in some instances but does not add any additional information to the acquired data.

Some workstations display the zoom (or magnification) factor so the radiologist knows what amount of data down-sampling or magnification is being displayed at any given time in a hanging protocol [16].

Another significant problem is the orientation of images. Images are hung correctly in display protocols when both the acquisition unit and the workstation use the correct orientation tag. Several types of images have a potentially confusing orientation, such as superolateral-to-inferomedial obliques, caudocranial (from below) views, and cleavage views. Without proper use of this information, any view (but especially the three mentioned) will be hung incorrectly, potentially leading to misinterpretation by the radiologist.

Another problem is the different shape of the window width/window level curve (called the "volume of interest lookup table"). Some vendors produce images that are meant to be displayed using a sigmoidal curve; others use a linear slope. If the workstation cannot apply the correct curve, the image will be degraded significantly (Fig. 5). This incompatibility is an example of the problems that result when systems evolve in a proprietary way. Along the same lines, any workstation that cannot identify skin line will not be able to keep the area around the breast dark if the radiologist manually increases the window level and or widens the window width. In this situation, the area around the breast becomes increasingly brighter, and image contrast is degraded (Fig. 6).

Processing algorithms

To a large degree, the appearance of a digital mammogram results from the image processing that is applied to it. Currently, most manufacturers offer no choice in processing and change their algorithms from time to time. These changes can alter the appearance of the mammogram significantly (Fig. 7). In addition, users have little or no information available to them about the algorithms that they are using. The radiologist faces the challenge of relearning what normal tissue looks like each time the algorithm is changed or each time a different vendor's equipment is purchased.

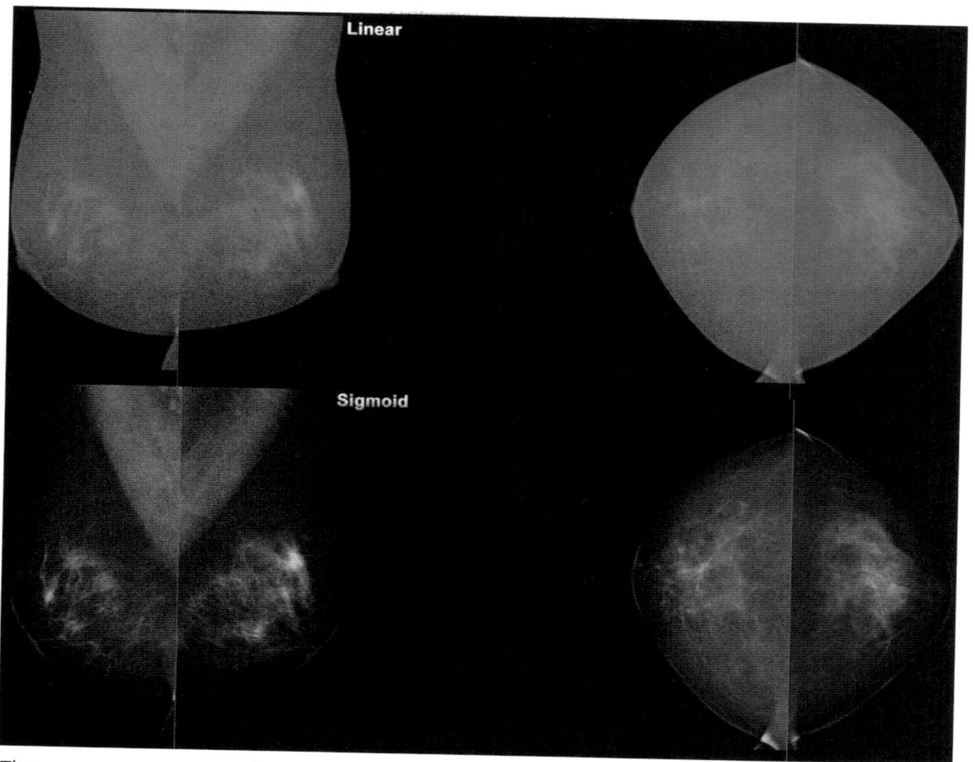

Fig. 5. The same mammogram (all for-presentation images) is displayed correctly on the bottom with the sigmoid lookup table and incorrectly on the top with a linear lookup table.

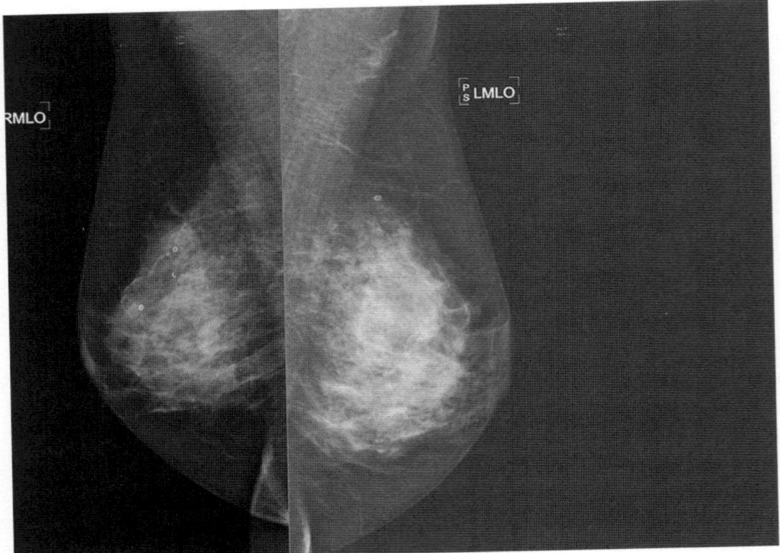

Fig. 6. The right mediolateral oblique view (RMLO) is shown as it originally appears on the diagnostic workstation. In the left mediolateral oblique view (LMLO) view, the window width and the window level have been increased at the diagnostic workstation. This common manipulation has changed the blackness of the image around the breast, thus decreasing the apparent contrast in the breast tissue and degrading the image.

The differences in processing algorithms, along with the sizing issues already discussed, make comparisons between years difficult (Fig. 8). Several authors have shown that different processing algorithms may be better or more preferred, depending on the particular tasks, lesions, and systems [11–13,17–20]. Two vendors currently offer more than one processing algorithm for interpretation. With these systems, the radiologist must choose which algorithm is preferable, because, to date, there has been no study showing that one kind of processing has superior diagnostic quality than another. Even if a facility chooses to purchase all acquisition units from the same vendor, that facility still must contend with images from almost every vendor, because patients bring prior digital images from the outside for comparison.

Prior mammograms

Several options exist for displaying prior mammograms. If the prior studies are analog, the radiologist must decide if the images should be hung on an

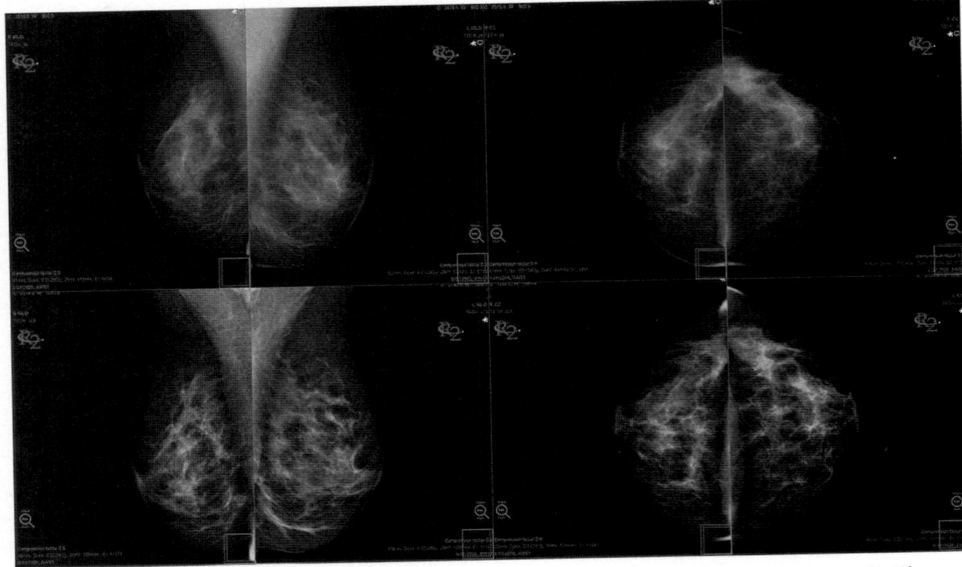

Fig. 7. The same patient was imaged 2 consecutive years on the same digital mammogram unit. The processing algorithm changed in the interval, resulting in a different look to the mammogram.

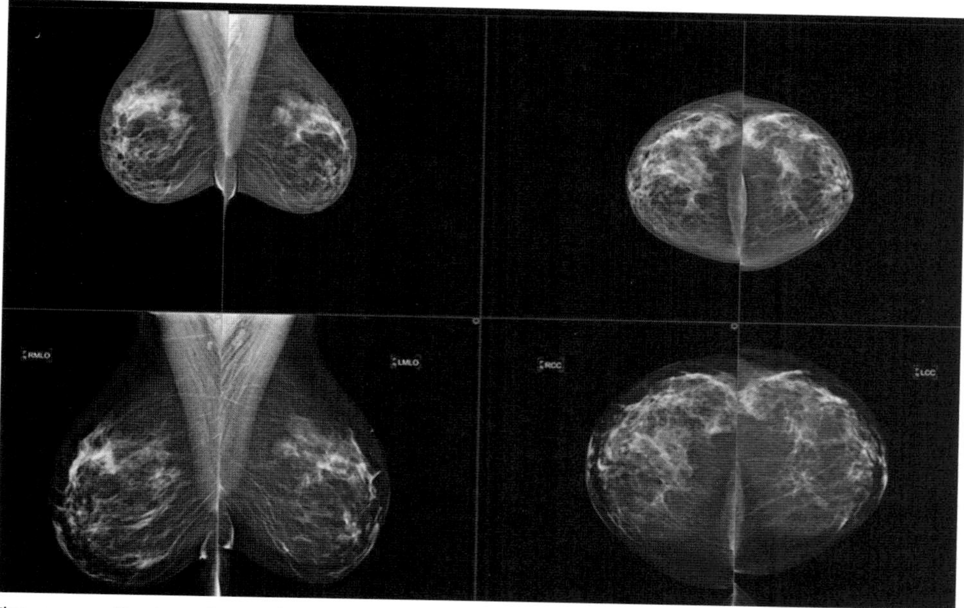

Fig. 8. The same patient was imaged in 2 consecutive years. On the top, the images were acquired at 50 microns. On the bottom, the images were acquired at 70 microns. The workstation is displaying the images in the fit-to-viewport mode but cannot scale the images to the same size. That difference, along with the disparate processing between vendors, makes comparison of this patient's mammogram very difficult.

alternator adjacent to the diagnostic workstation or if the images should be digitized and placed in a hanging protocol for soft-copy comparison. The advantage of digitization is that the prior images will be in much closer proximity to the current digital mammogram. Also, all of the luminance issues surrounding the difference in light output between traditional alternators and computer monitors are solved with digitization and soft-copy display of prior images. Analog digitizers typically produce a 50-micron image, so all the sizing problems discussed previously apply to these images as well. The algorithms that process the digitized analog images are evolving rapidly. These images are not FDA approved for primary interpretation and do not replace the original analog images for medical-legal purposes or for American College of Radiology requirements.

Integrating the Health care Enterprise profiles

To ensure that any digital mammogram can be displayed correctly, the Mammography Image Profile is necessary [16]. This profile, written in 2006, was developed to resolve the display problems that are nearly ubiquitous when mammography images are displayed on third-party workstations. For example, it allows images of different pixel sizes to be scaled to the same size for display so that the radiologist can evaluate changes in lesion size or developing asymmetries. It also clearly defines image orientation to solve the common problem of left images hanging like right images, as well as addressing the window width/window level lookup table differences and the background blackness maintenance. This profile also addresses CAD display issues, annotations, and problems with printer integration.

Storage considerations

Image sizes

Both short-term and long-term storage needs for digital mammography are significant, for several reasons. First, because the pixel sizes are small, and the matrices large, the images are big, ranging in size from 8.8 to 52 megabytes per view. Therefore, a standard four-view mammogram can be up to 208 megabytes. Second, as discussed previously, both for-processing and for-presentation data sets are produced for every image. If a facility elects to store both types of images, storage needs double. CAD files are small, so the decision to store them in the long-term archive is more a medical-legal decision than a storage-space decision. Similarly, if annotations are stored as a DICOM overlay, the storage added is insignificant. If the workstation allows annotated images to be saved and stored only as a screen capture, however, then each of these images is the same size as the original view and should be considered in the calculation of storage requirements.

Compression

Currently, visually lossless compression is acceptable for storage. These ratios typically range from 1.5 to 3:1, so only moderate savings in storage space are realized. Lossy compression ratios higher than 3 or 4:1 currently are not recommended, mainly because of concerns about the possible inability to evaluate subtle calcifications at these higher ratios [21]. To date, several studies have shown that far higher compression ratios (up to 80:1) might not result in loss of diagnostic information [22–24]. Studies evaluating the ability to detect and characterize lesions accurately with lossy compression ratios are still needed to answer this clinical question with confidence. Until that time, because of the medical-legal issues surrounding the maintenance of the originally interpreted data and the important need in mammography to have diagnostic-quality prior images for comparison, lossy compression is not recommended [21]. Therefore, if a practice produces 100 digital mammograms per day, stores both for-presentation and for-processing data, and the images, on average, are compressed 2.5:1, the storage needs range from 7 gigabytes to more than 16 gigabytes per day.

Prior studies

Prior analog images are one of the most important considerations in determining storage requirements. For workflow purposes, many facilities digitize the prior analog mammograms so that they can be displayed in soft copy immediately adjacent to the current digital study. Currently, these digitizers produce 50-micron images, with image sizes of 35 to 58 megabytes per view, depending on the size of the film. If these images are stored in the archive, the storage space required again increases by a factor of two for each prior year that is digitized. If a facility produces 20,000 digital mammograms per year and digitizes and stores two prior analog studies using a lossless compression ratio of 2.5:1, the long-term storage requirements for that facility range from 6.3 to 13.4 terabytes per year,. The file sizes also affect short-term storage. To maximize workflow efficiency, having prior studies readily available is critical because multiple prior images often are reviewed in the course of interpretation of a mammogram. As facilities accumulate years of digital mammograms or digitize multiple prior years of analog studies, the ability to have many (or all) prior studies quickly accessible will be important. Therefore the required on-line storage space will increase over time, and the ability of the system to retrieve many old studies quickly (pre-fetch capability) must be robust. In facilities in which the on-line storage and/or the pre-fetch capabilities of the pre-existing picture archive and communication system (PACS) cannot meet the workflow needs of digital mammography, a mini-PACS solution can be implemented. The disadvantage of a mini-PACS solution is that it continues to isolate digital mammography from the rest of the system so that, to view a digital mammogram, a workstation must be networked to it. If that workstation also functions as a multimodality workstation, it also might have to be networked to the main PACS and even to the radiology information system (RIS).

Push versus pull

The configuration of how the images arrive at the diagnostic workstation also influences the amount of storage necessary. Several systems follow a "push" model of moving data in which the images are sent either by a predetermined mechanism or manually to each workstation. In a facility with multiple acquisition units and multiple diagnostic workstations, all of the images from every unit and the prior images from off-line storage may be pushed to every workstation. Such a model creates a lot of network traffic and requires more on-line storage space for each workstation. If a "pull" model is used, the images are pulled to the diagnostic workstation, again either by a predetermined specification or manually. From a storage standpoint, this model is more efficient than the push model but could have some effects on display speed. Many systems use a combination of push and pull models to maximize the benefits of both.

Network issues

Hand-in-hand with storage needs are transmission concerns. The bandwidth of the network can affect display speed, and therefore radiologist workflow, significantly. For example, if a facility has an Ethernet 100-base T network, a four-view mammogram with lossless compression can be transmitted in approximately 1 minute. If the facility uses a cable network, several minutes may be needed to transmit the study. These transmission times are long, and the amount of bandwidth necessary to move mammography images affects the transmission of all the rest of the data moving through the system. To avoid congestion in the network and avoid workflow slowdowns, many facilities pre-fetch prior studies to on-line storage before the radiologist logs on to read.

Clinical and ergonomic issues to consider in converting to digital mammography

General clinical considerations

Factors that must be considered in converting a busy breast-imaging practice from film to digital mammography include how many digital mammography units to acquire, whether mammography is performed in more than one site, the number of sites at which mammography is interpreted, and whether a practice PACS system is already in existence.

The more mammographic units there are in the practice, and the more sites there are where mammography is performed and interpreted, the more complex the issues around conversion become. Early in the process decisions must be made about how many units to convert, if all units are to be converted eventually, and how quickly to make the conversion . If only one unit is converted at one or at multiple sites for a period of time, issues may arise as to which patients are examined on the digital versus the film units. Patients and referring physicians may request or even demand one type of examination.

If the practice has more than one site, another issue that will occur is whether all units at one site are converted first or if a partial conversion to digital mammography is made at each site. The speed of conversion to an all-digital practice, if that is the goal, will depend very much on the funding available from the practice administration, both within the radiology department itself and within the hospital or medical group. As many radiologists can testify, slower conversion is more painful, because one still must be able to interpret film as well as digital mammographic examinations. Some of the advantages of a digital system, such as decrease in, and eventual elimination of, the necessity for a film storage area and associated personnel, lack of need of a dark room and processor, and ease of transmission of the images will not be realized fully until a practice converts completely to all-digital mammography.

If not all the units at a single site are converted within 1 year, some patients still will be getting film examinations, prolonging the time during which both digital and film examinations must be interpreted. Some practices store current examinations, after interpretation, as digital images on their departmental PACS using one of the CAD system digitizers to convert the film images [25]. This method provides digital comparisons with back up of the films if needed the next year. If the choice is to convert one site before converting the others, patients and referring physicians may want to send patients only to the site where the digital units are available. The goal should be to convert all the units at all sites as quickly as possible to take advantage of digital conversion.

Once a practice has decided on the general speed of conversion to digital mammography, a decision as to which digital units to purchase must be made. Although radiologists and administrators are used to buying whichever film mammography unit is available at the best price with the add-ons they want at that particular time, this process is less of an option with digital units. Film units produce a common viewable image that is very similar, no matter which manufacturer's equipment is used. As explained in detail previously, digital mammographic images are not as easily interchangeable and comparable [26].

Patient throughput issues

In addition, the decision whether to use the digital unit or units for screening or diagnostic mammography or both may have to be made. Because throughput of patients is typically faster on the digital systems than on film units, and because the cost of the digital unit is much higher, the decision often is made to use the digital unit in the screening setting to ensure maximum usage of the digital units. If digital mammography is used for screening, additional imaging may be performed with film mammography or digitally. This process can lead to difficulties in evaluation of current additional views and comparison of studies at 6-month or yearly follow-up. Differences in display size will affect the evaluation of calcifications and masses, and different processing algorithms can make it difficult even to see the same area of concern, particularly if it is a vague area of asymmetry or a cluster of calcifications. Careful attention to these factors is required.

Whether the digital units are used for screening, diagnostic, or both types of examinations, the type of patients examined on the digital units when there also are film units in the system becomes an issue. Some patients and their referring physicians may insist on digital imaging, whether or not the DMIST results indicate that digital imaging will improve detection of malignancy. If the practice has only a limited number of digital units, or digital units at only one site, a scheduling nightmare can result. Even if the practice protocol is to prescreen patients in an attempt to use digital imaging only for patients shown in the DMIST to have benefited from digital imaging or whose last examination was a digital one, inefficiencies in running the daily schedule of patients for examination can occur if there are not enough digital units within the practice.

Many practices that already have begun to acquire digital mammography units have placed these units in the screening rather than the diagnostic setting. The speed with which patients can be imaged and the examinations checked by the technologist using the digital radiography units is such that patient room-time for a screening examination can be as low as 5 minutes. Thus, there is the potential to use fewer mammographic units to produce the same number of studies. It has been reported that one digital radiography unit can replace two film units [27]. With computed radiography units, because the images must be processed and reviewed afterwards, the throughput of patients is similar to that for film units, although film-handling times are eliminated after completion of the examination. Newer and improved computed radiography mammography systems do produce images faster and at a much lower cost [28].

The use of digital mammographic units in the diagnostic area also can result in increased throughput. Again, the main speed advantage is realized only with the use of digital radiography (not computed radiography) units. Images can be checked immediately to ensure that they include the area of concern that is being evaluated and can be repeated without having to take the patient out of the room and then brought back in. Needle-localization procedures can become almost real time, with localizations taking as little at 10 to 15 minutes from initial imaging to completion of the procedure [25]. Because the technologist does not have to leave the room to develop the films, there is added patient safety, because there always are two people in the room throughout the procedure. Although computed radiography units take longer, some time is saved if the image processor is in the room, and, again, two people can remain within the room for added patient safety.

Ductograms can be performed more easily with digital imaging because patients do not have to hold still with the needle in place nearly as long. The decision to inject more contrast can be made easily, and additional views to demonstrate the area better can be obtained quickly. The use of digital magnification can help in interpreting these studies, without having to move the patient to set up for a direct magnification view with its attendant greater risk for needle displacement.

Newer imaging techniques can be incorporated more easily into practice. Tomosynthesis using digital imaging is possible already, although it is not yet available for purchase. Contrast-enhanced imaging also can be performed more easily, although the clinical utility of this technology has not yet been proven.

Speed of conversion

How fast a practice can convert to all-digital mammography depends on human factors as well as financial ones. Technologists, radiologists, and physicists must learn new quality-control methods. Currently these methods are different for each manufacturer's equipment, a factor that, again, may encourage the use of only one type of digital unit [29]. Efforts are under way to recommend a more uniform approach to digital quality control, which will reduce time and confusion.

Technologists must learn to use digital units to acquire images, although this is not a time-consuming issue. For digital radiography units they also must learn and be encouraged to use all the tools available to review the images before the patient leaves the room. Because the acquisition monitors used by technologists often are of lower resolution than work (interpretation) monitors, and because there is a relatively high level of ambient light in the examination room, technologists should be provided with adequate time to review the images under the best possible viewing conditions to check for positioning, compression, and lack of artifacts. Technologists also must be familiar with the ability to enlarge the images and change the brightness and contrast of the images on the acquisition station.

If more than one image in each view is necessary to cover the whole breast, the order of obtaining the images becomes important in some of the digital radiography systems. Radiologists, for example, want to compare the two images for each side. If the technologist obtains the upper and more posterior breast in the mediolateral oblique (MLO) projection on one side first, then acquires the more anterior and inferior portion, and does the opposite on the second side, the images when pulled up for review on the workstation may show the first image of each side obtained in MLO projection; then the second view either shows up automatically or must be dragged manually into the viewing position. For these systems, training all the technologists always to obtain the views in the same sequence will reduce the image-manipulation time for the radiologist.

Although the technologist needs less time to acquire the mammograms with digital and especially with digital radiography units, radiologist needs longer to interpret them, especially initially. Clearly, with experience, this time can be decreased [27]. Manipulating the digital image, including magnifying the image and inverting it, takes more time than reviewing a film image, even if one uses a magnifying glass and a bright light. Initially, radiologists report that interpreting a digital mammogram takes about twice as long as interpreting a film mammogram. With experience, this time decreases. Those experienced in digital interpretation say that with optimal system set-up and reading or hanging protocols on the workstations, and with experience, the time needed for interpretation of film and digital examinations can be similar. It is also faster when one has old digital images for comparison, rather than film images [30,31].

Interpretation of digital mammography must be performed on a workstation to take full advantage of the benefits. Practices that routinely print the digital images limit interpretation benefits and increase the costs of imaging handling, because these printed images must be hung and removed by a person, and the images must be stored in film jackets, requiring the retention of file room space and personnel. Printing images does allow the radiologist to mark areas of concern, so that the technologist has this marked image in the room if the patient needs to be called back for additional imaging . The radiologist can save these marks electronically, however, and the technologist can pull the marked images onto the acquisition monitor.

Optimization of interpretation time requires that hanging protocols be developed to review the digital images as efficiently as possible. These protocols must be adjusted for more than two views of each breast for screening and to allow review of the current images quickly, with the ability to compare the two sides and the craniocaudal (CC) and MLO views of one side simultaneously. Protocols must allow comparison of several old studies in sequence, ideally without having to drag and drop every image. For diagnostic imaging, all the images should be viewable at full resolution. Ideally, protocols to display routine diagnostic views should be set up and easily retrievable for use during interpretation.

All these protocols should be radiologist specific. Standardized hanging protocols are helpful initially, but most experienced mammographers have their own preferences on how to review and compare examinations, and systems should be easily programmable and adaptable for individual readers. Manufacturer-provided training should include enough time to set up these specific protocols and should include a second training visit that allows refinement of radiologist-specific protocols after a few weeks of operation.

Where to interpret studies

If mammography is performed at only one site, and only a small volume is performed, interpretation can be performed at one workstation. Depending on the volume of screening and diagnostic examinations, about two to three mammographic units require one workstation for efficient use of radiologist time. With a higher volume of diagnostic studies, or if the practice is reading screening examinations on-line, more workstations are needed, because interrupting the interpretation of a digital examination to look at images from another ongoing examination may be more disruptive than with film examinations. Workstations for interpretation of diagnostic and screening examinations can be separated, and this model is recommended for greater radiologist efficiency, because it already in place for interpretation of film examinations at many breast centers.

If the practice has several sites at which examinations are performed, digital mammography allows images to be interpreted more easily off-site, although this benefit may not be realized for a couple of years after digital imaging is first adopted because of the need for comparison with old film examinations. Initially, the patient's old films must be transported to the interpretation site and hung for comparison with the new digital studies. This process, of course, will not be an issue for practices that digitize prior examinations.

Interpretation, particularly of screening mammograms, can be performed off-site with images transmitted electronically rather than transported and hung by practice personnel. Radiologists, who are in limited supply, do not need to waste time traveling to different sites. For remote locations, even diagnostic examinations can be interpreted on-line with immediate transmission of the images to the radiologist, who can communicate need for additional images to the technologist by telephone or fax and give the patient the results immediately by telephone [32]. This ability is a major benefit of digital mammography but may be limited to diagnostic examinations that do not include ultrasound.

Practices that perform mammography at several sites may need more than one place to interpret studies. Which studies are to be interpreted at each site must be determined. Screening examinations can be interpreted at a central site for more efficiency, and diagnostic cases could be performed separately at each site, possibly only on specific days. For radiologists reading at separate sites, consulting with one other on difficult cases is much easier than with films, if digital examinations are sent to departmental or breast imaging–specific PACS. This ability to obtain second opinions quickly clearly benefits the patient as well as the radiology practice.

How to configure reading rooms

Breast imaging typically has been relegated to small corners of the department with small reading rooms. Although film alternators and computers with multiple monitors eventually will not be needed, most practices will need them for 2 to 3 years during the transition period from film to digital mammography. Reading rooms must accommodate this equipment. Also, the high-intensity lights required on the film mammography alternators and the number of computers and monitors required will create a large amount of heat within the reading room. Planning the ideal reading rooms should include the engineering department, so that adequate cooling is available within the reading rooms for optimal functioning of the computers and for the radiologists' comfort. Ambient lighting in these rooms must be controlled easily, and there must be adequate shielding and easy control of the lights on the film alternators so that digital mammograms can be viewed simultaneously nearby on soft-copy display. There also must be some indirect lighting so that paperwork can be reviewed and keyboards can be seen and so personnel can safely move around the room. PACS monitors and RIS system monitors should have dark backgrounds or be easy to turn on and off, to avoid the light reflecting off the workstation monitors. If more than one reading station is in the room, separation of the reading areas is necessary. A convenient way to create separation is with a dark curtain reaching almost to the ceiling, because traditional moveable panels as used in many departments do not extend high enough to block lights.

Typically, a reading space for mammography interpretation needs a film alternator for the old films set at a right angle to the three monitor workstations for digital interpretation and at least one other computer monitor for connection to RIS and departmental PACS so that ultrasounds, MR images, and other pertinent studies and reports can be available. In a diagnostic breast imaging reading room, PACS access for interpretation of breast ultrasound and MR imaging must be readily available. If CAD is used, a computer for this function also is needed in the reading room, but no separate monitor is needed for mammography. For for MR imaging, some systems require a dedicated monitor in addition to a computer; other systems may use a departmental PACS monitor. The workspace also needs a telephone and possibly a dictation system. If voice recognition is used, the keyboard for the system where the reports will be reviewed must be easily accessible.

Careful attention to ergonomic issues in setting up the workspace is recommended. For years, mammographers have leaned forward to see the images up close and to review them with a magnifying glass. This setting leads to significant neck and back strain. Film alternators never have been at the correct height for all radiologists who read mammograms. The optimal distance for viewing images on the digital workstations differs slightly for each radiologist, but optimal image distance averages 30 to 60 cm, with the radiologist looking straight ahead, not up or down. The use of adjustable ergonomic tables and chairs that can accommodate all the radiologists in the group is important to reduce eye, neck, and back strain. Keyboards need to be at a height that will reduce wrist and arm strain. This factor is especially important if radiologists are using a mammography dictation program that generates the report and statistics immediately.

Clinical issues regarding image storage and retrieval

Images need to be retrieved when patients return for additional diagnostic studies or interventional procedures and when they return for short-interval follow-up or for yearly examinations. Images also need to be retrieved for conferences or tumor boards, for teaching, for consultation with other radiologists within the practice, and for review by other physicians at the time of an appointment or treatment. Issues regarding retrieval vary with the type of system being used for interpretation—a manufacturer-specific workstation or a PACS system—and how images are stored. Clearly, if digital mammography is to be useful, images must be stored electronically and be readily retrievable. Who is responsible for image retrieval will vary with the type of image storage being used. Some ancillary staff, technologists, and radiologists must know how to retrieve prior images. Clearly, if reading is done on a general PACS system with a dedicated mammography FDA-approved workstation, this expertise is less of an issue.

For a truly digital system to work, the surgeons and other physicians who are accustomed to reviewing mammograms when they see the patients in their offices and operating rooms must be given access to digital monitors so they can see the images, unless a practice wants to continue to print a lot of images (which can be quite expensive). Other physicians do not need high-resolution monitors; once the radiologist has marked and saved the pertinent images, other providers will be able to see the vast majority of the findings well enough to work from them with lower-resolution display systems. Radiologists will have to spend some time training other practitioners on how to look at the images on digital monitors, however. Surgeons will be able to see specimen radiographs quickly through the system-wide PACS, if the images are obtained digitally.

Consideration must also be given as to how images will be sent out when requested by other sites for comparisons or second opinions. Another consideration is how the practice will review digital images from other practices. Will the radiologist reviewing the case have to open it on a regular RIS computer, or can or should the images be loaded into a workstation or PACS and reviewed on a mammography-approved workstation? The latter method, rather than printed digital images, is the best way to review outside images. Programs to allow one to copy digital images onto a compact disc (CD) and to open these images are available, and such a program should be selected for the practice. As with the rest of digital radiology, CDs or DVDs of the images may be given to patients or sent outside for review or comparison.

Digital mammography and paperwork

With a PACS system, requests for examinations can be provided on-line rather than on paper. History sheets, often completed by patients, can be quite helpful in providing information pertinent to the mammography interpretation and also are helpful in medicolegal situations. These sheets can be digitized and stored, or the same data can be collected using a tablet personal computer [33]. To the authors' knowledge, not one of the currently available digital mammography workstations can display this sort of data currently.

Summary

There are many issues to consider in converting a busy breast imaging practice from film to digital mammography, but the authors believe that the clear benefits to the practice and to many patients make this effort worthwhile. If the technical, ergonomic, and clinical issues can be addressed in a satisfactory manner, breast imaging clinics can be part of a fully digital radiology practice.

References

[1] Shtern F. Digital mammography and related technologies: a perspective from the National Cancer Institute. Radiology 1992;183:629–30.

[2] Lewin JM, Hendrick RE, D'Orsi CJ, et al. Comparison of full-field digital mammography with screen-film mammography for cancer detection: results of 4,945 paired examinations. Radiology 2001;218(3):873–80.

[3] Lewin JM, D'Orsi CJ, Hendrick RE, et al. Clinical comparison of full-field digital mammography and screen-film mammography for detection of breast cancer. AJR Am J Roentgenol 2002;179:671–7.

[4] Cole E, Pisano ED, Brown M, et al. Diagnostic accuracy of Fischer Senoscan Digital Mammography versus screen-film mammography in a diagnostic mammography population. Acad Radiol 2004;11:879–86.

[5] Skaane P, Young K, Skjennald A. Population-based mammography screening: comparison of screen-film and full-field digital mammography with soft-copy reading–Oslo I study. Radiology 2003;229:877–84.

[6] Skaane P, Skjennald A. Screen-film mammography versus full-field digital mammography with soft-copy reading: randomized trial in a population-based screening program—the Oslo II study. Radiology 2004;232:197–204.

[7] Pisano ED, Gatsonis C, Hendrick E, et al. DMIST Investigators Group. Diagnostic performance of digital vs. film mammography for breast-cancer screening. N Engl J Med 2005;353(17):1773–83.

[8] Rosenberg RD, Yankaskas BC, Abraham LA, et al. Performance benchmarks for screening mammography. Radiology 2006;241(1):55–66.

[9] Pisano ED, Gatsonis C, Yaffe M, et al. The American College of Radiology Imaging Network (ACRIN) digital mammographic Imaging screening trial (DMIST): objectives and methodology. Radiology 2005;236:404–12.

[10] Keen JD. Digital and film mammography. N Engl J Med 2006;354(7):765–7.

[11] Pisano E, Cole E, Hemminger B, et al. Image processing algorithms for digital mammography: a pictorial essay. Radiographics 2000;20:1479–91.

[12] Sivaramakrishna R, Obuchowski N, Chilcote W, et al. Comparing the performance of mammographic enhancement algorithms: a preference study. AJR Am J Roentgenol 2000;175:45–51.

[13] Pisano E, Cole E, Major S, et al. Radiologists' preferences for digital mammographic display. Radiology 2000;216:820–30.

[14] Channin D. Integrating the healthcare enterprise: a primer, part 2. Seven brides for seven brothers: the IHE integration profiles. Radiographics 2001;21:1343–50.

[15] Integrating the healthcare enterprise. Available at: www.ihe.net. Accessed January 27, 2007.

[16] IHE technical framework. Available at: www.ihe.net/Technical_Framework/index.cfm. Accessed January 27, 2007.

[17] Cole E, Pisano E, Kistner E, et al. Diagnostic accuracy of digital mammography in patients with dense breasts who underwent problem-solving mammography: effects of image processing and lesion type. Radiology 2003;226:153–60.

[18] Singh S, Bovis K. An evaluation of contrast enhancement techniques for mammographic breast masses. IEEE Trans Inf Technol Biomed 2005;9(1):109–19.

[19] Cole E, Pisano E, Zeng D, et al. The effects of gray-scale image processing on digital mammography interpretation performance. Acad Radiol 2005;12(5):585–95.

[20] Qian W, Lihua L, Clarke L, et al. Digital mammography: comparison of adaptive an nonadaptive CAD methods for mass detection. Acad Radiol 1999;6:471–80.

[21] Avrin D, Morin R, Piraino D, et al. Storage, transmission, and retrieval of digital mammography, including recommendations on image compression. J Am Coll Radiol 2006;3:609–14.

[22] Penedo M, Souto M, Tahoces P, et al. Free-response receiver operating characteristic

evaluation of lossy JPEG2000 and object-based set partitioning in hierarchical trees compression of digitized mammograms. Radiology 2005;237: 450–7.

[23] Suryanarayanan S, Karellas A, Vedantham S, et al. Detection of simulated lesions on data compressed digital mammograms. Radiology 2005;236:31–6.

[24] Sung M, Kim H, Kim E, et al. Clinical evaluation of JPEG2000 compression for digital mammography. IEEE Trans Nucl Sci 2002;49(3):827–32.

[25] Harris C. Digital mammography hits the tipping point. Health Imaging and IT 2006;4:6262–8.

[26] Siegel E. Digital mammography image quality: image display. J Am Coll Radiol 2006;3:615–27.

[27] Smith R. The FFDM crucible. Imaging Economics 2005;18:25–34.

[28] Freiherr G. CR mammography could split diagnostic marketplace. Technology advisor (supplement to Diagnostic Imaging) 2006;17–32.

[29] Williams M, Yaffe M, Maidment A, et al. Digital mammography image quality—image acquisition. J Am Coll Radiol 2006;3:589–608.

[30] Pisano ED, Cole EB, Kistner EO, et al. Digital mammography interpretation: comparison of the speed and accuracy of softcopy versus printed film display. Radiology 2001;223: 483–8.

[31] Berns EA, Hendrick RE, Solan M, et al. Digital and screen-film mammography: comparison of image acquisition and interpretation times. AJR Am J Roentgenol 2006;187(1):38–41.

[32] Lou SL, Sickels EA, Huang HK, et al. Full-field direct digital telemammography: technical components, study protocols, and preliminary results. IEEE Trans Inf Technol Biomed 1997; 1(4):270–8.

[33] Khorasani R. You should eliminate paper from your PACS workflow: why and how? J Am Coll Radiol 2006;3:628–9.

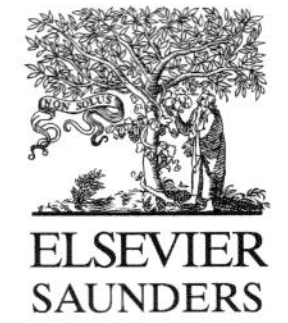
ELSEVIER
SAUNDERS

RADIOLOGIC
CLINICS
OF NORTH AMERICA

Radiol Clin N Am 45 (2007) 831–843

Digital Mammography: Novel Applications

Elizabeth A. Rafferty, MD[a,b,*]

The goal of radiographic mammography is the detection of breast cancer. Although the goal is easily stated, the task is not easy. The breast is markedly heterogeneous in its composition and varies markedly in appearance between individuals. This lack of a consistent "normal" appearance complicates the recognition of abnormal. To challenge the interpreter further, the object of interest—the cancer—is extremely close in radiographic attenuation to the surrounding normal parenchyma of the breast, and these normal structures can act as camouflage, hindering the radiologist in detecting malignancy. Thus, efforts over the years have focused on producing a "better" image—one that would exploit the differences between the normal and the abnormal, thereby facilitating the radiologist in detecting cancer. Since the 1960s, these efforts have been focused on developing dedicated mammography equipment, optimal screen-film combinations, and improved processing techniques that incrementally have refined the quality of the image produced for interpretation.

Efforts to optimize mammography proved fruitful from the outset. To validate the potential efficacy of mammographic screening in reducing deaths from breast cancer, several trials were undertaken. The Health Insurance Plan of New York Trial (HIP), undertaken in the 1960s, was the first randomized, controlled trial of mammographic screening. The demonstration of a reduction in the mortality rate from breast cancer of approximately 30% at 10-year follow-up [1] validated the hypothesis that the detection of malignancy within the breast at a subclinical stage would allow effective intervention and treatment, thus interrupting the natural course of the disease. More impressive, perhaps, is the

This work was supported by grants IDEA DAMD-97-1-7144 and CTR DAMD 17-98-8309 from the Department of Defense and by a research grant from Hologic, Inc.
[a] Department of Radiology, Harvard Medical School, Wang Building, Suite 240, 15 Parkman Street, Boston, MA 02114
[b] Avon Comprehensive Breast Center, Massachusetts General Hospital, Wang Building, Suite 240, 15 Parkman Street, Boston, MA 02114
* Department of Radiology, Division of Breast Imaging, Massachusetts General Hospital, Wang Building, Suite 240, 15 Parkman Street, Boston, MA 02114.
E-mail address: erafferty@partners.org

0033-8389/07/$ – see front matter doi:10.1016/j.rcl.2007.06.005
radiologic.theclinics.com

recognition that the reduction in breast cancer deaths achieved during the HIP trial occurred while mammographic technology was in its infancy and optimal imaging techniques had not yet been defined.

Similarly, the Two County Swedish Trial, the largest of the randomized, controlled trials, also confirmed a mortality benefit of approximately 30% for women invited to attend mammographic screening when compared with the noninvited controls. This achievement is more notable when one recognizes that the trial used only single mediolateral oblique views of each breast and offered evaluation at only 2- or 3-year intervals. In the ensuing years, efforts focused on perfecting equipment and techniques. As implementation of high-quality mammographic screening became more widespread, benefit continued to accrue. Tabar and colleagues [2] noted that an organized screening program with high levels of participation could achieve overall mortality reductions of 50% within the population, and a staggering 63% decrease in breast cancer deaths was observed in the women who actually availed themselves of the service [3,4].

Although mammography has proven invaluable in the early detection and diagnosis of breast cancer, it is widely recognized to be an imperfect test. Reported sensitivities of screening mammography range from 45% to 85% [5] with performance suffering as parenchymal density increases. Holland and colleagues [6] reported that 76% of missed cancers occurred in women who had dense breast tissue. The inverse relationship of breast density and mammographic sensitivity is not surprising when one recalls that the fundamental challenge of mammographic detection involves discerning the often subtle changes manifested by malignancy from a background of structures of minimally different attenuation.

Unfortunately, improving the performance limitations of mammography in dense breast tissue proved technically challenging. Although screen-film mammography (SFM) produces images of extremely high spatial resolution—critical for delineating the fine structural detail of the breast—the analog system can function only within a relatively narrow dynamic range to produce an image that is optimally exposed for radiologic interpretation; this constraint markedly reduces the degree of object contrast that can be depicted in the image.

For this reason, attention turned toward the development of digital platforms that could accomplish mammographic imaging. Adopting a digital system would allow the functions of image acquisition, display, and archiving to be decoupled, thus allowing their individual optimization. The practical result of this implementation would be a significant expansion of the dynamic range of contrast that could be captured in the mammographic image, potentially offsetting the effect of increasing breast density on the sensitivity of the examination. The advent of full-field solid-state digital detectors made digital mammography a reality, and many viewed the transition from the analog to the digital platform as an opportunity to improve the efficacy of mammography.

Initial studies were disappointing, however. In the first prospective comparison of SFM and full-field digital mammography (FFDM), Lewin and colleagues [7] found no statistically significant difference between the two modalities in the rate of cancer detection , although FFDM did result in a statistically significant reduction in the recall rate. Thus, the authors concluded that no difference in cancer detection rate existed between SFM and FFDM; however, FFDM may confer a relative advantage over the analog modality by decreasing recall rates at screening. The lack of detection advantage for the digital modality reported by Lewin and colleagues [7] was confirmed by Skaane and coworkers [8,9] in two separate clinical trials comparing the performance of SFM and FFDM.

For those who had anticipated that the transition to the digital platform would translate into dramatic improvements in mammographic performance, the results of these three clinical trials were disheartening and raised concern that radiographic imaging of the breast as a means of detecting preclinical malignancy had already achieved its maximum potential. Some suggested that perhaps additional efforts should be directed toward evaluation of alternative modalities to supplement or replace mammographic surveillance in breast cancer screening, particularly in women who have dense breasts. Although it was clear that the theoretical benefit of the enhanced dynamic range afforded by the digital modality had not yet been confirmed in clinical practice, the trials conducted at that point had been only modest in size. Perhaps a larger trial with more substantial statistical power would demonstrate advantages of digital mammography.

Across 33 sites, the Digital Mammographic Imaging Screening Trial (DMIST) enrolled 49,528 women to undergo both SFM and digital mammography [10]. Despite the additional statistical power, when the cohort was analyzed as a whole, no statistically significant difference was observed between the analog and digital modalities with respect to diagnostic accuracy, echoing the previous results of comparative studies.

In contrast to its predecessors, however, the DMIST trial had sufficient statistical power to permit subset analysis, and the results were noteworthy. Digital mammography had demonstrated significant advantage in detecting breast cancer in specific subsets of women: women under 50 years of age, women who were pre- or perimenopausal, and women who had heterogeneously dense or extremely dense breast tissue. Although some debate exists regarding possible explanations for this benefit, as well as its actual magnitude, the unifying characteristic suggested by these three groups is increased breast density. Postulation that dense breast parenchyma represents the common feature relating the subgroups exhibiting benefit from the digital modality also has intuitive appeal in affirming the relative value of an enhanced dynamic range in mammographic interpretation.

Are the relatively modest gains in cancer detection suggested by the DMIST study sufficient to prompt widespread adoption of the digital modality? Many would argue that they are not. Perhaps, however, the development of digital breast imaging does not constitute an end point but rather represents the beginning of a new era for mammography: an era in which the digital platform serves as the basis for development of innovative radiographic methods of imaging the breast, innovations that were not possible on the analog platform. This article explores some of the novel applications that are being investigated to capitalize on the strengths of the digital platform and to realize fully the potential benefits of enhanced detection anticipated from digital mammography.

Contrast-enhanced mammography

Malignant tumors have demonstrated the ability to incite the growth of new blood vessels, a phenomenon known as "tumor angiogenesis." Indeed, this process of neovascularization seems to be essential for tumors to grow beyond a few millimeters in size [11]. These malignant neovessels are characterized further by abnormalities of the basement membrane that manifest physiologically as an increase in vascular permeability, resulting in vessels that are "leaky." From an imaging perspective, the process of tumor angiogenesis provides the opportunity to use the biology of cancer growth to assist in detection and characterization of malignancy. Through the administration of contrast media, imaging can both facilitate the detection of tumors within the breast and capture the dynamic behavior of contrast within a lesion, providing potential insight into the probability of malignancy [12].

In attempting to enhance breast cancer detection and characterization, contrast-enhanced techniques have been evaluated in conjunction with CT [13,14] and, far more extensively, with MR imaging [15–17]. Breast imaging with both CT and MR imaging has several advantages beyond the ability to exploit the properties of angiogenesis. With both modalities the degree of inherent contrast resolution grossly surpasses that achievable with even digital mammography. Additionally, the cross-sectional nature of both modalities should allow more accurate delineation of tumoral size and extent and of the distribution of disease. MR imaging presents the additional advantage of imaging without associated radiation exposure.

Although contrast-enhanced breast imaging with both CT and MR imaging offers clear benefits in the assessment of breast abnormalities, these modalities also have drawbacks. The body of knowledge describing contrast-enhanced CT of the breast is relatively limited, and technique considerations and issues of interpretation are not well understood. The potential contribution of contrast-enhanced MR imaging in the diagnosis and treatment of breast disease has, on the other hand, been an active area of investigation for the past 15 years. Although the technique has demonstrated impressive sensitivity in the detection of invasive breast cancer [15,18], its lack of specificity has been problematic. A relative lack of sensitivity with respect to the diagnosis of ductal carcinoma in situ also has been cited as a disadvantage of MR imaging [19,20]. Issues of cost, access, and consistency of interpretation also present ongoing challenges.

A major limitation of both CT and MR imaging of the breast is the relative lack of spatial resolution associated with the examinations, particularly when compared with mammography. The ability to discern fine detail is fundamental in the analysis of lesions detected by mammography, providing much of the insight into assessing the malignant potential of the finding. The application of contrast enhancement to the mammographic examination holds the potential for adding significant object contrast to enhance the mammographic visibility of malignant lesions while retaining the advantage of exquisite image detail. In addition, the widespread availability and relative affordability of the mammographic platform hold obvious appeal.

Initial efforts at evaluating the feasibility of coupling contrast administration with radiographic imaging of the breast used an image intensifier system and fluoroscopic acquisition techniques [21–23]. Although these early reports described success in demonstrating rapid, avid enhancement and subsequent early washout of contrast in cancerous tumors, similar to the classic kinetic patterns of malignancy currently described in breast MR imaging analysis, the technique proved impractical for routine use. The introduction of the digital platform for mammographic imaging, with its attendant ability to acquire multiple sequential images quickly, rekindled interest in investigating the potential utility of contrast-enhanced mammography. To date, two basic techniques of accomplishing contrast-enhanced digital mammography have been described.

Contrast-enhanced digital mammography using sequential temporal acquisition

Jong and colleagues [24] described their initial clinical experience with contrast-enhanced mammography. Modifications to the mammographic equipment and adjustment of exposure factors were implemented to assure that a significant fraction of the X-ray beam had energies above the k-edge of iodine (33.2 keV) to achieve maximized object contrast. Imaging was conducted in the craniocaudal (CC) projection using light compression to minimize any patient motion and to avoid restriction of venous outflow that might limit the delivery of contrast agent. A mask image was obtained initially. After the injection of iodinated contrast material, multiple postcontrast images were obtained. Subtraction images were generated from the pre- and postcontrast acquisitions and analyzed for lesion visibility.

Jong and colleagues [24] successfully performed this technique in 22 patients, 10 of whom had malignant lesions and 12 of whom had benign lesions. They identified suspicious contrast enhancement in 8 of the 10 malignant lesions (80%); false-negative studies occurred in one case of ductal carcinoma in situ and in one low-grade invasive ductal carcinoma. Enhancement was also identified in 5 of the 12 benign lesions (42%). Of note was the investigators' observation that kinetic analysis of the temporal contrast enhancement did not prove reliable in distinguishing benign from malignant processes. The authors concluded that techniques of contrast-enhanced mammography warranted further development and potentially could offer an alternative imaging modality for indications currently investigated using breast MR imaging.

Subsequently, Dromain and colleagues [25] sought to assess the diagnostic accuracy of contrast-enhanced digital mammography and to correlate it to histologic quantification of microvessels. For the performance of the study, the investigators adjusted the X-ray spectra to energies just above the k-edge of iodine in a way similar to that described by Jong and colleagues [24] to enhance the visibility of contrast-avid lesions. Imaging was performed in the CC projection using light compression. Twenty consecutive patients who had a total of 22 suspicious lesions were enrolled in the study before undergoing biopsy. All lesions proved to be malignant on histologic evaluation. A mask image was obtained; then contrast was injected, and multiple sequential contrast-enhanced images were obtained. Image subtraction was performed, and the subtracted were sequences reviewed.

Sixteen of the 20 malignancies demonstrated contrast enhancement, yielding a sensitivity of 80% for the technique. The four malignant tumors that failed to demonstrate enhancement were all invasive ductal carcinomas; the two cases of ductal carcinoma in situ, and the two invasive lobular carcinomas demonstrated marked contrast uptake. This observation prompted the authors to suggest that the presence or degree of contrast enhancement observed did not seem to correlate in a predictable fashion with tumor histology. Again, additional investigation was considered to be warranted.

Contrast-enhanced digital mammography using dual-energy acquisition techniques

Dual-energy techniques involve the performance of low- and high-energy X-ray exposures of the breast during a single compression. Image-processing techniques then are used to subtract the images of differential energies, resulting in a significant negation of the native parenchymal density of the breast. Lewin and colleagues [26] reported on the feasibility of a contrast-enhanced technique of digital mammography using dual-energy acquisition. Dual-energy imaging was performed in the mediolateral oblique (MLO) projection after the administration of intravenous contrast. Exposure energies were manipulated to fall just below and just above the k-edge of iodine to allow significant object contrast for enhancing lesions. A theoretical advantage of the dual-energy technique over the temporal technique of contrast enhancement previously described is that the breast can be optimally compressed during the acquisition of the dual-energy pair, because both dual-energy acquisitions are obtained after the injection of the contrast medium. Thus, excellent image detail can be preserved without concern about the compromise of breast perfusion.

In their pilot investigation, Lewin and colleagues [26] evaluated 26 women who had suspicious breast lesions detected by imaging or palpation. Eleven of the 13 invasive cancers within the study population demonstrated strong enhancement; two of the invasive cancers and one case of ductal carcinoma in situ demonstrated only faint enhancement. Two of 12 benign lesions demonstrated contrast enhancement and constituted false-positive studies. Although this pilot was undertaken to evaluate the feasibility of applying dual-energy acquisition techniques to contrast-enhanced mammography, the sensitivity of this approach was similar to that of temporal subtraction techniques. Others have presented preliminary data evaluating the ability to perform dual-energy imaging for contrast-enhanced digital mammography using a single-shot electronic spectrum-splitting technique with a photon-counting detector to obviate the need for two separate exposures [27].

Breast tomosynthesis

Normal breast tissue can obscure malignancy from detection by the radiologist; this problem is one of the fundamental challenges in mammographic interpretation. Incremental improvements in image quality can be gained by refining the quantum performance of digital detectors, increasing their spatial resolution, and extending the limit of their dynamic range; however, the basic problem of structure overlap remains. Not only can adjacent structures decrease the visibility of cancers; they also can mimic abnormality through the summation of their radiographic attenuations. These summation artifacts are a well-recognized contributor to the false-positive rates of screening mammography. It is intuitive that the diagnostic accuracy of mammography could be improved by minimizing the impact of structure overlap within the breast.

Breast tomosynthesis: development and image acquisition

Tomosynthesis is a three-dimensional radiographic technique that allows review of unique planes of interest in isolation from adjacent planes to minimize the effects of structure overlap. Based on the work of Ziedes des Plantes [28], several investigators developed and described tomosynthesis applications [29,30]. Unfortunately, these film-based tomosynthesis systems proved too complex for practical use; not until the introduction of the full-field digital mammographic detector did breast tomosynthesis become clinically feasible.

To acquire a conventional digital mammogram, the breast is positioned and compressed on the imaging receptor. Photons generated by the X-ray tube pass through the compressed breast, strike the detector, and are read to produce the clinical image reviewed by the radiologist. In breast tomosynthesis, the digital mammography platform is modified to allow the X-ray tube to travel through a proscribed arc of excursion acquiring a fixed number of discrete projection images while the breast remains in compression (Fig. 1). The individual projection images are extremely low in dose, so the composite dose incurred during a tomosynthesis acquisition is comparable to a single-view mammogram.

Tomosynthesis: reconstruction techniques

Image reconstruction is a critical element to the successful implementation of tomosynthesis, transforming the raw projection image data captured during an acquisition sweep into a seamless cross-sectional data set suitable for interpretation. Niklason and coworkers [31] described a shift-and-add methodology for tomosynthesis reconstruction that simulated the simultaneous tube and detector motion encountered in conventional tomography. Although effective for minimizing structure overlap, this approach introduced an unacceptable degree of out-of-plane blurring. Filtered back-projection, a Fourier-based technique commonly used in CT reconstruction, also has proven successful in tomosynthesis reconstruction. This technique benefits from sharp image detail, but optimizing the reconstruction filter is critical to maintain acceptable signal-to-noise ratios. A maximum-likelihood iterative method for tomosynthesis reconstruction has been developed by Wu and colleagues [32]. This technique seeks to optimize feature contrast and sharpness while minimizing image noise, but the computationally dense nature of this method may present a challenge for commercial implementation.

Tomosynthesis: clinical applications

The ability of tomosynthesis to minimize the effects of structure overlap within the breast should enhance lesion detection (Fig. 2). In a pilot study, Rafferty and coworkers [33] evaluated radiologists' ability to identify suspicious breast lesions using conventional mammography and using tomosynthesis imaging. Forty-seven lesions were identified in 40 patients. The visibility of masses and areas of architectural distortion was deemed to be superior on tomosynthesis in 89% of cases. Notably, seven mammographically occult lesions presenting as palpable abnormalities were included in this pilot investigation; six of those seven lesions were detected using tomosynthesis imaging.

The superior visibility of masses and architectural distortion seen in this pilot evaluation did not translate to the identification of suspicious calcifications, however. In 71% of cases, in fact, calcifications were visualized better with conventional mammography than with tomosynthesis imaging [33]. The investigators hypothesized that the distributional component of calcifications was not being well depicted on tomosynthesis imaging because of the cross-sectional nature of the examination. To test this hypothesis, the digital data sets were reformatted into 1-cm volumetric units for presentation. Using this alternative volumetric review format, the readers judged calcifications to be more

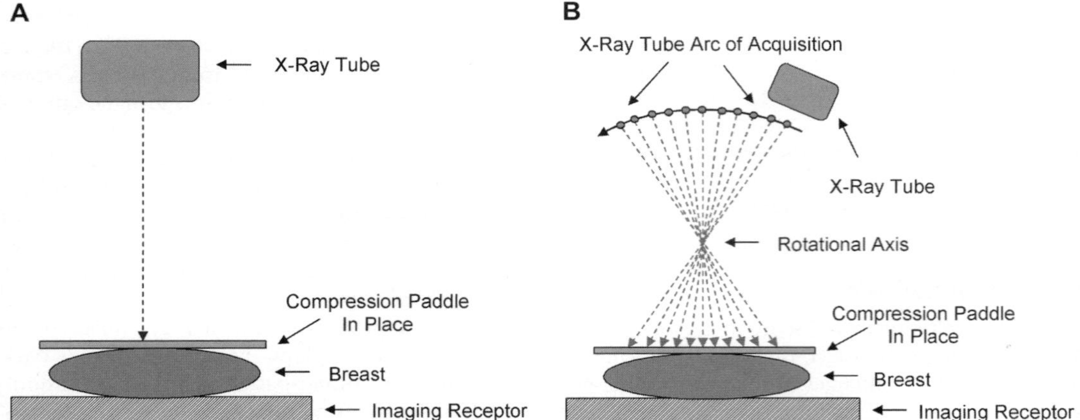

Fig. 1. Image acquisition. (*A*) In conventional mammography, the X-ray tube remains stationary. X-ray photons pass through the compressed breast and strike the digital detector producing a projection image. (*B*) In tomosynthesis imaging, the X-ray tube traverses a proscribed arc acquiring a series of low-dose projection images that subsequently are synthesized to produce a three-dimensional data set.

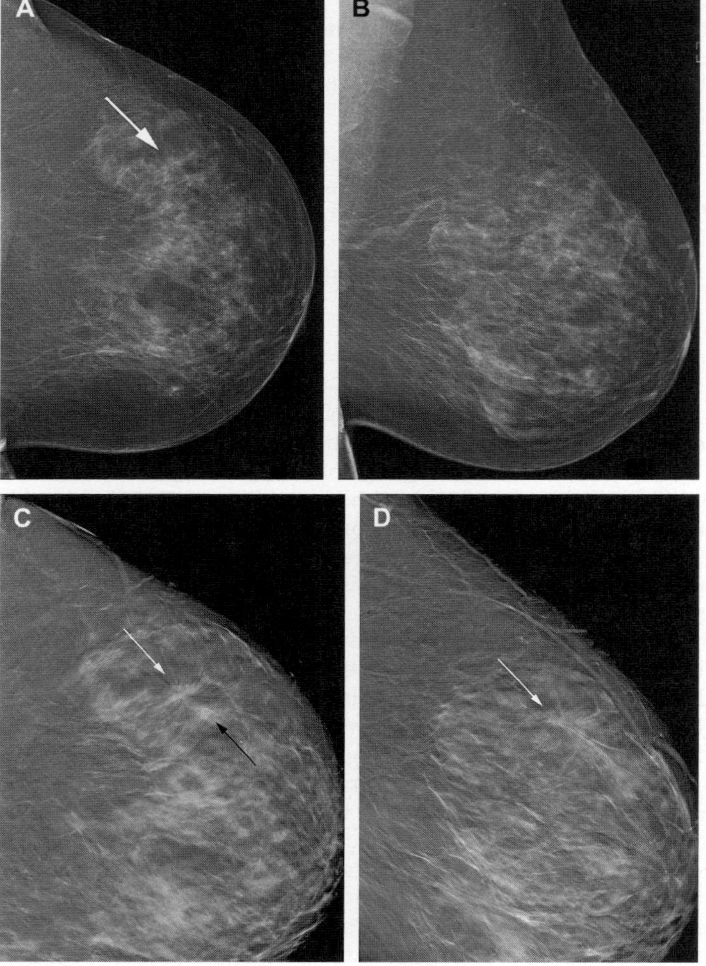

Fig. 2. Enhanced visibility of masses with tomosynthesis. (*A*) Conventional craniocaudal mammogram shows very subtle spiculated mass (*arrow*). (*B*) Conventional mediolateral oblique mammogram shows no abnormality. (*C*) Tomosynthesis slice in the craniocaudal position clearly shows spiculated mass (*white arrow*). Additionally, adjacent irregular mass is identified (*black arrow*). (*D*) Tomosynthesis slice in the mediolateral oblique position shows a spiculated mass (*arrow*) found on biopsy to be multifocal invasive ductal carcinoma.

conspicuous with tomosynthesis imaging than with conventional mammography in 88% of cases [34]. When investigation expanded to include evaluation of calcification conspicuity on a tomosynthesis prototype using an amorphous selenium-based digital detector, volumetric presentation of the data sets was not needed to visualize calcifications optimally (Fig. 3).

In addition to making lesions more visible, tomosynthesis, by eliminating the confounding information of structure overlap, also should facilitate the marginal analysis of mass lesions (Figs. 4 and 5). In a blinded review, three radiologists independently reviewed 47 lesions in 40 patients and estimated the probability of malignancy for each. All three readers classified lesions as benign or malignant more accurately when using tomosynthesis than when reviewing conventional mammography [35].

Summation artifacts are responsible for a substantial portion of recalls in a mammographic screening program. These artifacts result from normal breast structures in the two-dimensional mammographic image superimposing to mimic a possible lesion. An anticipated benefit of tomosynthesis is the potential to reduce the recall rate of mammographic screening by minimizing screening callbacks attributable to summation artifact (Fig. 6). In a blinded reader study designed to estimate the potential utility of tomosynthesis in decreasing false-positive recalls after mammographic screening, radiologists reviewed a mixed tomosynthesis case set comprised of normal subjects, patients documented to have summation artifact on conventional mammography, and patients who had undergone biopsy for Breast Imaging Reporting and Data System category 4 and 5 lesions [36]. In this pilot study of 60 patients, the readers decreased their false-positive screening recall rate by 83% when interpreting tomosynthesis studies, compared with their interpretations of the conventional mammographic studies, without any significant decrease in cancer detection.

Investigators initially hoped that the three-dimensional nature of the tomosynthesis examination would obviate the need to perform imaging evaluation in two positions. Indeed, when one considers the rationale for performing conventional mammography in two views—inclusion of the maximal amount of breast tissue, the ability to recognize potential summation artifact through interimage correlation, and the need to localize abnormalities in three-dimensional space to facilitate intervention—these goals theoretically should be accomplished with single-view MLO tomosynthesis provided that stringent positioning criteria are maintained. An initial pilot study seeking to confirm this hypothesis yielded surprising results, however. Rafferty and colleagues [37] performed tomosynthesis imaging in the MLO and CC positions in 34 women scheduled to undergo biopsy for suspicious breast lesions. The tomosynthesis data sets were reviewed, and the visibility of each lesion was rated independently for each acquisition. Twenty-two of the 34 lesions were deemed equally visible on both acquisitions. Twelve of the 34 lesions (35%), however, were more visible or were only visible on one of the two acquisitions. In 33% of cases, the MLO view yielded superior visualization; in 67% of cases, findings were more visible in the CC acquisition. In fact, three of the suspicious findings were visualized only in the CC tomosynthesis data set, and all three of these

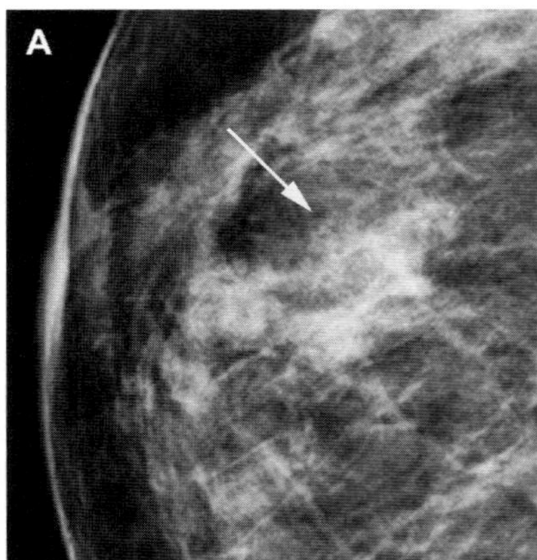

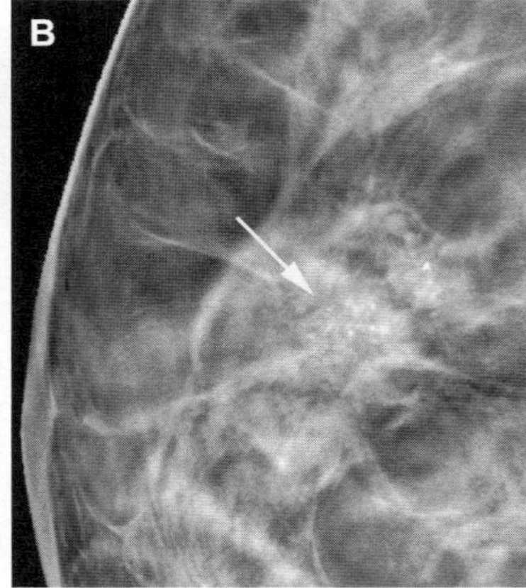

Fig. 3. Enhanced visibility of calcifications with tomosynthesis. (*A*) On a conventional craniocaudal mammogram, calcifications are difficult to visualize (*arrow*). (*B*) Tomosynthesis slice in the craniocaudal position clearly shows clustered pleomorphic calcifications (*arrow*) found on biopsy to ductal carcinoma in situ.

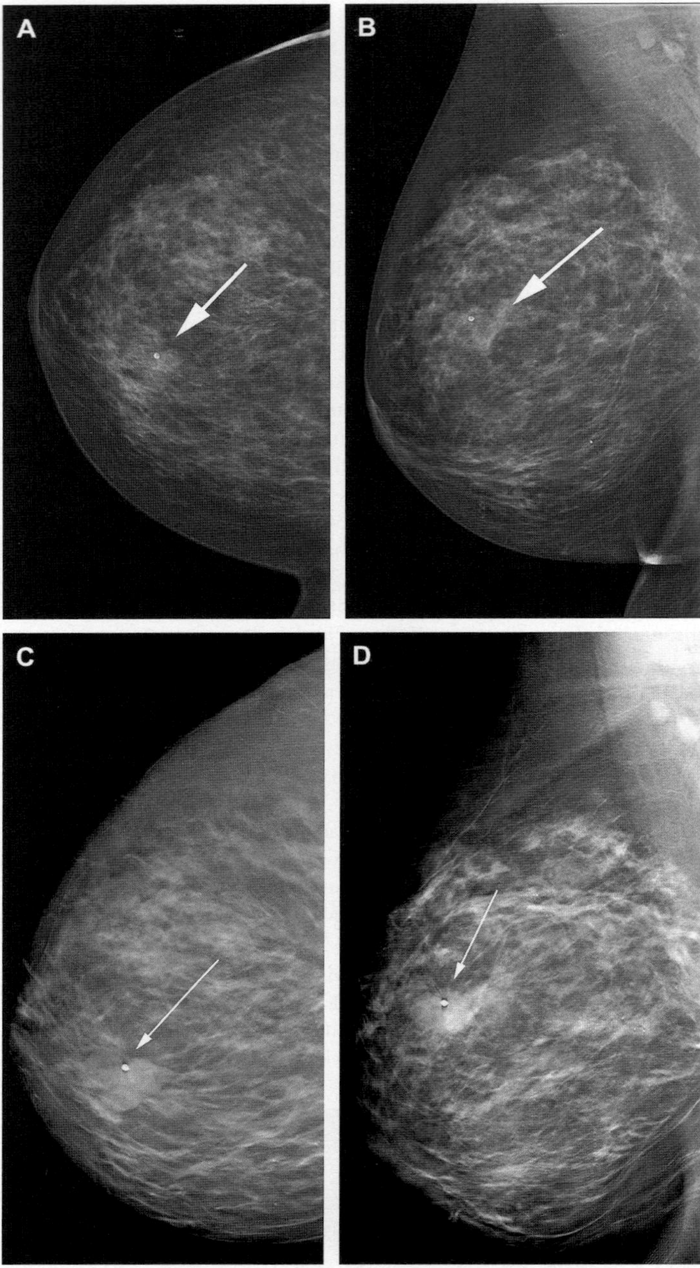

Fig. 4. Facilitation of margin analysis with tomosynthesis. (*A*) Conventional craniocaudal and (*B*) mediolateral oblique mammograms show developing asymmetry (*arrows*). Tomosynthesis slices in the (*C*) craniocaudal and (*D*) mediolateral oblique positions clearly demonstrate a mass with irregular and subtly spiculated margins (*arrows*) found on biopsy to be invasive ductal carcinoma.

lesions proved to be malignant. The investigators concluded that imaging in both the MLO and CC positions is desirable to visualize lesions optimally when performing tomosynthesis (Fig. 7).

Fusion technologies

Limitations of mammographic specificity stem from a combination of factors. Even when areas of interest are well visualized, the significant overlap in the appearance of benign and malignant processes in the breast limits specificity and often necessitates biopsy for certainty. Combining the fine anatomic detail of mammographic imaging with data from other imaging modalities could allow more precise characterization of breast lesions and result in enhanced diagnostic accuracy. The introduction of the digital mammography platform

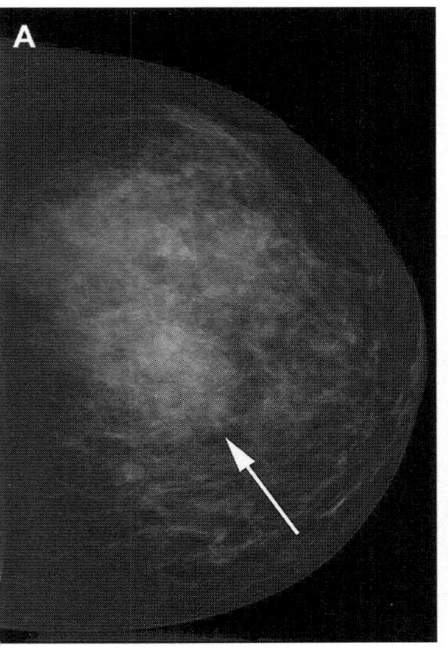

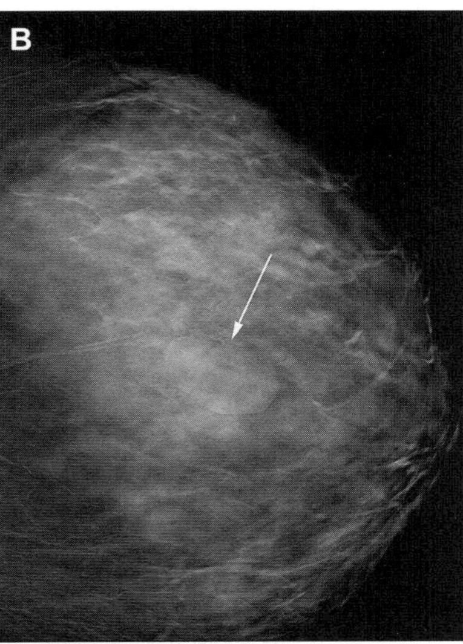

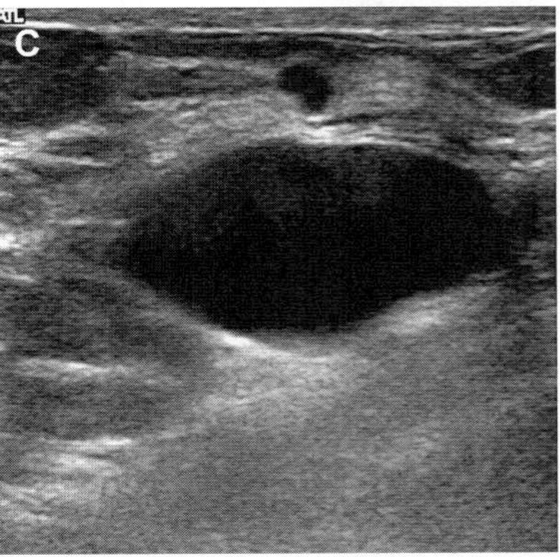

Fig. 5. Facilitation of margin analysis with tomosynthesis. (*A*) Conventional craniocaudal mammogram showing subtle mass with obscured rather than ill-defined margins (*arrow*). (*B*) Tomosynthesis slice in the craniocaudal position shows oval circumscribed mass (*arrow*) suggesting benign etiology. (*C*) Focused sonography confirms simple cyst correlating to the mammographic finding.

offers the opportunity to explore true fusion of imaging modalities through the superimposition of digital data sets. Although in the preliminary stages, attempts to fuse digital mammographic imaging with other imaging modalities have been explored.

Behrenbruch and colleagues [38] reported on efforts to fuse digital mammographic data with data from contrast-enhanced MR imaging. This undertaking holds inherent appeal when one realizes that a growing subset of women is undergoing breast MR imaging evaluation and that most of these women already have undergone mammography. Because correlation of the information obtained from the two modalities can sometimes prove challenging to the radiologist, successful fusion techniques would have value. Behrenbruch's initial work faced multiple challenges, however. Fusion of a two-dimensional data set—mammography—with a three-dimensional data set—MR imaging—is technically difficult. Additionally, mammographic imaging is acquired with the breast in compression in the upright position, whereas MR imaging typically is acquired in the pendent position without compression. These variables significantly complicate the process of registering the data to allow confident correlation of localized imaging findings. The clinical viability of the technique will depend on the development of computer models to permit this registration, an effort that remains ongoing.

Fewer technical challenges are encountered in the attempt to couple dual modalities on a common imaging platform. In one such endeavor, Williams and colleagues [39] evaluated the feasibility of adapting a scintimammography camera to a digital mammography gantry. Single gamma nuclear imaging of the breast may provide physiologic information regarding breast lesions that, in combination with the anatomic detail offered by mammography, might improve the specificity of the examination. The clear advantage of this prototype

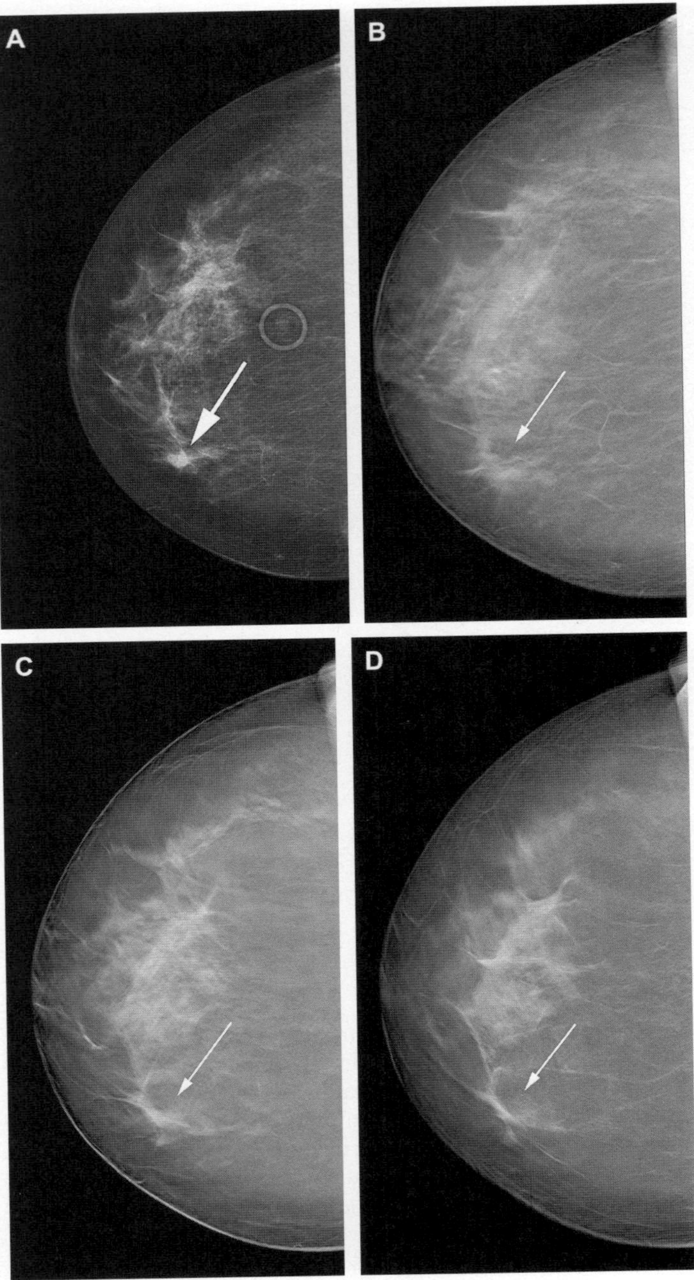

Fig. 6. Potential for tomosynthesis to reduce the recall rate from screening. (*A*) Conventional craniocaudal mammogram shows apparent mass in the medial aspect of the breast (*arrow*). (*B, C, D*) Slices from tomosynthesis acquisition in the craniocaudal position showing normal structures medially (*arrows*) that superimpose to form the summation artifact seen on conventional mammography.

design is that the breast can be imaged with the dual modalities without interval repositioning, thus facilitating registration of the data sets. To date the investigators have optimized the imaging platform using phantoms, and an initial pilot study of 10 patients has been performed. The sensitivity and specificity of the combined imaging technique are promising. Further investigation with prospective clinical trials will be necessary to confirm clinical utility.

Another effort to implement a dual-modality imaging platform was reported by Kapur and coworkers [40] who developed a prototype imaging system combining breast ultrasound with digital mammography. Recognizing that prior efforts to fuse mammographic and sonographic imaging data had suffered from limited image quality and the inability to coregister the data sets effectively, the investigators directed efforts toward the design of a compression paddle and coupling medium

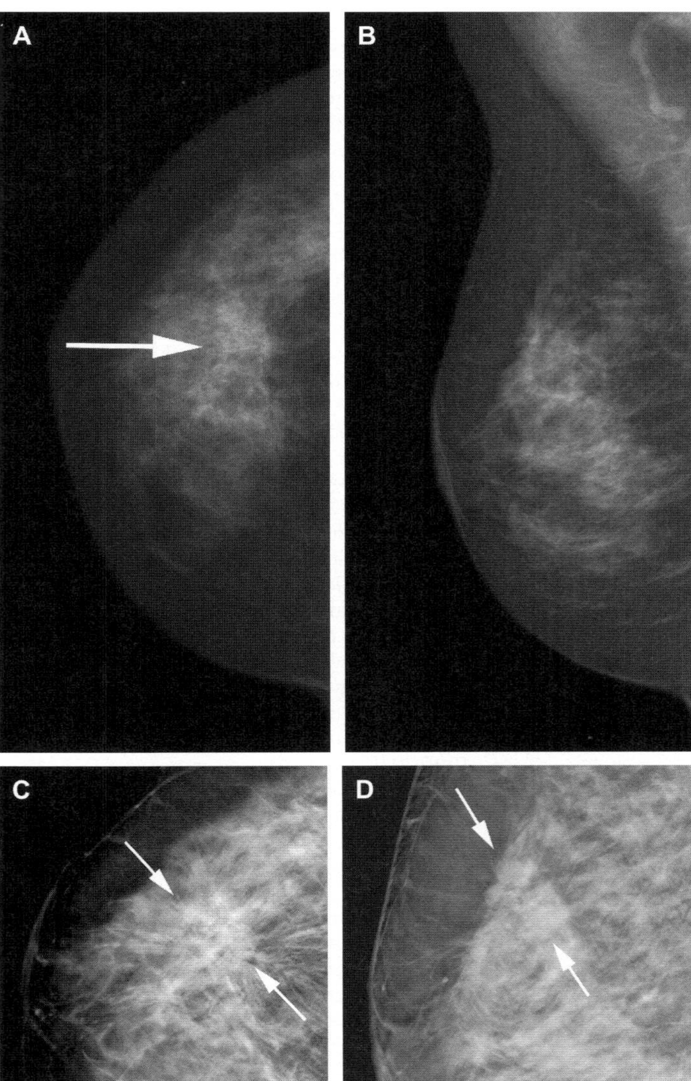

Fig. 7. Conspicuity of breast lesions on mediolateral oblique versus craniocaudal acquisitions. (*A*) Conventional craniocaudal mammogram shows subtle area of architectural distortion (*arrow*). (*B*) Conventional craniocaudal mammogram shows no abnormality. (*C*) Tomosynthesis slice in the craniocaudal position shows a spiculated mass with associated architectural distortion (*delineated by arrows*). (*D*) Tomosynthesis slice in the craniocaudal position shows focal increased density with subtle spiculation (*delineated by arrows*). The finding is more visible and its extent is clearer on the craniocaudal acquisition. Invasive ductal carcinoma was documented at biopsy.

that would allow excellent radiographic and sonographic imaging quality. Similarly, adaptation of a high-frequency ultrasound probe to allow automated scanning of the breast immediately following the mammographic exposure should improve reproducibility and facilitate registration of the data. Using data obtained from 48 initial clinical patients, further refinements to the prototype system have been implemented, and the authors anticipate a prospective clinical trial in the near future.

Summary

From the first reports of mammographic screening trials 25 years ago, mammography has proven its value in reducing breast cancer mortality, and this documented benefit has been sustained over the ensuing years. Little opportunity existed, however, to advance the analog modality further and to realize further gains in mortality reduction from mammography. With the introduction of the full-field digital detector with its superior contrast resolution, incremental gains in the diagnostic accuracy of mammography were anticipated. Although the DMIST trial ultimately did suggest enhanced detection capability for the digital modality in select subgroups of women, the gains were admittedly modest, leading some to suggest that mammography had already achieved its full potential. This view is shortsighted. Transition from the analog to the digital platform should not be seen as an end point, but rather as a necessary foundation to enable the development of additional radiographic imaging techniques of the breast. Some potential advanced applications in digital mammography, such as contrast-enhanced mammography, breast tomosynthesis, and dual-modality mammographic fusion, have been presented. By building on the prior successes of mammography, these innovative mammographic techniques may provide the opportunity to improve mammographic performance further and, in so doing, further reduce mortality from breast cancer.

References

[1] Shapiro S, Venet W, Strax P, et al. Ten to fourteen-year effect of screening on breast cancer mortality. J Natl Cancer Inst 1982;69(2):349–55.

[2] Tabar L, Fagarberg CJ, Gad A, et al. Reduction in mortality from breast cancer after mass screening with mammography. Lancet 1985;1(8433):829–32.

[3] Tabar L, Vitak B, Chen HH, et al. Beyond randomized controlled trials: organized mammographic screening substantially reduces breast cancer mortality. Cancer 2001;91(9):1724–31.

[4] Tabar L, Vitak B, Chen HH, et al. The Swedish Two-County Trial twenty years later. Updated mortality results and new insights from long-term follow-up. Radiol Clin North Am 2000;38(4):625–51.

[5] Fletcher SW, Black W, Harris R, et al. Report of the international workshop on screening for breast cancer. J Natl Cancer Inst 1993;85(20):1644–56.

[6] Holland R, Mravunac M, Hendriks JH, et al. So-called interval cancers of the breast. Cancer 1982;49(12):2527–33.

[7] Lewin JM, Hendrick RE, D'Orsi CJ, et al. Comparison of full-field digital mammography with screen-film mammography for cancer detection: results of 4,945 paired examinations. Radiology 2001;218(3):873–80.

[8] Skaane P, Young K, Skjennald A. Population-based mammography screening: comparison of screen-film and full-field digital mammography with soft-copy reading—Oslo I study. Radiology 2003;229(3):877–84.

[9] Skaane P, Skjennald A. Screen-film mammography versus full-field digital mammography with soft-copy reading: randomized trial in a population-based screening program—the Oslo II Study. Radiology 2004;232(1):197–204.

[10] Pisano ED, Gatsonis C, Hendrick E, et al. Diagnostic performance of digital versus film mammography for breast-cancer screening. N Engl J Med 2005;353(17):1773–83.

[11] Weidner N, Semple JP, Welch WR, et al. Tumor angiogenesis and metastasis—correlation in invasive breast carcinoma. N Engl J Med 1991;324(1):1–8.

[12] Kuhl CK, Mielcareck P, Klaschik S, et al. Dynamic breast MR imaging: are signal intensity time course data useful for differential diagnosis of enhancing lesions? Radiology 1999;211(1):101–10.

[13] Chang CH, Nesbit DE, Fisher DR, et al. Computed tomographic mammography using a conventional body scanner. AJR Am J Roentgenol 1982;138(3):553–8.

[14] Izzo L, Stasolla A, Basso L, et al. Characterization of tumoral lesions of the breast: preliminary experience with multislice spiral CT. J Exp Clin Cancer Res 2005;24(2):209–15.

[15] Heywang SH, Wolf A, Pruss E, et al. MR imaging of the breast with gd-DTPA: use and limitations. Radiology 1989;171(1):95–103.

[16] Buadu LD, Murakami J, Murayama S, et al. Breast lesions: correlation of contrast medium enhancement patterns on MR images with histopathologic findings and tumor angiogenesis. Radiology 1996;200(3):639–49.

[17] Orel SG, Schnall MD. MR imaging of the breast for the detection, diagnosis, and staging of breast cancer. Radiology 2001;220(1):13–30.

[18] Gilles R, Guinebretiere JM, Lucidarme O, et al. Nonpalpable breast tumors: diagnosis with contrast-enhanced subtraction dynamic MR imaging. Radiology 1994;191(3):625–31.

[19] Orel SG, Mendonca MH, Reynolds C, et al. MR imaging of ductal carcinoma in situ. Radiology 1997;202(2):413–20.

[20] Westerhof JP, Fischer U, Moritz JD, et al. MR imaging of mammographically detected clustered microcalcifications: is there any value? Radiology 1998;207(3):675–81.

[21] Ackerman LV, Watt AC, Shetty P, et al. Breast lesions examined by digital angiography. Work in progress. Radiology 1985;155:65–8.

[22] Watt AC, Ackerman LV, Shetty PC, et al. Differentiation between benign and malignant disease of the breast using digital subtraction angiography of the breast. Cancer 1985;56(6):1287–92.

[23] Watt AC, Ackermann LV, Windham JP, et al. Breast lesions: differential diagnosis using digital subtraction angiography. Radiology 1986;159(1):39–42.

[24] Jong RA, Yaffe MJ, Skarpathiotakis M, et al. Contrast-enhanced digital mammography: initial clinical experience. Radiology 2003;228(3):842–50.

[25] Dromain C, Balleyguier C, Muller S, et al. Evaluation of tumor angiogenesis of breast carcinoma using contrast-enhanced digital mammography. AJR Am J Roentgenol 2006;187(5):W528–37.

[26] Lewin JM, Isaacs PK, Vance V, et al. Dual-energy contrast-enhanced digital subtraction mammography: feasibility. Radiology 2003;229(1):261–8.

[27] Bornefalk H, Lewin JM, Danielsson M, et al. Single-shot dual-energy subtraction mammography with electronic spectrum splitting: feasibility. Eur J Radiol 2006;60(2):275–8.

[28] Ziedes des Plantes BG. [Eine Neue Methode Zur Diffenzierung in der Rontgenographie

(Planigraphie)]. Acta Radiol 1932;13:182–92 [in German].

[29] Garrison JB, Grant DG, Guier WH, et al. Three dimensional roentgenography. Am J Roentgenol Radium Ther Nucl Med 1969;105(4):903–8.

[30] Miller ER, McCurry EM, Hruska B. An infinite number of laminagrams from a finite number of radiographs. Radiology 1971;98(2):249–55.

[31] Niklason LT, Christian BT, Niklason LE, et al. Digital tomosynthesis in breast imaging. Radiology 1997;205(2):399–406.

[32] Wu T, Moore RH, Rafferty EA, et al. A comparison of reconstruction algorithms for breast tomosynthesis. Med Phys 2004;31(9):2636–47.

[33] Rafferty EA, Kopans DB, Georgian-Smith D, et al. Comparison of full-field digital tomosynthesis and conventional two view film screen mammography in lesion detection and assessment of lesion conspicuity [abstract]. In: Abstracts of the 103rd Annual Meeting of the American Roentgen Ray Society. San Diego (CA), May 4–9, 2003.

[34] Rafferty EA, Wu T, Moore RH, et al. Optimization of image acquisition and display algorithms to enhance visualization of microcalcifications during digital breast tomosynthesis [abstract E16–499]. In: Abstracts of the 89th Scientific Assembly and Annual Meeting of the Radiological Society of North America. Chicago, November 30–December 5, 2003.

[35] Rafferty EA, Georgian-Smith D, Kopans DB, et al. Comparison of full-field digital tomosynthesis with two view conventional film screen mammography in the prediction of lesion malignancy [abstract A14–135]. In: Abstracts of the 88th Scientific Assembly and Annual Meeting of the Radiological Society of North America. Chicago, December 1–6, 2002.

[36] Rafferty EA, Kopans DB, Georgian-Smith D, et al. Evaluation of the call-back rate for screening mammography using full-field digital tomosynthesis versus conventional film screen mammography [abstract]. In: Abstracts of the 103rd Annual Meeting of the American Roentgen Ray Society. San Diego (CA), May 4–9, 2003.

[37] Rafferty EA, Niklason LT, Jameson-Meehan L. Breast tomosynthesis: one view or two? [abstract SSG01–04]. In: Abstracts of the 92nd Scientific Assembly and Annual Meeting of the Radiological Society of North America. Chicago, November 26–December 1, 2006.

[38] Behrenbruch CP, Marias K, Armitage PA, et al. Fusion of contrast-enhanced breast MR and mammographic imaging data. Br J Radiol 2004;77 Spec No 2:S201–8.

[39] Williams MB, More MJ, Narayanan D, et al. Combined structural and functional imaging of the breast. Technol Cancer Res Treat 2002;1(1): 39–42.

[40] Kapur A, Carson PL, Eberhard J, et al. Combination of digital mammography with semi-automated 3D breast ultrasound. Technol Cancer Res Treat 2004;3(4):325–34.

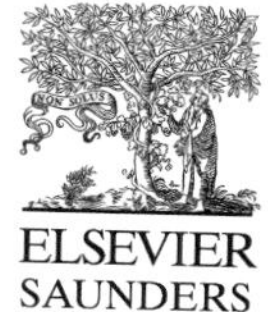

ELSEVIER
SAUNDERS

RADIOLOGIC
CLINICS
OF NORTH AMERICA

Radiol Clin N Am 45 (2007) 845–861

Diagnostic Breast Ultrasound: Current Status and Future Directions

Wei Yang, MD*, Peter J. Dempsey, MD

As with many modalities eventually used in medicine, the basic technology of diagnostic medical ultrasound became available after being released by the military after the end of World War II. High-frequency ultrasound had been used to detect flaws in metal surfaces. Almost 60 years later, it has matured into an integral facet of the breast imaging armamentarium. Despite developments in MR imaging and positron emission tomography (PET), ultrasound remains the most cost effective, accurate, and useful of the adjunctive breast imaging tools and is available in virtually every practice. It clearly is the instrument of choice for image-guided breast biopsies and preoperative needle localizations and has revolutionized diagnostic breast evaluation by providing rapid, cheap, and accurate guidance for breast intervention. Mindful of the range of breast imaging practices throughout the United States, Europe, and Asia, this article documents the currently accepted uses for breast ultrasound and suggests fruitful areas for further development and application. Particular emphasis is given to potentially

Division of Diagnostic Imaging, Department of Diagnostic Radiology, The University of Texas, M.D. Anderson Cancer Center, P.O. Box 301439 – Unit 1350, Houston, TX 77230, USA
* Corresponding author.
E-mail address: wyang@di.mdacc.tmc.edu (W. Yang).

radiologic.theclinics.com
doi:10.1016/j.rcl.2007.06.009

useful aspects of breast ultrasound, color Doppler, and power Doppler imaging, that are seldom highlighted in the clinical literature.

Established areas of progress

Breast Imaging Reporting and Data System nomenclature

To assimilate the impact of the expanded role of breast ultrasound and to underscore the integral role breast ultrasound plays in evaluating clinical breast problems, the Breast Imaging Reporting and Data System (BI-RADS) lexicon for reporting breast ultrasound findings was developed to correlate exactly with the terms that have been used for several years in radiographic mammography. This lexicon provides a unified method for reporting all breast imaging findings, highlighting for clinicians the overall impression of the study and clearly indicating the clinical management recommended. Several recent studies have evaluated the sensitivity and positive and negative predictive values of the BI-RADS lexicon for ultrasound [1–3]. The general consensus is that it creates a uniform platform for communication of important information regarding sonographic findings among breast radiologists and primary physicians including surgeons, medical oncologists, family practitioners, and gynecologists. One of the most important features of the BI-RADS lexicon for lesion characterization is margin analysis.

Limitations

Operator dependency

Despite several attempts during the past 25 years to automate the image acquisition process, the standard throughout the country remains the use of hand-held transducers, relying on the operator's experience, technical proficiency, and clinical acumen to differentiate true abnormalities from normal structures [4]. With this practice it is easy to create false-positive findings, leading to misinterpretation and misdiagnosis. Some companies are seeking to minimize this operator dependency by automating the process with a high-frequency, multidetector sweep-scanning device that permits precise localization and correlation in two planes within the breast and allows reconstruction of the images in the coronal plane, similar to methods available in CT and MR imaging.

Equipment dependency

The initial rudimentary machines did not have scan converters, and not until approximately 1974 was true gray-scale imaging technically possible. Resolution was limited by transducer technology. Initial units used for breast employed transducers using frequencies of 3.5 or 5 mHz, which, although allowing deep tissue penetration, severely limited resolution. Technical advances found newer ways to achieve the necessary depth of penetration while improving resolution capability. Currently, 10- to 15-mHz transducers are the norm and achieve excellent resolution without sacrificing the necessary depth of penetration. Extended-field-of-view imaging, available on most current ultrasound scanners, allows simple and elegant demonstration and measurement of large lesions that extend beyond the width of the transducer footprint (Fig. 1).

Need for a recent mammogram

Although an American College of Radiology Imaging Network trial to assess the possibilities of breast

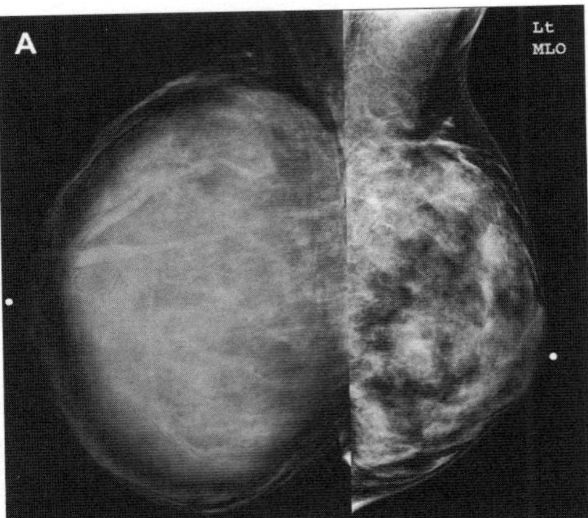

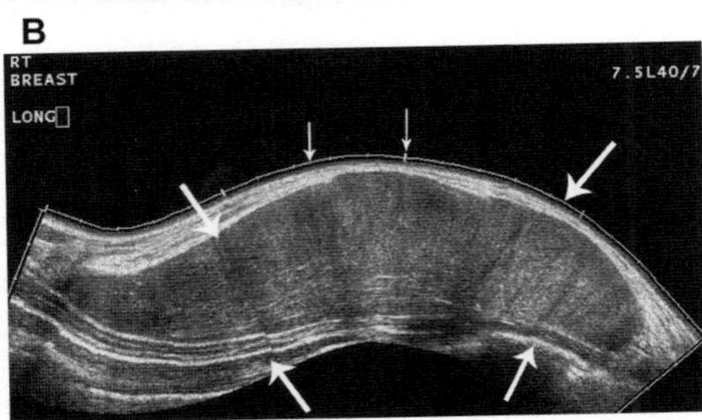

Fig. 1. (*A*) A 17-year-old-female presents with an enlarging mass in her right breast. Bilateral mediolateral oblique mammograms show global asymmetry of the right breast. (*B*) Sagittal extended-field-of-view ultrasound image demonstrates a solid homogeneously hypoechoic mass with circumscribed margins and a pseudocapsule (*thick arrows*). The centimeter markers superficial to the mass (*thin arrow*) allow a simple estimate of the dimensions of this mass. Surgical excision with reconstruction confirmed a giant fibroadenoma.

ultrasound as a screening instrument is in progress, to date breast ultrasound has been used as an adjunctive tool, not as a screening modality [5–8]. The exception is in young patients (in their teens or early 20s); in these patients breast ultrasound often can reach a definitive diagnosis for a clinically palpable finding. As a general rule for daily clinical practice, performing a breast ultrasound without an accompanying mammogram is dangerous and can lead to erroneous conclusions and missed cancer diagnoses.

Erroneous conclusions resulting from the use of image-processing algorithms without understanding the electronic principles

Recently, various manufacturers have developed several different image-processing methods (eg, tissue harmonic imaging, spatial compound imaging) in the laudable effort to make diagnosis of lesions easier for the breast imager [9–11]. Employing these methods without understanding their basis in physics, however, is dangerous. The goal has been to improve the conspicuity of real lesions while reducing the possibility for false-positive findings.

Changing indications for biopsy

In earlier years, biopsies were done to avoid the risk of a false-negative result when the imaging findings were inconclusive or indeterminate. With the marked improvement in resolution coupled with a greater understanding of breast pathology, imaging findings often are sufficient to make a confident diagnosis of a benign lesion, thus avoiding an unnecessary biopsy [12]. A common example is the detection and diagnosis of small and perhaps multiple fibroadenomas in younger patients. Ultrasound often can depict them confidently as circumscribed, ovoid lesions with specular echoes typical of fibroadenomas (Fig. 2). With an experienced sonographer using good equipment and technique, further invasive procedures often are unnecessary.

Current indications

Adjunct to mammography and clinical breast examination

Although entities such as summation artifacts seen on one view of a screening mammogram are always best investigated first by work-up mammography, diagnostic breast ultrasound is effective in the clarification of many positive findings on both mammography and clinical examination. Except for summation artifacts, the ultrasound examination can establish whether a lesion is present at all or if the finding previously noted is simply a normal parenchymal variation. The combination of a negative diagnostic mammogram and a negative diagnostic ultrasound has a sufficiently high negative predictive value that biopsy of a low-suspicion palpable lesion is not indicated [13–16]. If a lesion does exist, ultrasound is capable of further characterization and, more importantly, of indicating whether an ultrasound-guided biopsy is appropriate. Fig. 3 shows a clinically palpable finding not seen mammographically that was imaged easily and biopsied under ultrasound guidance and proved to be a cancer. On the other hand, one of

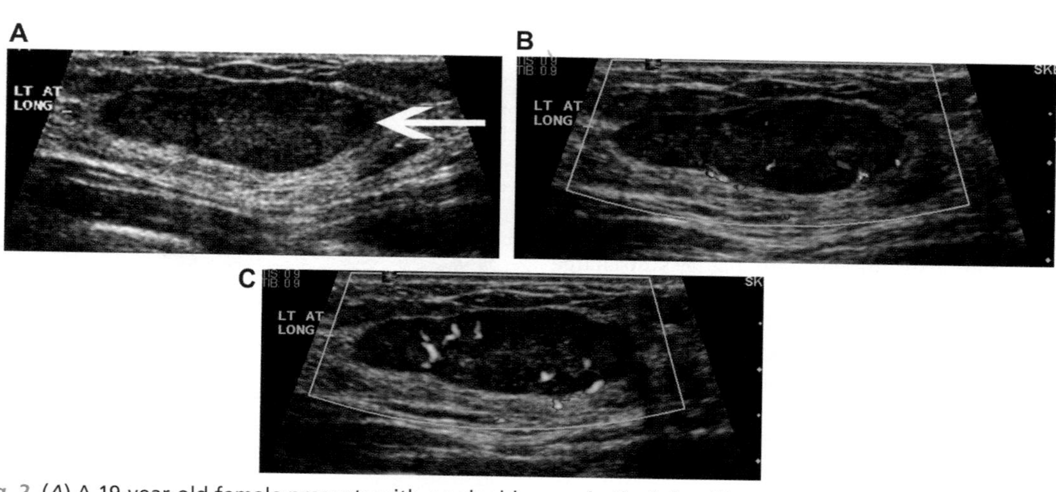

Fig. 2. (*A*) A 19-year-old female presents with a palpable mass in the left axillary tail. Transverse gray-scale ultrasound shows typical features of a fibroadenoma, comprising an oval solid hypoechoic circumscribed mass with a pseudocapsule (*arrow*). (*B*) Color Doppler ultrasound image shows weak peripheral and central vascularity associated with this mass. (*C*) Power Doppler ultrasound image shows longer segments of vessels in the periphery and center of this mass.

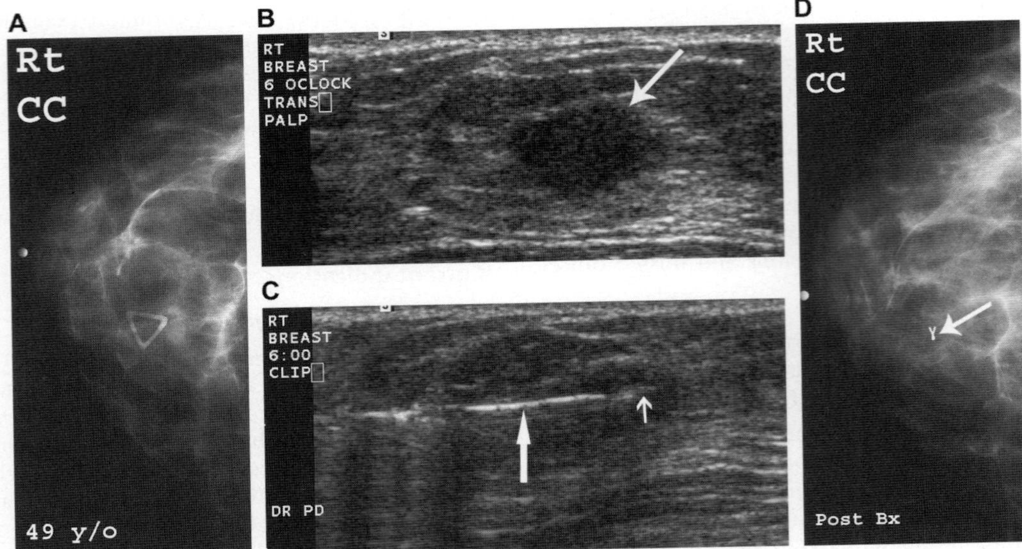

Fig. 3. (*A*) Right craniocaudal mammogram of a 44-year-old woman who presents with a palpable mass and a negative diagnostic mammogram. The triangle skin marker demonstrates the site of the palpable mass. (*B*) A transverse sonogram shows an irregular, solid, hypoechoic nodule corresponding to the palpable mass at the right 6 o'clock position (*arrow*). (*C*) A transverse ultrasound image during ultrasound guided clip placement within this mass. The long arrow indicates the needle shaft, and the short arrow indicates the clip. (*D*) Postbiopsy right craniocaudal mammogram shows clip marking the site of mammographically occult palpable cancer (*arrow*).

the common benign findings of a clinically palpable area is a prominent fat lobule (Fig. 4). A physician can use the real-time sonographic image viewed on the screen as an effective display tool for the patient and allay the patient's fears quite effectively.

Primary methodology for young patients

Quite frequently a palpable finding in a young patient is a fibroadenoma (see Fig. 2) (and its variants), a breast abscess (Fig. 5), or changes best described as "developmental anomalies" (macromastia, micromastia) [17–21]. Healthy adolescent girls, rarely, may present with painless discharge from around the nipple and a periareolar mass. Ultrasound is a useful tool in the diagnosis of this condition (Fig. 6) [22] and in this clinical setting is the primary imaging tool. Ultrasound intuitively seems advantageous in this group of patients because of the homogeneously dense parenchyma and the reported increased radiosensitivity of breast tissue in these young women [23]. Technically well-performed ultrasound in young girls can be the key to preventing the devastating mistake of excision of a normally developing breast bud (Fig. 7) resulting in the complete lack of development of that breast.

Initial imaging modality for pregnant patients who have clinical symptoms

Unfortunately, young women, and especially young pregnant women, are not immune to breast cancer. Because of the patient's young age and the hormonal environment in pregnancy, these cancers tend to be high grade and rapidly growing, so prompt and accurate diagnosis is critical for therapy to be initiated. These cancers may be mammographically occult because of dense parenchyma, but they can be detected and evaluated effectively

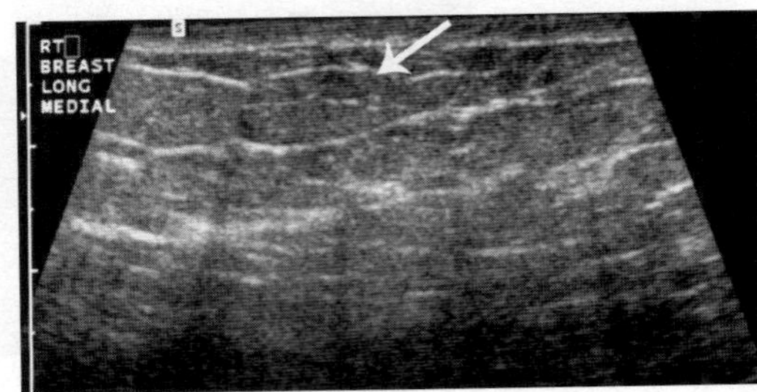

Fig. 4. Transverse sonogram of the medial right breast at a site of palpable concern in a 60-year-old woman demonstrates a benign fat lobule (*arrow*), without suspicious findings.

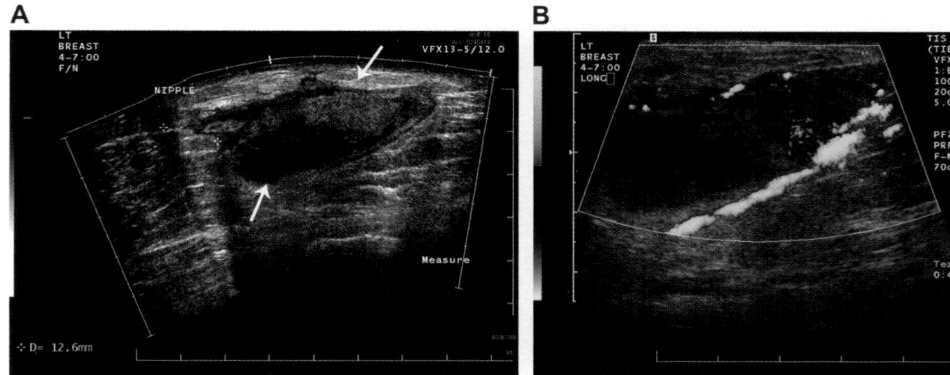

Fig. 5. (*A*) 56-year-old woman presents with a painful left breast mass associated with fever. Transverse sonogram shows a complex oval mass with mixed solid and cystic components and a partially defined capsule (*arrows*), highly suggestive of abscess formation. (*B*) Power Doppler sonography in the same patient shows peripheral rimlike vascularity in this biopsy-proven abscess that later underwent ultrasound-guided drainage and catheter placement.

with sonography (Fig. 8) [24]. With recently documented advances, pregnant women who have breast cancer can be treated effectively with specific chemotherapy regimens and have a full-term, successful outcome of the pregnancy [25,26]. After delivery, definitive surgery can be performed.

Fortunately, in most pregnant patients referred for ultrasound examination of palpable findings, findings are benign; entities such as fibroadenomas enlarging in the hormonal environment of pregnancy, lactating adenomas, and galactoceles are common (Fig. 9).

Infection

Infection happens frequently in the postoperative and the postpartum setting, when the patient may present with an enlarged, red, and tender breast with or without associated overlying skin changes. The clinical dilemma is to exclude an underlying abscess that requires intervention (either imaging-guided or surgically guided) or an early inflammatory breast carcinoma [27,28]. Ultrasound is the imaging modality of choice because the breast frequently is too tender for compression with mammography. Careful and gentle scanning provides valuable information regarding the presence or absence of an underlying fluid collection (including abscess or galactocele in the postpartum setting or abscess or progressive tumor after surgical treatment of breast cancer). When an abscess is identified (see Fig. 6), imaging-guided drainage is swift and efficacious.

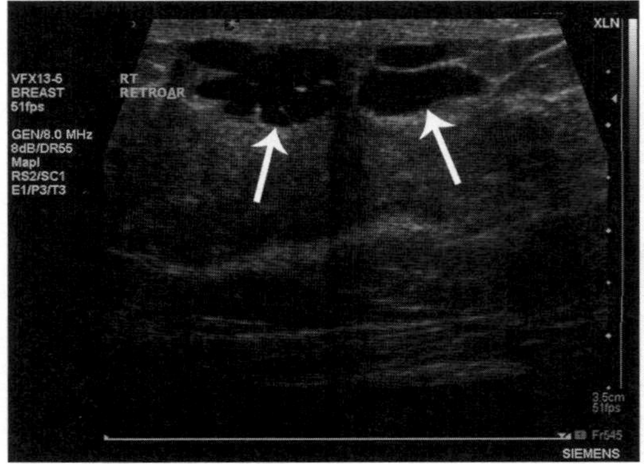

Fig. 6. A 13-year-old female presents with discharge from the Montgomery tubercles and a palpable right periareolar mass. Transverse right sonogram shows prominent retroareolar ducts (*arrows*) consistent with fibrocystic change. No suspicious findings were noted. The patient's symptoms resolved spontaneously after 3 months.

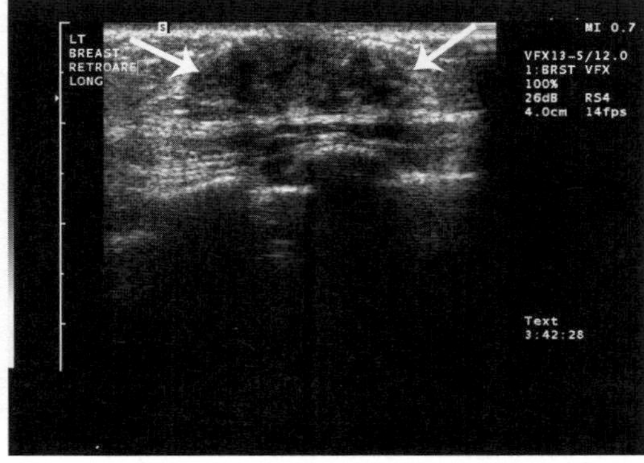

Fig. 7. A 13-month-old female presents with a palpable asymmetric right breast mass. Transverse sonogram demonstrates a normal breast bud in the retroareolar position with normal fibroglandular parenchyma (*arrows*).

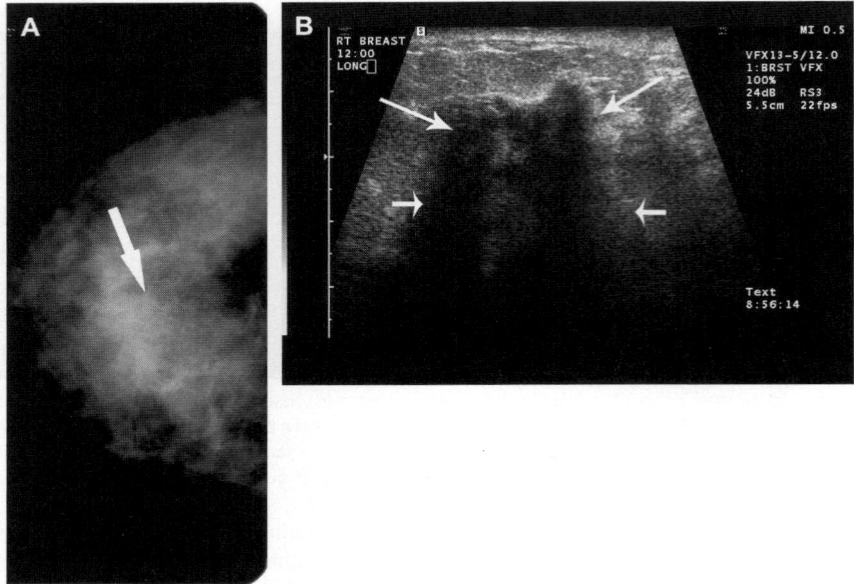

Fig. 8. (*A*) A33-year-old woman at 26 weeks' gestation presents with a palpable breast mass in the right breast. Right craniocaudal mammogram demonstrates a vague focal asymmetry in the central 12 o'clock position (*arrow*). (*B*) Transverse sonogram of the right 12 o'clock position demonstrates an irregular solid hypoechoic mass (*long arrows*) with an echogenic boundary and posterior acoustic shadowing (*short arrows*). Core-needle biopsy showed high-grade invasive ductal carcinoma.

Ultrasonography of the male breast

Although male breast cancer is uncommon, there are multiple indications for imaging the male breast with sonography. These indications include a palpable mass in the breast or axilla, particularly in males who have a known primary tumor, including melanoma, prostate cancer, or lymphoma. Ultrasound often can characterize such masses and offer immediate pathologic confirmation using ultrasound-guided fine-needle aspiration biopsy. Men who have chronic liver disease and men taking long-term antihypertensive medication who

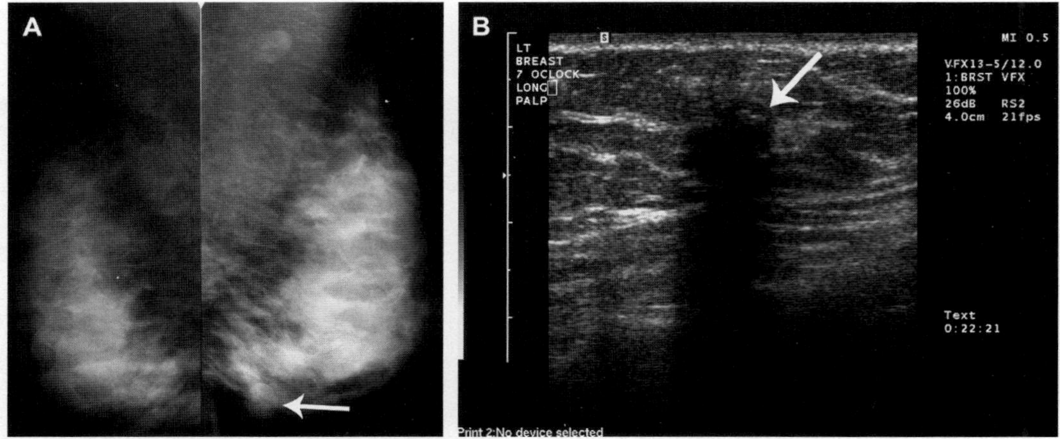

Fig. 9. (*A*) Bilateral mediolateral mammograms in a 33-year-old woman at 32 weeks' gestation demonstrates an oval mass in the inferior left breast (*arrow*) corresponding to a palpable finding. Global increased breast density bilaterally is consistent with gestational and lactation change. (*B*) Transverse sonogram demonstrates an irregular solid hypoechoic mass (*arrow*) that was avascular (not shown) and demonstrates marked posterior acoustic shadowing. Core biopsy showed galactocele with inflammatory change and no evidence of malignancy. This lesion had resolved spontaneously at 12-month follow-up.

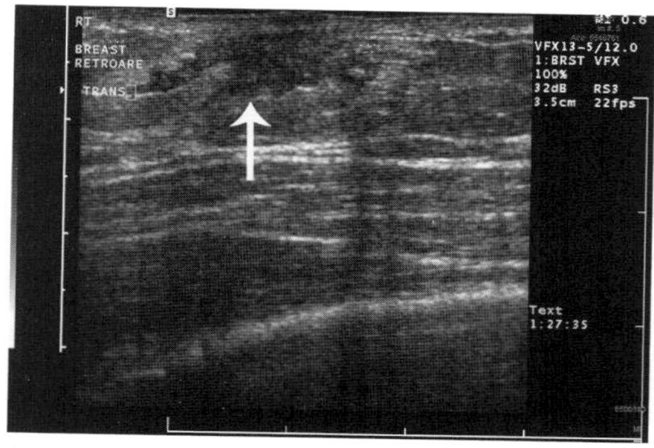

Fig. 10. Transverse sonogram of the right retroareolar region shows hypoechoic nodular gynecomastia (*arrow*) in a 16-year-old male who presented with a palpable mass.

present with palpable swelling of the breast(s) have a clinical diagnosis of gynecomastia. The sonographic features of gynecomastia include prominent glandular tissue in the acute nodular hypoechoic form (Fig. 10) or the chronic hyperechoic dendritic form [29]. This finding is distinct from the solid or complex cystic mass in the subareolar position that is typical for male breast carcinoma (Fig. 11) [30,31].

Imaging guidance for interventional procedures

It is now commonplace for needle biopsies using either fine-needle aspiration or core technique to be done with ultrasound guidance, if technically feasible. Even vacuum-assisted biopsies can be done in this fashion, although resorting to this more aggressive method is not always necessary. If a diagnosis

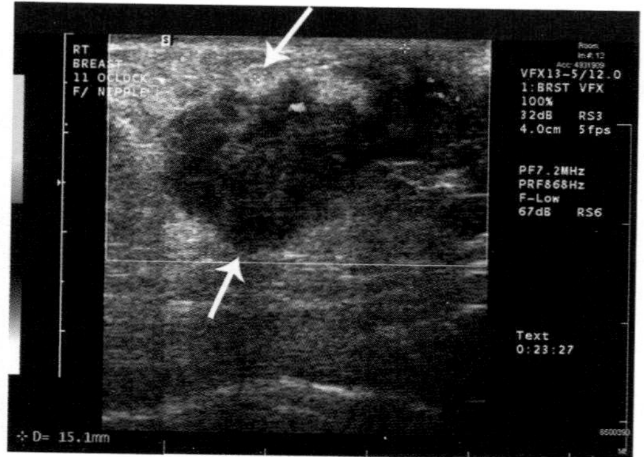

Fig. 11. Transverse sonogram in a 71-year-old man who presented with a palpable mass shows an eccentric mass at 11 o'clock in the right breast that is irregular in shape and has microlobulated margins and internal hypervascularity (*arrows*). Pathology showed grade 2 invasive ductal carcinoma.

of cancer is established, and if preoperative neoadjuvant chemotherapy is to be employed, a metallic (titanium) tumor marker can be placed percutaneously into the epicenter of the tumor at the time of biopsy (see Fig. 3; Fig. 12) [32–35]. Up to 30% of these tumors undergo complete clinical response, and thus the marker would be the only way that an accurate pre-excision localization could be performed.

Any cancer easily visible on ultrasound is a candidate for preoperative localization by this method. Careful preprocedure scrutiny should be used, however, because any segmental areas of microcalcifications associated with the cancer are better localized mammographically with a bracketing technique.

At a few institutions, such as the University of Texas M.D. Anderson Cancer Center, preoperative localization using ultrasound is actually performed in the operating room after the patient has been anesthetized and positioned for surgery [36]. Some surgeons appreciate the real-time demonstration of the perpendicular distance from the overlying skin to the center of the tumor (Fig. 13). This method also obviates the need for an additional procedure requiring local anesthesia and needle placement in the conscious patient.

Second-look study after a positive breast MR imaging or positron emission tomography study

At the M.D. Anderson Cancer Center, as at many institutions, ultrasound has been used effectively to investigate possible areas of significance that have been detected on either breast MR imaging or PET/CT scan. Even if the patient has had a previous breast ultrasound, the second-look procedure allows attention to be focused on targeted areas whose localities have been documented on the MR imaging or PET/CT roadmap. If successfully imaged and localized by ultrasound, the area can be biopsied quickly and accurately, and a clip can be placed in both a time-effective and cost-effective manner (Fig. 14) [37–39]. Otherwise, a separate MR imaging–guided procedure, which is much more expensive and technically more complicated, must be scheduled.

Breast cancer imaging

Definitive surgery, as the name indicates, should be a planned curative procedure based on the most accurate anatomic information available concerning the precise area of breast cancer involvement. When the surgery is performed and undiagnosed metastatic nodes are present in the infraclavicular, internal mammary, supraclavicular, or low neck region(s), the ultimate clinical outcome will be less than ideal.

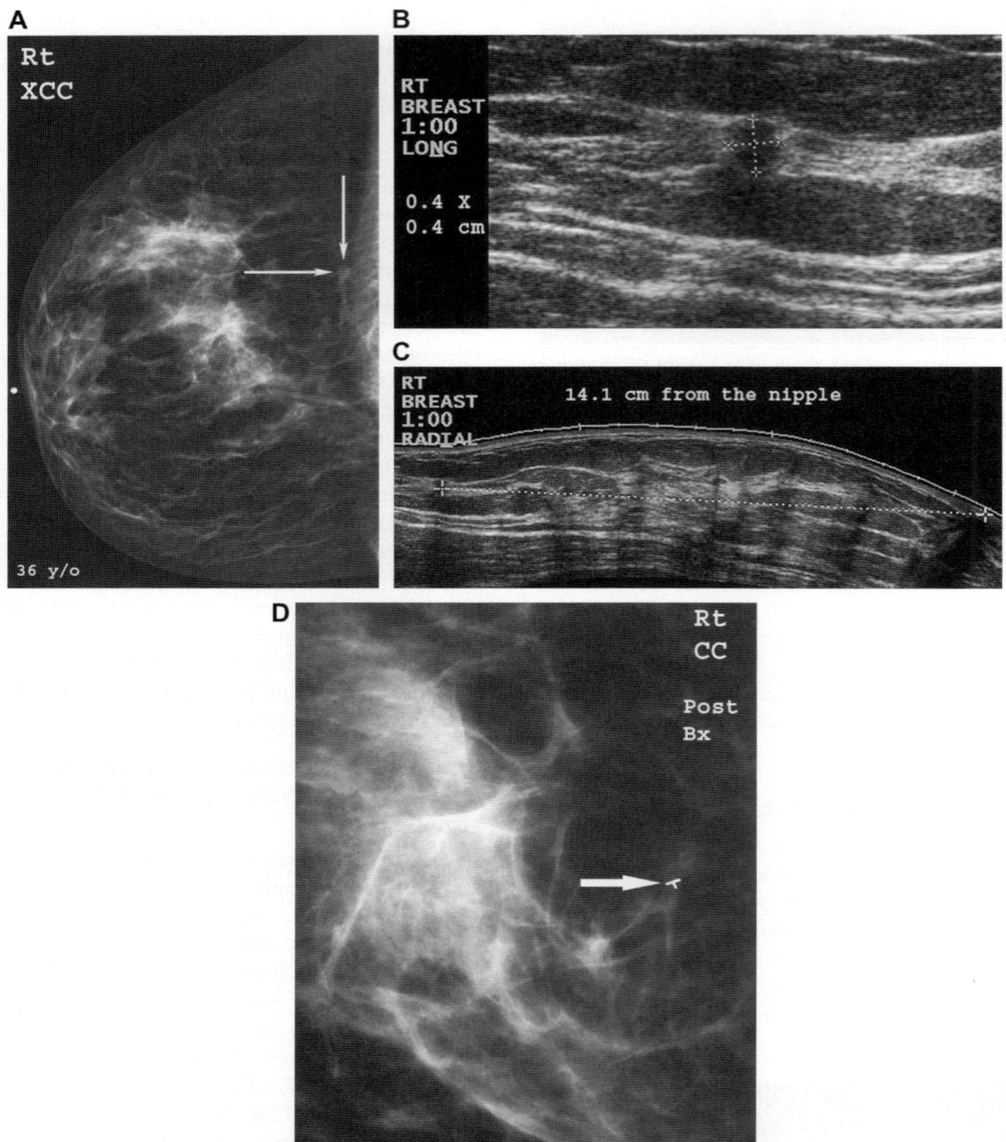

Fig. 12. (*A*) Exaggerated right craniocaudal mammogram of a 36-year-old woman demonstrates a suspicious 4-mm irregular nodule (*arrows*) detected on screening mammography. (*B*) Longitudinal ultrasound demonstrates a solid hypoechoic mass (marked by dotted cross) with irregular margins and no posterior acoustic phenomena. (*C*) Longitudinal extended-field-of-view view ultrasound image accurately documents distance of the lesion from the nipple, confirming sonographic–mammographic correlation of this abnormality. (*D*) Postbiopsy right craniocaudal mammogram demonstrates the postbiopsy clip within the mass (*arrow*).

At the M.D. Anderson Cancer Center, ultrasound is used regularly for staging purposes. It is surprising how frequently unsuspected nodal metastases can be easily imaged, biopsied, and histologically proven (by fine-needle aspiration), thus providing more accurate TNM staging and, ultimately, the best patient care. The authors believe that many cases reported as early recurrences are undoubtedly patients who were treated conservatively and who had unsuspected metastatic disease at the time of initial diagnosis.

Many recent papers cite MR imaging as the best initial staging method for breast cancer [8,40,41]. Although the sensitivity of MR imaging is superb, the detection of additional "enhancing lesions" poses the problem of obtaining quick, inexpensive

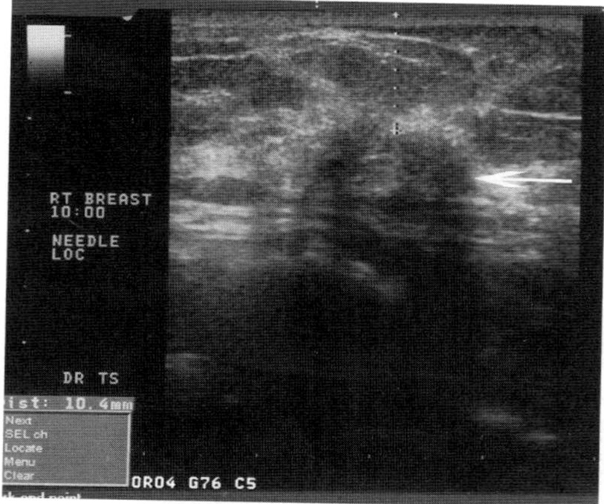

Fig. 13. Transverse intraoperative ultrasound image demonstrates known cancer (*arrow*) at the 10 o'clock position in the right breast, and the perpendicular distance of the cancer from the skin measured by calipers (10.4 mm).

histologic proof of their significance. Furthermore, assessment of all regional nodal basins is not possible with MR imaging, whereas ultrasound allows assessment of multifocality (Fig. 15) and multicentricity (Fig. 16); histologic proof can be obtained inexpensively at the time of the study. In addition, all regional nodal basins can be assessed and biopsied as needed with fine-needle aspiration biopsy [42–45].

At the M.D. Anderson cancer center, patients who have been diagnosed as having breast cancer by needle or excisional biopsy undergo an ultrasound of the ipsilateral breast and axillary, internal mammary, and infraclavicular nodal basins. If suspicious nodes are seen in any of these sites, the supraclavicular area is scanned as well (Fig. 17). Histologic verification is achieved by immediate fine-needle aspiration biopsy beginning with the highest-order suspicious node detected. This procedure is appropriate in a primary cancer institution where the N stage affects overall staging and determines eligibility for various chemotherapy protocols [46]. Additionally, these sites of disease can be used to assess response in patients undergoing neoadjuvant chemotherapy.

Older literature focused entirely on the presence of a fatty hilum [47–50]. If it was present, the node was considered benign. More recent experience demonstrates this assumption is not true. Because the afferent lymphatic channels enter the node through the periphery of the cortex, it is in this area that early changes of metastatic disease become manifest. Specifically, very subtle cortical nodularity can be seen as the first sign of metastatic involvement, even when a prominent fatty hilum is still present (Fig. 18). These nodular areas may be perceived as somewhat hypoechoic relative to the rest of the nodal cortex, but this observation is predicated on the most meticulous technique. When doing a biopsy, it is critical to direct the needle tip to these nodular areas and not to the hilar regions or the cortical regions as yet unaffected sonographically.

Ultrasound also is used effectively to assess tumor response after the initiation of chemotherapy protocols. Volume measurements of a mass by ultrasound are obtained by taking measurements in three orthogonal planes and applying a volumetric formula for an ellipsoid, thus rendering ultrasound a particularly facile and cost-effective tool. In addition, should a marked positive response to chemotherapy be noted with significant reduction in tumor volume, a metallic tumor marker can be placed at the time of the examination.

Benign versus malignant: the goal of lesion characterization

Since the first papers reporting the use of breast ultrasound were published in the early 1950s, one of the principal goals of its use has been distinguishing benign from malignant tumors using a variety of sonographic criteria. A frequently cited article regarding tissue characterization was published in 1995 by Stavros and colleagues [51]. Based on a large volume of data derived from the study of 750 breast nodules, the acoustic characteristics of benign and malignant lesions were enumerated and described in detail. Although the ultimate reference standard for the distinction between benign and malignant lesions remains histologic, this article helped decrease the "gray areas" in interpretation.

Use and interpretation of color Doppler and power Doppler imaging

Neoangiogenesis is believed to be caused by the protein angiogenin that is produced by tumor cells [52] and has been shown to correlate with rapid tumor growth and metastasis [53]. Tumoral vessels frequently are irregular, tortuous, and variable in caliber, forming reticular networks with arteriovenous shunts and dichotomous branching [54]. Doppler ultrasound requires a high-frequency transducer; usually, a 7- to 13-MHz annular array or broadband linear array is used. Ideally, the technique should be able to evaluate flow signals of very small vessels with diameters below 0.1 mm and with low flow velocity. Successful Doppler-based assessment requires standardization of technique, evaluation, and analysis [55–57]. The different

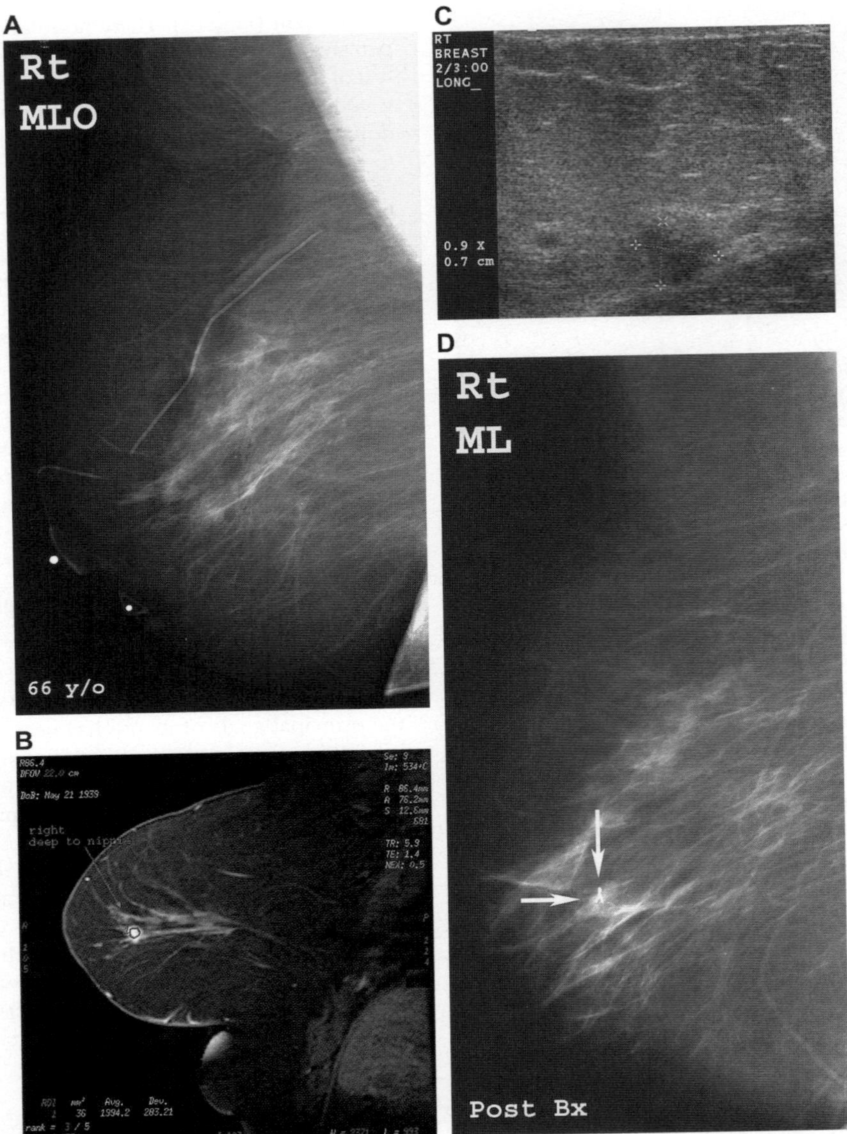

Fig. 14. (*A*) Right mediolateral oblique mammogram of a 66-year-old woman who presents with a palpable nodule denoted by radiopaque skin marker. No definite lesion is seen mammographically. A previous benign surgical biopsy site is marked with an opaque, linear scar marker. The palpable nodule was sonographically occult (not shown). (*B*) Sagittal, dynamic, contrast-enhanced MR image of the right breast demonstrates a small, enhancing lesion with malignant-type washout kinetics (not shown) corresponding to site of the palpable nodule (*purple arrow*). (*C*) A second-look ultrasound demonstrated an irregular, solid, hypoechoic nodule measuring 9 mm by 7 mm. Ultrasound-guided core biopsy showed intermediate-grade invasive ductal carcinoma. (*D*) Post-biopsy lateral right mammogram demonstrates postbiopsy clip (*arrows*) without corresponding mammographic abnormality corresponding to the lesion visualized on MR imaging.

forms of Doppler imaging include color Doppler, spectral Doppler, and power Doppler. Color Doppler and spectral Doppler imaging employ instruments to visualize the mean intravascular frequency shift caused by Doppler effects of flowing blood corpuscles that are frequency modulated.

Advances in technology and ultrasound equipment have led to improved detection of blood flow with Doppler sonography in all solid masses, benign and malignant, thus improving the sensitivity and specificity [58,59]. The proof of or extent of tumor vascularity alone is no longer a sufficient criterion

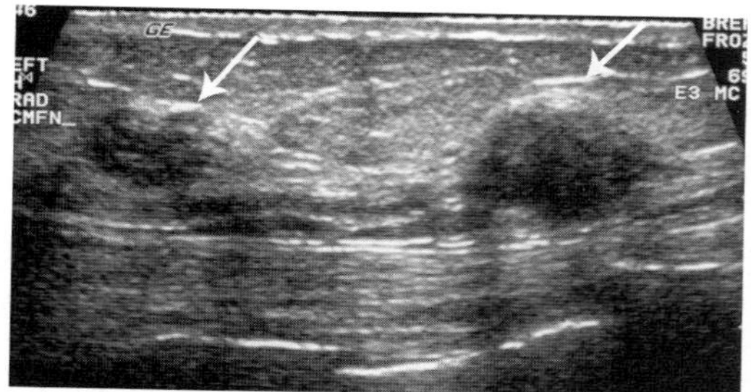

Fig. 15. Transverse sonogram in a 26-year-old woman shows two masses in the left breast (*arrows*) consistent with multifocal invasive carcinoma.

in the differential diagnosis of breast lesions [60–64]. Additional useful criteria include structural characteristics of tumor vessels correlating to histologic patterns. Characteristics of malignant tumors include hypervascularity (92%–9%), irregular abnormal vascularity (54.2%), and more than one vascular pole [65] (Fig. 19A–C). Benign lesions tend to have one vascular pole, weak, peripheral vascularity (Fig. 20), and no central vessels (Fig. 21) [66]. Color Doppler imaging is less helpful in the differential diagnosis of breast lesions, such as mucinous and in situ carcinomas, and of invasive ductal carcinoma less than 9 mm in diameter, which often may show avascularity [65]. Benign lesions that display a false-positive malignant-type hypervascularity include hypervascularized,proliferating, juvenile phyllodes tumors and fibroadenomas (Fig. 22). These hypervascularized masses require biopsy.

Spectral Doppler imaging is less useful than color Doppler imaging in differentiating benign from malignant masses [66,67]. The large variation of velocities within cancers presumably is caused by the tortuous vessels and arteriovenous shunts that are typical of malignant neovascularization [68,69]. The formation of arteriovenous shunts and thin-walled vessels lacking smooth muscle, as seen in malignant tumors, results in high-velocity and high-pulsatility flow [70] with significantly higher peak systolic Doppler frequency shifts in malignant than in benign lesions ($P < .01–<.0001$) [62,71]. A wide overlap of parameters prevents spectral Doppler imaging from being a valuable tool in the differentiation of breast lesions [71,72].

Power Doppler imaging depicts the intensity of energy of the Doppler signal and is based on the amplitude of Doppler shift [73,74]. The wider dynamic range of power Doppler imaging makes it more sensitive in detecting small vessels and low flow. Power Doppler imaging is independent of the Doppler angle and therefore is not subject to aliasing; power Doppler also may depict longer segments of smaller vessels because of the increased signal-to-noise ratio (see Fig. 2). Disadvantages of power Doppler imaging include reduced temporal resolution, lack of directional or velocity information, a high number of color artifacts, and the inability to differentiate between arteries and veins. Power Doppler imaging has a sensitivity of 74.5% and a specificity of 74.6% that is useful in the depiction of small cancers that are less than 5 mm in size [75]. One study found that penetrating vessels were more likely to be present in malignant tumors [76,77]. Typical power Doppler signs of malignancy include central, borderline penetrating, branching, disordered, and intratumoral vessels (see Figs. 19–21) [75–77].

Doppler imaging may be useful in differentiating postoperative changes from recurrent tumor. In the

A

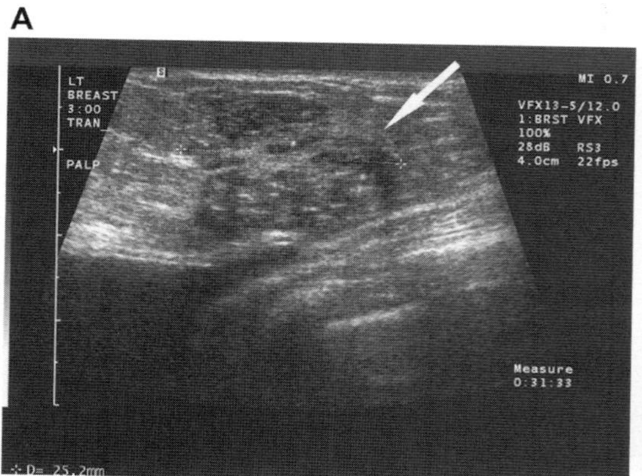

B

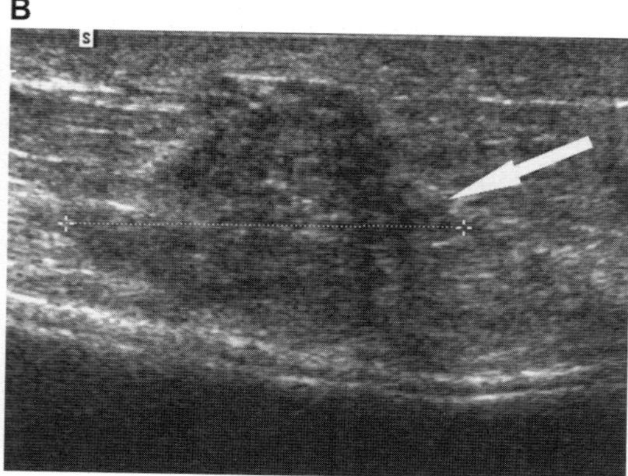

Fig. 16. (*A*) Transverse sonogram in a 29-year-old woman shows an irregular, solid, hypoechoic mass in the 3 o'clock position in the left breast with indistinct margins and internal microcalcifications (*arrow*) corresponding to a palpable finding. Pathology from ultrasound-guided core-needle biopsy showed high-grade ductal carcinoma in situ. (*B*) A second nonpalpable mass with similar features (*arrow*) was detected in the 9 o'clock position in the left breast, consistent with multicentric disease.

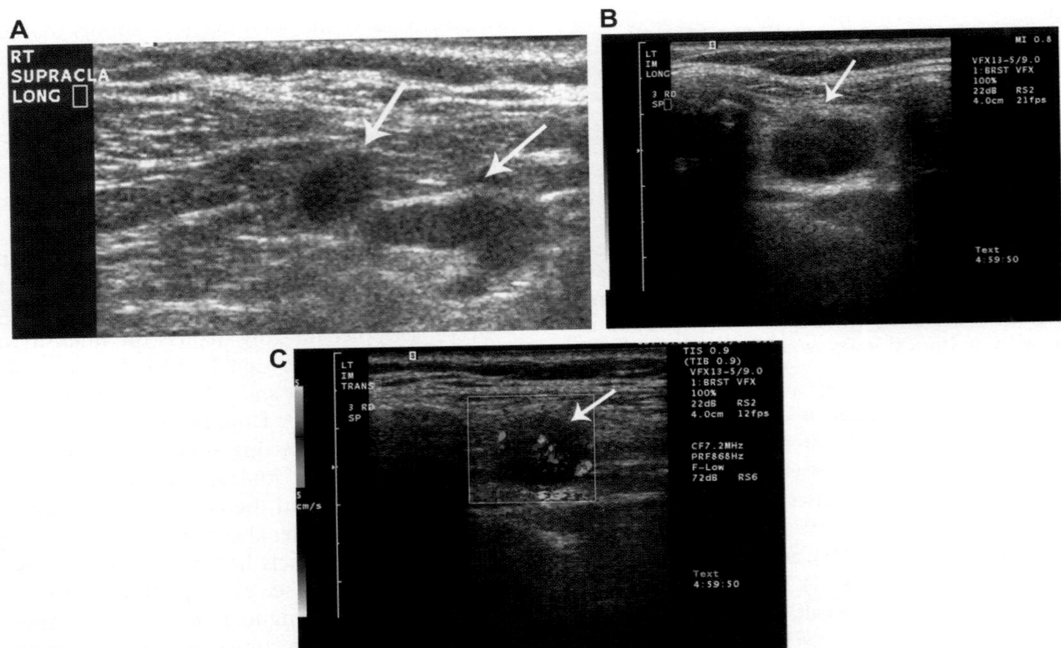

Fig. 17. (*A*) Transverse sonogram of the right supraclavicular fossa shows two abnormal nodes with eccentric cortical hypertrophy (*arrows*). (*B*) Transverse sonogram in left third internal mammary lymph node space shows an abnormal oval solid hypoechoic nodule (*arrow*) consistent with internal mammary lymphadenopathy. (*C*) Color Doppler ultrasound image of this node demonstrates internal hypervascularity (*arrow*).

first 18 months, nodular scars or granulomas also may be hypervascularized, although the likelihood of hypervascularity decreases as the age of the scar increases. Criteria include the number and regularity of vessels [78]. Postsurgical scars usually are slightly or not vascularized, whereas all malignant lesions tend to display increased and irregular vascularity [78].

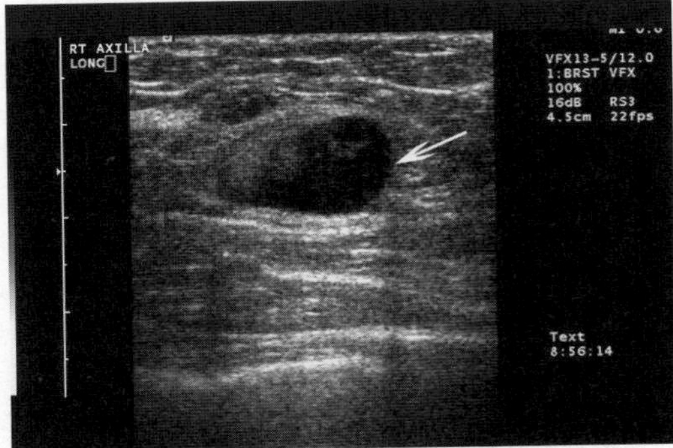

Fig. 18. Transverse ultrasound image of right axillary node in a 36-year-old woman who had documented right breast cancer shows focal eccentric cortical hypertrophy (*arrow*). Ultrasound-guided fine-needle aspiration biopsy confirmed metastatic carcinoma.

Future directions

Elastography in breast imaging

Because malignant lesions tend to be "harder" than benign lesions, several groups have suggested and investigated the application of elastography to evaluate breast lesions visualized on ultrasound. The major problems have been in the exact quantification of these results. Three distinct methods of measurement have been proposed and tested, with varying degrees of success: spatial correlation, phase-shift tracking, and combined autocorrelation.

The major drawbacks can be summarized under the general heading of operator dependency. This limitation involves the technique of pressure application, the experience of the investigator(s), and the very involved manual tracing of lesion boundaries. In its present form, the use of elastography in routine clinical practice does not seem feasible [79–81].

Breast ablation techniques

In other organs, such as prostate, liver, and kidney, the possibility of avoiding open surgical intervention by the ablation of small tumors has received much attention. Ablative techniques for benign

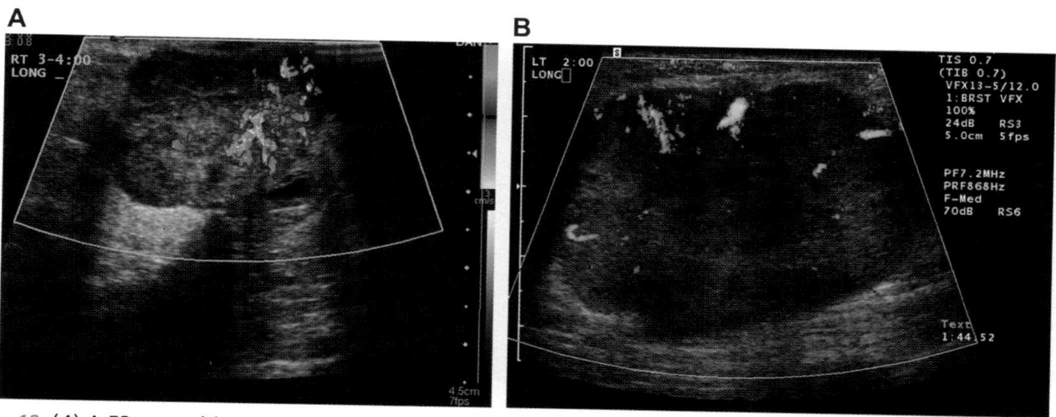

Fig. 19. (*A*) A 53-year-old woman with a history of ductal carcinoma in situ 5 years ago presents with a palpable finding at the segmentectomy site in the right breast at 4 o'clock position. Color and power Doppler ultrasound images show marked internal hypervascularity within a recurrent invasive ductal cancer that extends to the overlying dermis. Note the chaotic pattern of branching vascularity and vessels of varying caliber. (*B*) A 57-year-old woman presents with a palpable left breast mass. The power Doppler ultrasound image shows internal hypervascularity (vessels of varied caliber) within an invasive metaplastic cancer.

(fibroadenomas) and malignant breast tumors have reached the stage of clinical testing, and early results seem encouraging. Numerous forms of possible tumor ablation have been examined, including chemical, thermal (radiofrequency, laser, cryoablation), microwave, and ultrasound [82]. The two techniques most widely tested and used thus far are cryoablation and ablation using radiofrequency currents. Both modalities are directed and confined to a highly localized area to avoid collateral tissue damage.

The cryoablation technique that has been used for both benign and malignant tumors employs a disposable, air-gap–insulated cryoablation probe 2.4 mm in diameter. In some cases, multiple probes have been used for larger masses. As ablation takes place, an ice ball is formed, the diameter of which is monitored with ultrasound [83,84].

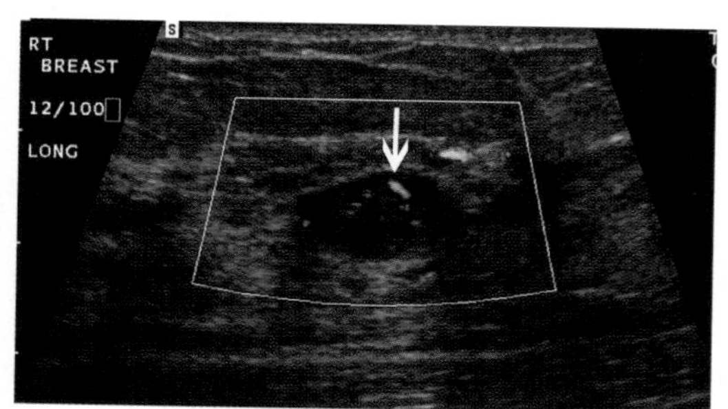

Fig. 20. A 41-year-old woman presents with a palpable finding in the right breast at 12 o'clock position. Transverse power Doppler ultrasound shows a single peripheral vessel (*arrow*) associated with a biopsy-proven fibroadenoma.

With radiofrequency ablation, the initial device inserted is a 15-gauge probe through which multipronged expandable electrodes are inserted and then deployed. Ablation progress is monitored both by constant temperature recording from the electrode tips as well as with ultrasound imaging [85].

If ablation is used as the only therapy for potentially malignant neoplasms, without subsequent surgical removal, the greatest potential drawback is the inability to assess tumor margins. This assessment always has been the primary measure of successful cancer surgical therapy, and loss of the ability to document tumor margins carefully will invariably leave an element of doubt.

Three-dimensional sonography

The advantages of three-dimensional sonography compared with those of conventional sonographic imaging remains controversial. Some single-institution studies have demonstrated superior image quality on three-dimensional sonography [86,87], but the diagnostic accuracy of this method was not statistically significant [88]. Three-dimensional sonography as an adjunct to conventional sonography requires further evaluation in larger clinical trials to determine clinical relevance and efficacy in diagnostic breast imaging.

Summary

Breast ultrasound remains a critical and reliable adjunctive modality in the detection and diagnosis of benign and malignant entities within the breast parenchyma and in the surrounding regional nodal

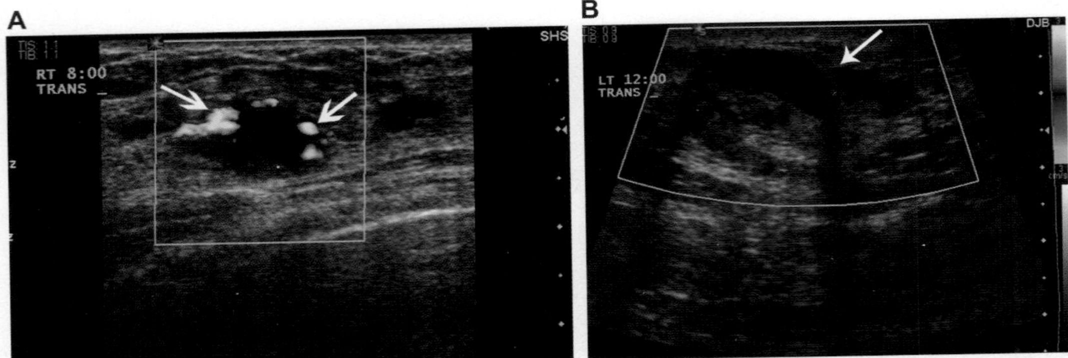

Fig. 21. (*A*) A 44-year-old woman who had a biopsy-proven left breast cancer presents with an exquisitely tender mass in the right breast. The power Doppler ultrasound image shows marked peripheral hypervascularity (*arrows*) associated with a densely inflamed cyst that was aspirated and showed benign ductal cells, with no evidence of malignancy. Note lack of central vascularity. (*B*) A 39-year-old woman presents with a palpable finding after transverse rectus abdominus myocutaneous reconstruction of the left breast. The color Doppler ultrasound shows an avascular mixed cystic and solid mass (*arrow*). Fine-needle aspiration biopsy confirmed fat necrosis.

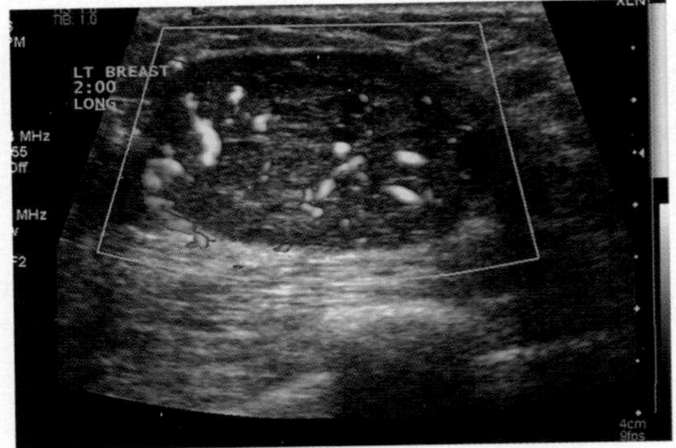

Fig. 22. A 27-year-old woman presents with a palpable mass in the left upper outer quadrant. Power Doppler ultrasound shows multiple internal vessels in a biopsy-proven phyllodes tumor.

basins. It is established as the first-line guidance modality for percutaneous biopsy, preoperative localization, and tumor marker placement procedures. Although operator-dependent, it nonetheless is accurate, patient friendly, and cost effective when used properly. It is a modality that seems destined for continued growth in both technical innovations and clinical use.

References

[1] Hong AS, Rosen EL, Soo MS, et al. BI-RADS for sonography: positive and negative predictive values of sonographic features. AJR Am J Roentgenol 2005;184(4):1260–5.

[2] Lazarus E, Mainiero MB, Schepps B, et al. BI-RADS lexicon for US and mammography: interobserver variability and positive predictive value. Radiology 2006;239(2):385–91.

[3] Costantini M, Belli P, Lombardi R, et al. Characterization of solid breast masses: use of the sonographic breast imaging reporting and data system lexicon. J Ultrasound Med 2006;25(5):649–59.

[4] Baker JA, Soo MS, Rosen EL. Artifacts and pitfalls in sonographic imaging of the breast. AJR Am J Roentgenol 2001;176(5):1261–6.

[5] Kolb TM, Lichy J, Newhouse JH. Occult cancer in women with dense breasts: detection with screening US—diagnostic yield and tumor characteristics. Radiology 1998;207(1):191–9.

[6] Berg WA. Rationale for a trial of screening breast ultrasound: American College of Radiology Imaging Network (ACRIN) 6666. AJR Am J Roentgenol 2003;180(5):1225–8.

[7] Berg WA. Supplemental screening sonography in dense breasts. Radiol Clin North Am 2004;42(5): 845–51, vi.

[8] Berg WA, Gutierrez L, NessAiver MS, et al. Diagnostic accuracy of mammography, clinical examination, US, and MR imaging in preoperative assessment of breast cancer. Radiology 2004; 233(3):830–49.

[9] Szopinski KT, Pajk AM, Wysocki M, et al. Tissue harmonic imaging: utility in breast sonography. J Ultrasound Med 2003;22(5):479–87.

[10] Haerten R, Lowery C, Becker G, et al. "Ensemble™ Tissue Harmonic Imaging": the technology and clinical utility. Electromedica 1999;1:50–6.

[11] Cha JH, Moon WK, Cho N, et al. Differentiation of benign from malignant solid breast masses: conventional US versus spatial compound imaging. Radiology 2005;237(3):841–6.

[12] Gordon PB, Gagnon FA, Lanzkowsky L. Solid breast masses diagnosed as fibroadenoma at fine-needle aspiration biopsy: acceptable rates

of growth at long-term follow-up. Radiology 2003;229(1):233–8.
[13] Harvey JA. Sonography of palpable breast masses. Semin Ultrasound CT MR 2006;27(4): 284–97.
[14] Mendelson EB. Problem-solving ultrasound. Radiol Clin North Am 2004;42(5):909–18, vii.
[15] Soo MS, Rosen EL, Baker JA, et al. Negative predictive value of sonography with mammography in patients with palpable breast lesions. AJR Am J Roentgenol 2001;177(5):1167–70.
[16] Shetty MK, Shah YP, Sharman RS. Prospective evaluation of the value of combined mammographic and sonographic assessment in patients with palpable abnormalities of the breast. J Ultrasound Med 2003;22(3):263–8.
[17] Hall FM. Mammography and sonography in young symptomatic women. AJR Am J Roentgenol 2003;181(5):1424 [author reply 1424–5].
[18] Morrow M, Wong S, Venta L. The evaluation of breast masses in women younger than forty years of age. Surgery 1998;124(4):634–40 [discussion: 640–1].
[19] Jackson VP, Reynolds HE, Hawes DR. Sonography of the breast. Semin Ultrasound CT MR 1996;17(5):460–75.
[20] Brand IR, Sapherson DA, Brown TS. Breast imaging in women under 35 with symptomatic breast disease. Br J Radiol 1993;66(785):394–7.
[21] Bock K, Duda VF, Hadji P, et al. Pathologic breast conditions in childhood and adolescence: evaluation by sonographic diagnosis. J Ultrasound Med 2005;24(10):1347–54.
[22] Rogerson T, Ingram D, Sterrett G, et al. Areolar discharge and peri-areolar breast cysts in adolescent females. Breast 2002;11(2):181–4.
[23] Feig SA. Radiation risk from mammography: is it clinically significant? AJR Am J Roentgenol 1984; 143(3):469–75.
[24] Yang WT, Dryden MJ, Gwyn K, et al. Imaging of breast cancer diagnosed and treated with chemotherapy during pregnancy. Radiology 2006; 239(1):52–60.
[25] Foxcroft LM, Evans EB, Porter AJ. The diagnosis of breast cancer in women younger than 40. Breast 2004;13(4):297–306.
[26] Hahn KM, Johnson PH, Gordon N, et al. Treatment of pregnant breast cancer patients and outcomes of children exposed to chemotherapy in utero. Cancer 2006;107(6):1219–26.
[27] Whitman GJ, Kushwaha AC, Cristofanilli M, et al. Inflammatory breast cancer: current imaging perspectives. Seminars in Breast Disease 2001;4:122–31.
[28] Gunhan-Bilgen I, Ustun EE, Memis A. Inflammatory breast carcinoma: mammographic, ultrasonographic, clinical, and pathologic findings in 142 cases. Radiology 2002;223(3):829–38.
[29] Caruso G, Ienzi R, Piovana G, et al. High-frequency ultrasound in the study of male breast palpable masses. Radiol Med (Torino) 2004; 108(3):185–93.
[30] Yang WT, Whitman GJ, Yuen EH, et al. Sonographic features of primary breast cancer in men. AJR Am J Roentgenol 2001;176(2):413–6.
[31] Chen L, Chantra PK, Larsen LH, et al. Imaging characteristics of malignant lesions of the male breast. Radiographics 2006;26(4):993–1006.
[32] Edeiken BS, Fornage BD, Bedi DG, et al. US-guided implantation of metallic markers for permanent localization of the tumor bed in patients with breast cancer who undergo preoperative chemotherapy. Radiology 1999; 213(3):895–900.
[33] Dash N, Chafin SH, Johnson RR, et al. Usefulness of tissue marker clips in patients undergoing neoadjuvant chemotherapy for breast cancer. AJR Am J Roentgenol 1999;173(4):911–7.
[34] Alonso-Bartolome P, Ortega Garcia E, Garijo Ayensa F, et al. Utility of the tumor bed marker in patients with breast cancer receiving induction chemotherapy. Acta Radiol 2002;43(1): 29–33.
[35] Nurko J, Mancino AT, Whitacre E, et al. Surgical benefits conveyed by biopsy site marking system using ultrasound localization. Am J Surg 2005; 190(4):618–22.
[36] Snider HC Jr, Morrison DG. Intraoperative ultrasound localization of nonpalpable breast lesions. Ann Surg Oncol 1999;6(3):308–14.
[37] Obdeijn IM, Brouwers-Kuyper EM, Tilanus-Linthorst MM, et al. MR imaging-guided sonography followed by fine-needle aspiration cytology in occult carcinoma of the breast. AJR Am J Roentgen 2000;174(4):1079–84.
[38] LaTrenta LR, Menell JH, Morris EA, et al. Breast lesions detected with MR imaging: utility of histopathologic importance of identification with US. Radiology 2003;227(3):856–61.
[39] Sim LS, Hendriks JH, Bult P, et al. US correlation for MRI-detected breast lesions in women with familial risk of breast cancer. Clin Radiol 2005; 60(7):801–6.
[40] Pavic D, Koomen MA, Kuzmiak CM, et al. The role of magnetic resonance imaging in diagnosis and management of breast cancer. Technol Cancer Res Treat 2004;3(6):527–41.
[41] Blair S, McElroy M, Middleton MS, et al. The efficacy of breast MRI in predicting breast conservation therapy. J Surg Oncol 2006;94(3):220–5.
[42] Krishnamurthy S, Sneige N, Bedi DG, et al. Role of ultrasound-guided fine-needle aspiration of indeterminate and suspicious axillary lymph nodes in the initial staging of breast carcinoma. Cancer 2002;95(5):982–8.
[43] Khan A, Sabel MS, Nees A, et al. Comprehensive axillary evaluation in neoadjuvant chemotherapy patients with ultrasonography and sentinel lymph node biopsy. Ann Surg Oncol 2005; 12(9):697–704.
[44] Mathijssen IM, Strijdhorst H, Kiestra SK, et al. Added value of ultrasound in screening the clinically negative axilla in breast cancer. J Surg Oncol 2006;94(5):364–7.

[45] Somasundar P, Gass J, Steinhoff M, et al. Role of ultrasound-guided axillary fine-needle aspiration in the management of invasive breast cancer. Am J Surg 2006;192(4):458–61.

[46] Greene FL, Page DL, Fleming ID, et al. American Joint Cancer Committee cancer staging manual. 6th edition. New York: Springer-Verlag; 2002. p. 221–40.

[47] Yang WT, Ahuja A, Tang A, et al. High resolution sonographic detection of axillary lymph node metastases in breast cancer. J Ultrasound Med 1996;15(3):241–6.

[48] Pamilo M, Soiva M, Lavast EM. Real-time ultrasound, axillary mammography, and clinical examination in the detection of axillary lymph node metastases in breast cancer patient. J Ultrasound Med 1989;8(3):115–20.

[49] Yang WT, Ahuja A, Tang A, et al. Ultrasonographic demonstration of normal axillary lymph nodes: a learning curve. J Ultrasound Med 1995; 14(11):823–7.

[50] Feu J, Tresserra F, Fabregas R, et al. Metastatic breast carcinoma in axillary lymph nodes: in vitro US detection. Radiology 1997;205(3):831–5.

[51] Stavros AT, Thickman D, Rapp CL, et al. Solid breast nodules: use of sonography to distinguish between benign and malignant lesions. Radiology 1995;196(1):123–34.

[52] Hartmann A, Kunz M, Kostlin S, et al. Hypoxia-induced up-regulation of angiogenin in human malignant melanoma. Cancer Res 1999;59(7): 1578–83.

[53] Srivastava A, Hughes LE, Woodcock JP, et al. Vascularity in cutaneous melanoma detected by Doppler sonography and histology: correlation with tumour behaviour. Br J Cancer 1989; 59(1):89–91.

[54] Less JR, Skalak TC, Sevick EM, et al. Microvascular architecture in a mammary carcinoma: branching patterns and vessel dimensions. Cancer Res 1991;51(1):265–73.

[55] Foster FS, Burns PN, Simpson DH, et al. Ultrasound for the visualization and quantification of tumor microcirculation. Cancer Metastasis Rev 2000;19(1–2):131–8.

[56] Donnelly EF, Geng L, Wojcicki WE, et al. Quantified power Doppler US of tumor blood flow correlates with microscopic quantification of tumor blood vessels. Radiology 2001;219(1): 166–70.

[57] Cosgrove D, Eckersley R, Blomley M, et al. Quantification of blood flow. Eur Radiol 2001;11(8): 1338–44.

[58] Ozdemir A, Ozdemir H, Maral I, et al. Differential diagnosis of solid breast lesions: contribution of Doppler studies to mammography and gray scale imaging. J Ultrasound Med 2001; 20(10):1091–101.

[59] Mehta TS, Raza S, Baum JK. Use of Doppler ultrasound in the evaluation of breast carcinoma. Semin Ultrasound CT MR 2000;21(4): 297–307.

[60] Peters-Engl C, Frank W, Leodolter S, et al. Tumor flow in malignant breast tumors measured by Doppler ultrasound: an independent predictor of survival. Breast Cancer Res Treat 1999;54(1): 65–71.

[61] Lee WJ, Chu JS, Huang CS, et al. Breast cancer vascularity: color Doppler sonography and histopathology study. Breast Cancer Res Treat 1996; 37(3):291–8.

[62] Madjar H, Sauerbrei W, Prompeler HJ, et al. Color Doppler and duplex flow analysis for classification of breast lesions. Gynecol Oncol 1997; 64(3):392–403.

[63] McNicholas MM, Mercer PM, Miller JC, et al. Color Doppler sonography in the evaluation of palpable breast masses. AJR Am J Roentgenol 1993;161(4):765–71.

[64] del Cura JL, Elizagaray E, Zabala R, et al. The use of unenhanced Doppler sonography in the evaluation of solid breast lesions. AJR Am J Roentgenol 2005;184(6):1788–94.

[65] Giuseppetti GM, Baldassarre S, Marconi E. Color Doppler sonography. Eur J Radiol 1998; 27(Suppl 2):S254–8.

[66] Lee WJ, Chu JS, Houng SJ, et al. Breast cancer angiogenesis: a quantitative morphologic and Doppler imaging study. Ann Surg Oncol 1995; 2(3):246–51.

[67] Chao TC, Lo YF, Chen SC, et al. Color Doppler ultrasound in benign and malignant breast tumors. Breast Cancer Res Treat 1999;57(2): 193–9.

[68] Schor AM, Schor SL. Tumour angiogenesis. J Pathol 1983;141(3):385–413.

[69] Strickland B. The value of arteriography in the diagnosis of bone tumours. Br J Radiol 1959; 32:705–13.

[70] Taylor KJ, Ramos I, Carter D, et al. Correlation of Doppler US tumor signals with neovascular morphologic features. Radiology 1988;166(1 Pt 1): 57–62.

[71] Sahin-Akyar G, Sumer H. Color Doppler ultrasound and spectral analysis of tumor vessels in the differential diagnosis of solid breast masses. Invest Radiol 1996;31(2):72–9.

[72] Rettenbacher T, Hollerweger A, Macheiner P, et al. Color Doppler sonography of normal breasts: detectability of arterial blood vessels and typical flow patterns. Ultrasound Med Biol 1998;24(9):1307–11.

[73] Rubin JM, Bude RO, Carson PL, et al. Power Doppler US: a potentially useful alternative to mean frequency-based color Doppler US. Radiology 1994;190(3):853–6.

[74] Bude RO, Rubin JM. Power Doppler sonography. Radiology 1996;200(1):21–3.

[75] Kook SH, Park HW, Lee YR, et al. Evaluation of solid breast lesions with power Doppler sonography. J Clin Ultrasound 1999;27(5):231–7.

[76] Raza S, Baum JK. Solid breast lesions: evaluation with power Doppler US. Radiology 1997;203(1): 164–8.

[77] Milz P, Lienemann A, Kessler M, et al. Evaluation of breast lesions by power Doppler sonography. Eur Radiol 2001;11(4):547–54.
[78] Baz E, Madjar H, Reuss C, et al. The role of enhanced Doppler ultrasound in differentiation of benign vs. malignant scar lesion after breast surgery for malignancy. Ultrasound Obstet Gynecol 2000;15(5):377–82.
[79] Moon WK, Chang RF, Chen CJ, et al. Solid breast masses: classification with computer-aided analysis of continuous US images obtained with probe compression. Radiology 2005;236(2):458–64.
[80] Regner DM, Hesley GK, Hangiandreou NJ, et al. Breast lesions: evaluation with US strain imaging – clinical experience of multiple observers. Radiology 2006;238(2):425–37.
[81] Itoh A, Ueno E, Tohno E, et al. Breast disease: clinical application of US elastography for diagnosis. Radiology 2006;239(2):341–50.
[82] Goldberg SN, Grassi CJ, Cardella JF, et al. Image-guided tumor ablation: standardization of terminology and reporting criteria. Radiology 2005; 235(3):728–39.
[83] Littrup PJ, Freeman-Gibb L, Andea A, et al. Cryotherapy for breast fibroadenomas. Radiology 2005;234(1):63–72.
[84] Roubidoux MA, Sabel MS, Bailey JE, et al. Small (<2.0-cm) breast cancers: mammographic and US findings at US-guided cryoablation—initial experience. Radiology 2004;233(3):857–67.
[85] Fornage BD, Sneige N, Ross MI, et al. Small (< or = 2-cm) breast cancer treated with US-guided radiofrequency ablation: feasibility study. Radiology 2004;231(1):215–24.
[86] Watermann DO, Foldi M, Hanjalic-Beck A, et al. Three-dimensional ultrasound for the assessment of breast lesions. Ultrasound Obstet Gynecol 2005;25(6):592–8.
[87] Cho KR, Seo BK, Lee JY, et al. A comparative study of 2D and 3D ultrasonography for evaluation of solid breast masses. Eur J Radiol 2005; 54(3):365–70.
[88] Cho N, Moon WK, Cha JH, et al. Differentiating benign from malignant solid breast masses: comparison of two-dimensional and three-dimensional US. Radiology 2006;240:26–32.

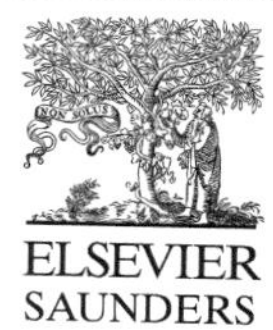

ELSEVIER
SAUNDERS

RADIOLOGIC
CLINICS
OF NORTH AMERICA

Radiol Clin N Am 45 (2007) 863–880

Diagnostic Breast MR Imaging: Current Status and Future Directions

Elizabeth A. Morris, MD

Breast MRI has become an integral and necessary component of any breast imaging practice. The performance and clinical uses of breast MRI are now standardized and much more defined than they were several years ago. In the past few years, great strides have been made by societies in the realm of defining indications and findings on breast MRI [1–3]. The most important development, however, of the past few years was made in the area of breast intervention: new biopsy coils and a choice of MR-compatible biopsy needles are now available, making percutaneous biopsy of a suspicious MR lesion a possibility [4]. Additionally, more imaging sequences are now available from manufacturers with an increase in both image quality and speed of acquisition [5]. Breast MRI is now available in many practices and is one of the fastest growing areas in radiology. In fact, many of our current algorithms in the detection and treatment of breast cancer have been changed by the availability of breast MRI.

The basic strength of breast MRI lies in the detection of cancer that is occult on conventional imaging such as mammography and sonography. Many studies have shown that breast MRI is best used in situations where there is a known cancer, suspected cancer, or a high probability of finding cancer. For example, in the preoperative evaluation of the patient with a known cancer, the ability of MRI to detect multifocal (within the same quadrant of the breast) and multicentric (within different quadrants) disease that was previously unsuspected

Memorial Sloan-Kettering Cancer Center, 1275 York Avenue, New York, NY 10021, USA
E-mail address: morrise@mskcc.org

radiologic.theclinics.com

doi:10.1016/j.rcl.2007.07.002

(Fig. 1) facilitates accurate staging [6–9]. Incidental synchronous contralateral carcinomas have also been detected when screening the contralateral breast in patients with known cancer and may be the most compelling reason for performing breast MRI in the preoperative setting (Fig. 2) [10–12]. In the patient with positive margins following an initial attempt at breast conservation (where MRI was not performed preoperatively), MRI can detect residual disease (Fig. 3) [13]; and in the patient with inoperable locally advanced breast cancer, MRI may provide information to assess response to neoadjuvant chemotherapy (Fig. 4) [14–17]. Suspected recurrence can be confirmed with MRI in the previously treated breast (Fig. 5) [18] and breast MRI is absolutely indicated in the patient

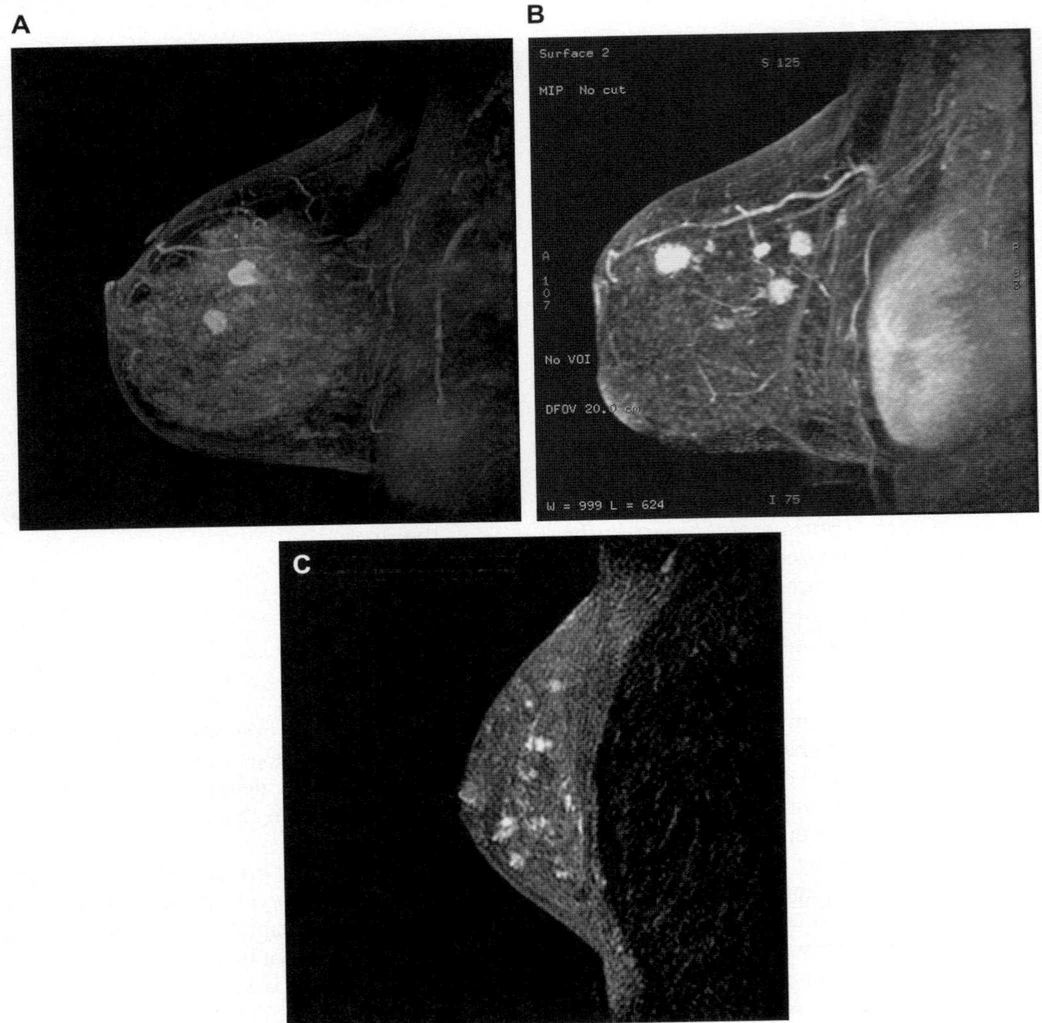

Fig. 1. Extent of disease evaluation. (*A*) Multifocal 43-year-old woman had routine mammography that was negative. Because of extreme breast density she underwent screening sonography, which demonstrated a suspicious lesion in the upper outer quadrant that subsequently was biopsied yielding invasive cancer. MRI demonstrates an additional invasive cancer inferiorly in the same quadrant compatible with multifocal disease. The patient underwent wide excision with negative margins. (*B*) Multicentric 45-year-old woman had negative mammography demonstrating dense breasts. Due to palpable fullness she underwent ultrasound that demonstrated two adjacent solid masses that were aspirated yielding suspicious cells. MRI demonstrates multiple masses extending over 8 cm suspicious for multicentricity. Biopsy of two lesions separated by a large distance was performed to confirm the need for mastectomy at initial surgery. (*C*) 46-year-old woman with prior contralateral mastectomy has routine screening MRI that demonstrated multiple suspicious masses in the remaining breast that proved to represent multicentric contralateral cancer. Mammography was dense and negative.

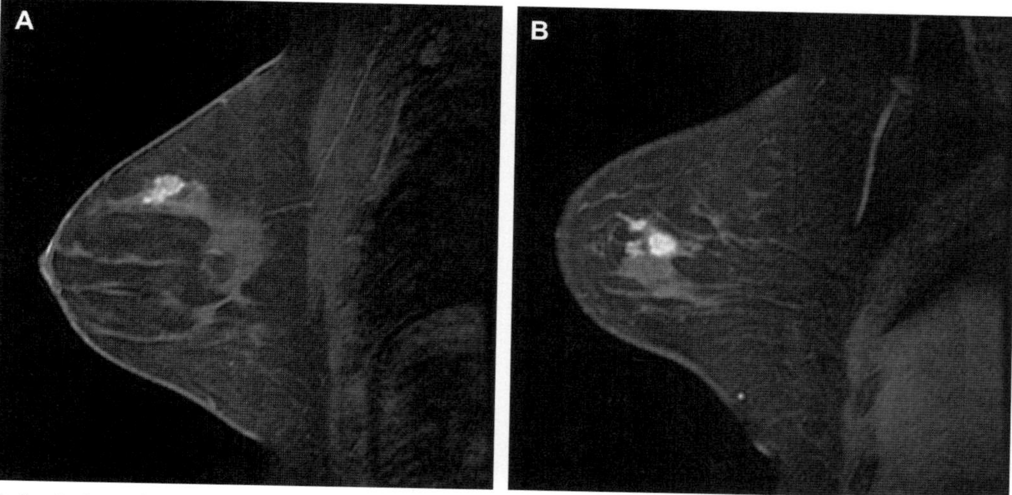

Fig. 2. Contralateral screening of a 35-year-old woman who presented with a palpable mass in the left breast at 12 o'clock. Mammogram was negative but a directed ultrasound demonstrated a mass that was biopsied yielding invasive carcinoma. (*A*) Left breast with known 1.5-cm poorly differentiated invasive ductal carcinoma. Sentinel node was positive. (*B*) Contralateral right breast with unsuspected lesion identified at targeted ultrasound proved to represent 1.6-cm poorly differentiated invasive ductal carcinoma with negative sentinel nodes. The patient elected to undergo bilateral mastectomy with immediate reconstruction.

with axillary node metastases with unknown primary (Fig. 6) [19,20]. The final important indication is the use of MRI for screening in certain high-risk patients (Fig. 7) [17,21–27], which will be discussed elsewhere in this book.

Recent guidelines and recommendations

During the past few decades, as breast MRI has been incorporated into the clinical evaluation of the breast, it became apparent that standardization of image acquisition and terminology is extremely important. The American College of Radiology (ACR) Committee on Standards and Guidelines has published a document for the indications and performance of breast MRI in 2004. Recently, the Breast Imaging Reporting and Data System (BI-RADS) lexicon [2] has added a section regarding breast MRI that has already been revised and further revisions are in progress. These efforts have been important in establishing the standards of reporting and the standards for patient selection. The existence of standardized guidelines in image acquisition and interpretation has helped disseminate this technology from academic centers into the community. Furthermore, the ACR is supporting efforts to establish a voluntary accreditation process for performing breast MRI. This will further standardize the acquisition of the MRI examination and provide high-quality imaging to women at those centers that are accredited. The revised recommendations for high-risk screening from the American Cancer

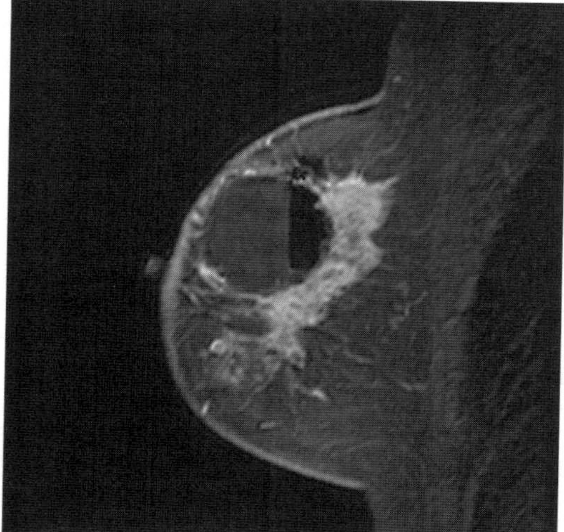

Fig. 3. Residual disease in a patient with positive margins. A 42-year-old patient desiring breast reduction surgery saw her plastic surgeon, who palpated a mass. Excisional biopsy confirmed invasive lobular carcinoma with positive margins. Mammography was unremarkable. MRI demonstrates a fresh postoperative seroma cavity with an air-fluid level and extensive residual masslike enhancement around the cavity compatible with residual disease. Targeted ultrasound was able to biopsy the adjacent hypoechoic area next to the seroma to confirm the presence of residual disease. At mastectomy, 7 cm of residual tumor was identified.

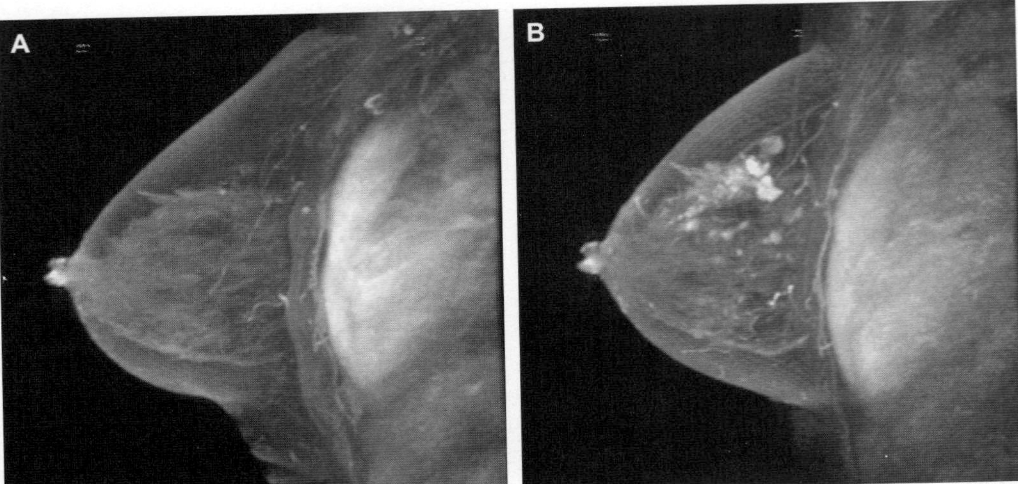

Fig. 4. Complete neoadjuvent chemotherapy response. (*A*) A 48-year-old woman with 4-cm invasive ductal carcinoma moderately to poorly differentiated underwent dose-dense adriamycin and cytoxan, paclitaxel to shrink the tumor for possible conservation. (*B*) Three months later following a full course there is no residual enhancement. Surgery however did demonstrate multiple foci of residual invasive disease; therefore, the MRI overestimated response. The patient was however able to achieve breast conservation therapy with negative margins.

Society (ACS) will no doubt accelerate this important accreditation process.

The ACS recently made a modification in the recommended screening guidelines to recommend annual screening MRI examination for certain high-risk women, which will be discussed briefly in this chapter.

Sensitivity and specificity issues in breast MR imaging

Breast MRI for cancer detection relies almost exclusively on the neovascularity associated with invasive carcinomas. The administration of an intravenous contrast agent such as gadolinium-diethylenetriamine pentaacetic acid (Gd-DTPA) allows these lesions to be well visualized, particularly if subtraction imaging or chemical fat suppression sequences are used. Leaky capillaries and arterio-venous shunts allow contrast agents to leave the lesion rapidly over time resulting in the characteristic washout time intensity curves that can be seen with most but not all malignancies [28]. Detection of invasive breast carcinoma is extremely reliable on MR imaging as the sensitivity approaches 100%. As the sensitivity for cancer detection is high, the negative predictive value of breast MRI is high. If no enhancement is present in the breast, and any possible technical mishap such as intravenous contrast extravasation has been excluded, there is an extremely high likelihood that no invasive carcinoma is present. Specificity is lower than sensitivity and therefore false positives can pose a problem in interpretation. False positives can be caused by high-risk lesions such as lobular carcinoma in situ (LCIS), atypical ductal hyperplasia (ADH), and atypical lobular hyperplasia (ALH), as well as benign masses such as fibroadenomas, papillomas, and lymph nodes. Additionally, fibrocystic changes, sclerosing adenosis, duct hyperplasia, and fibrosis can result in a benign biopsy. With experience,

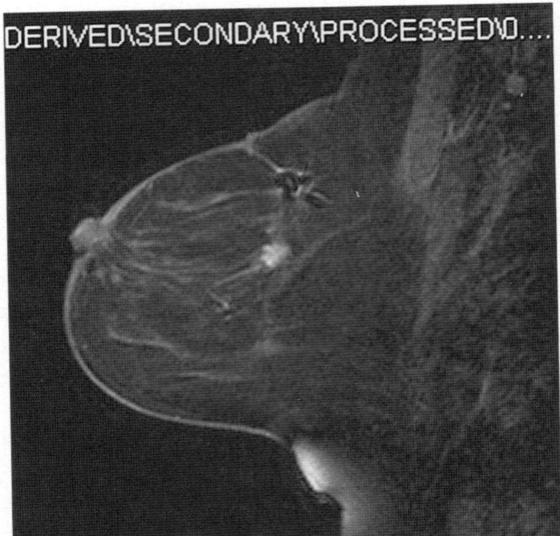

Fig. 5. Recurrence. A 68-year-old woman status post–breast conservation 2 years earlier for 0.6-cm invasive with an extensive intraductal component. Margins at initial surgery clear at 3 mm. First postsurgical MRI demonstrates suspicious mass compatible with recurrence. Completion mastectomy was performed.

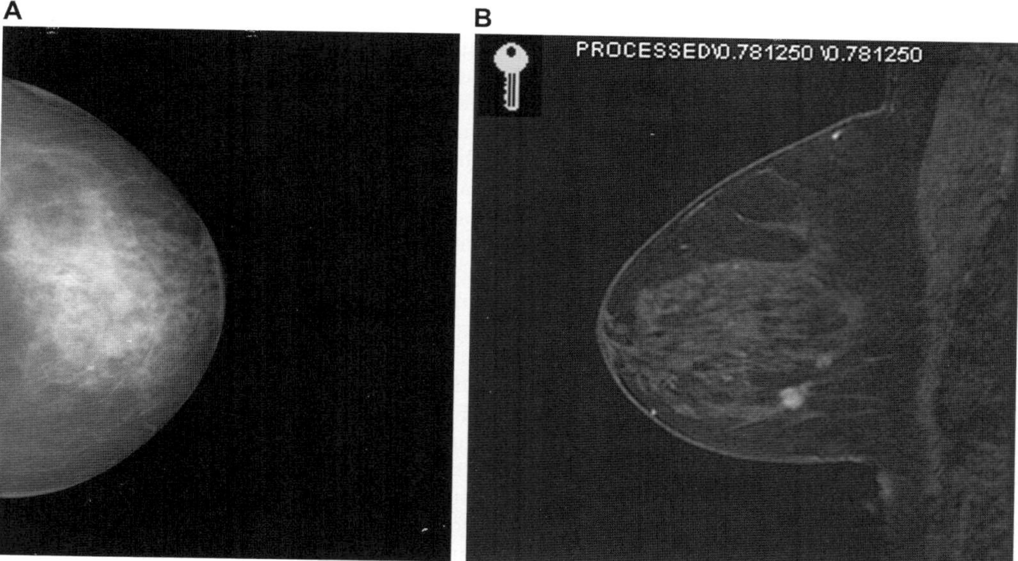

Fig. 6. Unknown primary. A 47-year-old woman presented with left axillary adenopathy with (*A*) negative mammogram and clinical examination. (*B*) MRI demonstrated an irregular mass in the lower breast that was not visible on ultrasound. MR needle localization was performed and pathology was 1-cm invasive ductal carcinoma.

many of these lesions can be diagnosed as benign; however, false positives will always be an issue on MRI as they are on mammography and sonography.

Despite the reputation of high detection of cancer, false negative examinations with MRI do exist. It should be noted that false negatives have been reported with some well-differentiated invasive ductal carcinomas as well as invasive lobular carcinoma [29]. Moreover, not all DCIS is detected on MRI. Although the sensitivity is very high for invasive carcinoma, the sensitivity DCIS has been reported in prior literature to be somewhat lower, possibly secondary to more variable angiogenesis associated with DCIS lesions and the variable

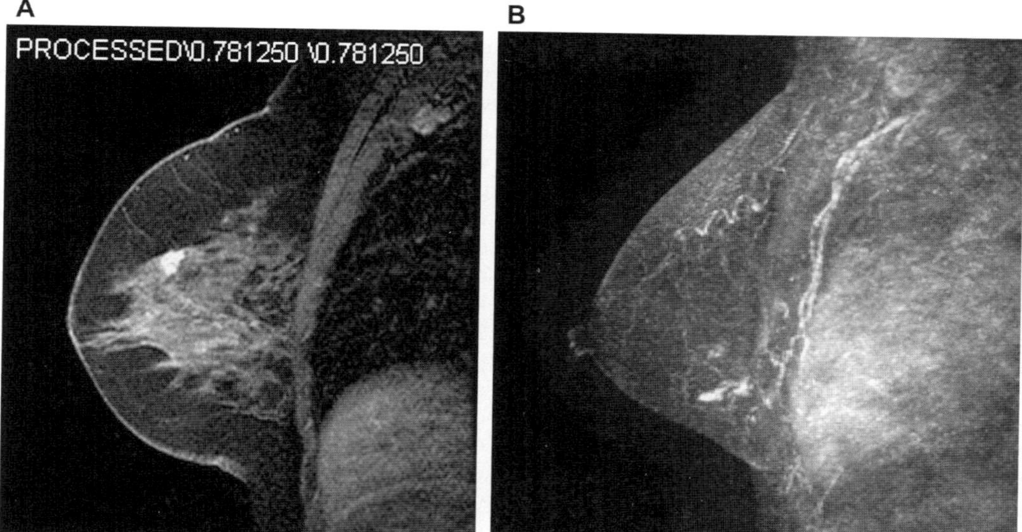

Fig. 7. High-risk screening. (*A*) Small node-negative invasive ductal cancer in a 34-year-old woman with a strong family history of breast cancer (two first-degree relatives). (*B*) Ductal carcinoma in situ in a 52-year-old patient with a personal history of contralateral invasive ductal carcinoma 8 years earlier. New linear enhancement on MRI was biopsied under MR guidance yielding DCIS.

appearance. But, more recent evidence suggests that the sensitivity for DCIS detection may actually be higher than previously reported now that high-resolution scanning techniques are more available and widely used and the patterns of DCIS on MRI are more recognized [30,31]. Morphology may be more important than kinetics in the evaluation of DCIS; thus, a slightly modified interpretation approach is taken when evaluating for DCIS. Although more work needs to be performed in the MR assessment of in-situ disease, MRI does not currently have as high a negative predictive value for DCIS as with invasive cancer. Therefore, MRI is not able to exclude DCIS with current technology and cannot be used to exclude the need for biopsy of suspicious calcifications. Nevertheless, MRI can detect mammographically occult DCIS and is able to play a valuable role possibly in the preoperative assessment of DCIS, where extent of disease may be underestimated by mammography.

Because of the potential issue of a false negative examination, a negative MRI examination should not deter biopsy of a suspicious lesion (BIRADS 4 or 5) on mammography or ultrasound. Mammographically suspicious findings, such as suspicious calcifications, spiculated masses, or areas of distortion warrant appropriate biopsy, regardless of a negative MR examination. The MRI should ideally be interpreted in conjunction with all other pertinent imaging studies such as mammograms and ultrasounds to arrive at the best treatment option for the patient. With these limitations, breast MRI is best used as an adjunct test to conventional imaging, complementing but never replacing basic mammography and sonography.

Preoperative staging

Background

Over the past 30 years, surgical treatment for breast cancer has evolved from total mastectomy in all cases to breast conservation therapy (BCT) in most cases. BCT has moved from being an experimental treatment to the mainstay of surgical therapy as observational studies and randomized controlled trials have demonstrated similar survival between the BCT and mastectomy groups. This has occurred with considerable refinement in patient selection, surgical technique with emphasis on clear margins, and postsurgical radiation and chemotherapy. To arrive at a point where BCT followed by radiation and chemotherapy has resulted in recurrence rates of approximately 10% or greater is remarkable given that is has been known all this while that residual disease is left in the breast. Elaborate treatment algorithms have evolved based on extent of disease evaluation based on clinical and mammographic examination. Surgeons and oncologists have accepted and become comfortable with the probability of recurrence in a significant but small number of patients. When these important studies were taking place, film screen mammography, which has significant limitations, was the standard of care. These days we now have better methods of evaluating tumor load in the breast with MRI, which is far superior to mammography. Controversy arises because the treatment of breast cancer is working well enough and clinicians who are vested in the treatment algorithm do not want to consider the extra information that MRI has to offer. Additionally, MRI has not undergone the rigorous evaluation and study design that these prior studies, many of them randomized controlled trials, have undergone. Certainly, the aim of incorporating breast MRI into the evaluation of cancer would not be to unnecessarily increase the mastectomy rate but rather triage those patients to the more appropriate therapy with full knowledge of the tumor load up front instead of having to guess.

If used carefully, breast MRI has the potential to decrease positive margin rates and recurrence rates in patients with newly diagnosed breast cancer who are candidates for BCT. Breast MRI may also help identify those patients in whom positive margins are likely to arise if surgery is undertaken and those patients who may best benefit from mastectomy as the first-line therapy.

Traditional preoperative planning for breast cancer involves clinical examination and mammogram. Assessment of lesion size, presence of multifocality or multicentricity, and involvement of adjacent structures such as pectoralis muscles and chest wall is therefore dependent on a modality that has limitations and is imperfect. It has been well documented that while mammography has benefits in overall screening of the average-risk population, it is less promising when certain individual groups of women are analyzed, such as women with dense breast tissue. Dense tissue is common, especially in younger women. It has been shown that 62% of women in their 30s, 56% of women in their 40s, 37% of women in their 50s, and 27% of women in their 60s had at least 50% density on mammography [32]. Aside from the inherent increased risk of breast cancer associated with increased density, mammographic detection of cancer is decreased [33,34] where up to 50% of cancer in some series can go undetected, particularly in young women who are at increased risk. This observation that breast density can hinder evaluation of additional disease is important in the realm of preoperative staging.

Breast MRI can give helpful information for staging on tumor size [35,36] and presence or absence of multifocal or multicentric disease, as well as whether the chest wall or pectoralis muscle is invaded [37]. It has been well documented that MR defines the anatomic extent of disease more accurately than mammography. Many studies have shown that MRI is able to detect additional foci of cancer in the breast that has been overlooked by our conventional techniques. Several investigators have shown that MRI is able to detect additional foci of disease (Fig. 8) in up to one third of patients, possibly resulting in a treatment change [7,38–41]. MRI can potentially provide valuable information for preoperative planning in the single-stage resection of breast cancer. By using breast MRI as a complementary test to the conventional imaging techniques, more precise information can be obtained about the extent of breast cancer, improving patient care. There is no evidence that the additional cancer found by MRI is any different or less significant that the cancer found by mammography, ultrasonography, or physical examination [42].

Contraindications to breast conservation therapy

A joint committee of the American College of Surgeons, American College of Radiology, and College of American Pathologists published standards for breast conservation in1992, which have been routinely updated. Absolute contraindications include inability of the surgeon to obtain negative margins after a reasonable number of surgeries, first or second trimester pregnancy, inability to undergo radiation (prior chest radiation, lupus, scleroderma, and so forth), and clinical or mammographically detected multicentric cancer.

Multicentric cancer detected on mammography or clinical examination occurs in approximately 10% or less of cases of breast cancer. MRI is able to detect multicentricity in 13% to 37% of patients. As multicentricity on mammography is a contraindication to BCT, one could extrapolate that additional disease on MRI would obviate BCT. If one compares the type of tumor that is detected as multicentric disease on MRI, it is no different from that detected by mammography. By all measurable standards they appear to be the same. Therefore why would we put more emphasis on the additional cancer that was detected by one modality as opposed to the other? Because the treatment trials were performed with mammography.

Presumably some of this multicentric disease results in recurrence at a later date. Even if we could identify 5% to 10% of patients who harbor additional multicentric disease that could presumably cause a recurrence, this would justify the use of preoperative MRI.

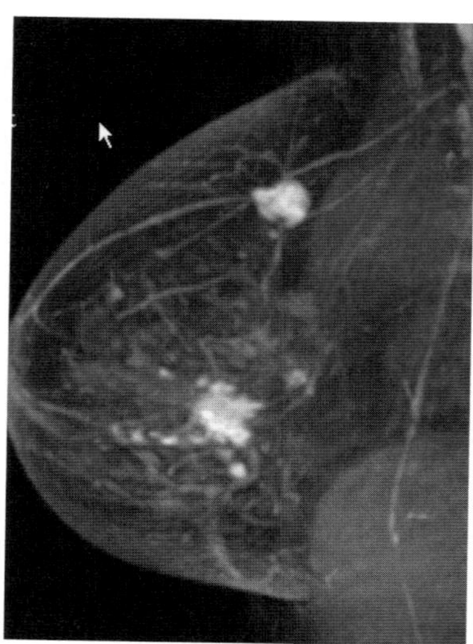

Fig. 8. Extent of disease evaluation. A 54-year-old woman with documented spiculated mass on mammography in the superior breast that was biopsied under ultrasound guidance yielding invasive ductal carcinoma. Additional disease not suspected on mammography or clinical examination in the inferior breast corresponded to a larger invasive ductal carcinoma with associated DCIS (note linear enhancement). Targeted ultrasound over this region with biopsy was able to document multicentric disease and the need for mastectomy as the first surgical procedure.

Recurrence

It has been long known that all disease is not eradicated by surgery alone. The rationale for delivering whole breast radiation (or even partial breast radiation) is that the surgeon has removed the bulk of the disease but that radiation is needed to treat remaining subclinical disease. It has been shown from a study of 282 mastectomy specimens [43] (performed for unifocal breast cancer, assessed clinically and mammographically) that the majority of breasts (63%) have additional sites of cancer that were undetected by clinical examination or mammography. Additional foci of cancer were found pathologically in 20% within 2 cm of the index cancer (multifocal disease) and in 43% more than 2 cm away from the index cancer (disease that may or may not require mastectomy). There were 7% who had additional foci of carcinoma more than 4 cm away from the index cancer, likely representing cancer within a separate breast quadrant (multicentric disease likely requiring mastectomy).

Breast radiation therapy developed to fill a need to treat residual disease and has become a mainstay of the treatment of breast conservation of most patients whether or not residual disease exists. It has been well documented that radiation reduces local recurrence. However, until the use of MRI, it has not been possible to reliably identify those patients who harbor additional multifocal or multicentric cancer and who may be at increased risk of recurrence. While there has been a large body of work showing that MRI can document this additional disease there is a relative paucity of data to document that the recurrence rates are decreased with the addition of MRI. There is only one published paper that has addressed the impact of preoperative MRI on recurrence rates [44]. It demonstrates that if MRI is performed, recurrence rates are lower. Unfortunately the study is flawed in that both groups of women (those that had MRI and those that did not) are not identical. Additionally, the tumor stage and types were different in the two groups. More studies examining this important issue need to be performed.

Positive surgical margins

One of the most important factors associated with local recurrence after lumpectomy is the status of the surgical margin. Standard surgical practice is to obtain clear margins even if this requires a second or sometimes third surgical procedure. It is assumed that reexcision to achieve clear margins is as effective as complete tumor removal in a single procedure.

In a significant percentage of patients, the surgeon may not get all the cancer at surgery. The imaging lesion on mammography or ultrasonography or the palpable lesion may be removed but the pathologic margins come back as close or positive. In these cases the surgeon usually recommends reexcision unless there is advanced age/comorbidities. The purpose of the return trip to the operating room is to further excise (usually blindly unless the postoperative mammogram shows residual calcifications) more tissue to hopefully get negative margins at the second surgery.

Positive margins increase the health care costs, as a return trip to the operating room is required as well as increasing anxiety and concern in the patient. Unless residual calcifications are identified, reexcision is usually performed blindly. Too little or too much tissue may be removed when there is no information about how much residual disease exists. Positive margin rates have been reported as high as 70%, although more conservative estimates report 30% to 50% of women undergoing breast conservation therapy may require additional surgery for positive margins. There is a real potential for MRI to aid the surgeon in mapping the amount of residual disease.

Controversies in using breast MR imaging in cancer staging

Controversy exists regarding the use of MRI to stage breast cancer [45]. Because breast cancer treatment has been successfully refined over the past decades there is appropriate concern about addition of MRI to the preoperative work-up of the known cancer [46]. The general argument is that with breast conservation surgery followed by radiation therapy, recurrence rates are low: reported recurrence rates at 10 years are conservatively 10% [47]. Early local recurrence is thought to be adversely related to patient outcome (likely reflecting residual disease not treated by surgery and radiation); however, recurrence that happens after 10 years is thought to probably not adversely affect patient outcome (likely a new primary).

In a study from Fox Chase Cancer Center [48] looking at Stage I and Stage II breast cancer treated with breast conserving therapy, axillary node dissection, and radiation therapy, the reexcision rate was 59%. Final margin status was negative in 77%, positive in 12%, and close (2 mm or less) in 11%. Recurrence rates at 5 years were not significantly different (negative 4%, positive 5%, close 7%); however, at 10 years there was a significant difference in recurrence rates (negative 7%, positive 13%, close 21%). First of all, these results underline the high proportion of patients undergoing a second surgery for margins that were not clear. Second, the importance of obtaining final negative margins is directly related to a low recurrence rate. Additionally, the results demonstrate that even from a specialty cancer center, recurrence rates can be significant.

Another controversial area in the performance of preoperative MRI has been the argument that MRI results in too many mastectomies and too many false positive biopsies. While it is true that before the advent of percutaneous MRI biopsy there were too many patients having mastectomies for MRI lesions that were not evaluated before surgery and later proved to be benign, the same cannot be said today. If one examines the literature of how preoperative MRI changed the surgical approach, MRI converts a patient to mastectomy approximately 15% of the time [38]. So it is the minority of patients undergoing preoperative evaluation who are converted to mastectomy. If you compare the number of MRI-prompted mastectomies with the number of women who have a recurrence at 10 years, they are surprisingly similar numbers. While there is no current evidence to directly suggest that MRI is detecting the disease that goes undetected, untreated, and ultimately results in a recurrence, it is an interesting question that warrants further examination. It is very likely in many cases that MRI is identifying disease that would likely cause a recurrence. Carefully designed studies are needed to evaluate this important question.

One recent study from Northwestern University in Chicago, Illinois [39], evaluated the impact of breast MRI on the surgical management of 155 women with newly diagnosed breast cancer. MRI identified 124 additional lesions in 73 patients. Change in surgical management occurred in 36 (23%) of 155. Lumpectomy was converted to mastectomy in 10 (6%) of 155. In 8 (80%) of 10 this was beneficial to the patient. In 2 (20%) 10 borderline lesions for BCT were converted to mastectomy on the basis of MRI where MRI overestimated disease. Overall, MRI resulted in a beneficial change in surgical management in 10% of newly diagnosed breast cancers. In these authors' estimation, the detection of additional ipsilateral and contralateral cancers justifies the role of preoperative breast MRI. They also found the specificity improved during the course of the study with refinements in MR technique and increase in radiologist expertise. In their estimation, 10 women must undergo breast MRI to result in a benefit to 1 patient. They compare this to the prophylactic mastectomy data where six women must undergo bilateral mastectomy to benefit one woman. Therefore, as women with newly diagnosed breast cancer are high risk, this seems like a reasonable number. They also note that additional cancer identified on MRI regardless of size should be considered important. If surgeons believe it is important to clear lumpectomy margins of microscopic disease with further surgery to minimize the risk of local recurrence, it would follow that small foci detected on MRI should be considered important and also warrant excision.

Issues to consider in relation to staging controversy

Recurrence rates and positive margin rates vary throughout the country between practices and individual surgeons. Recurrence rates are cited as being low and decreasing, although no standardization or auditing occurs in most surgical practices. Positive margin rates necessitating return to the operating room for further reexcision are also not audited or standardized. Unlike breast imaging where benchmarks are published and auditing of a practice is routine, breast surgical practice is not as scrutinized or regulated. The impact of breast MRI on an individual surgical practice will depend on the positive margin rate as well as the recurrence rate of that individual practice.

From the radiology perspective, these issues raise many questions, such as what lesion size can we safely ignore on MRI. If we are committed to using radiation on all patients, perhaps MRI is too sensitive in detecting cancer in general. For our current treatment algorithms that involve the use of radiation, MRI is likely detecting subclinical disease that radiation therapy would adequately treat. In general, it is recognized that disease 1 cm or less will be treated with radiation. On the other hand, MRI may detect additional disease that would not be treated with adjuvant therapy, particularly invasive cancers that are 1 cm or greater. If we desire to continue in the treatment algorithms that have evolved and that use postoperative radiation therapy, the challenge is identifying what is and what is not significant disease. At this time, identification of significant disease that will not be treated with radiation therapy is not possible and all additional disease is treated surgically. Performing breast MRI to possibly prevent recurrence may have benefit to a significant number of breast conservation patients, namely those who will recur (at least 10% by 10 years). Certainly it would be better to prevent recurrence with the attendant health care and personal costs if one could. Trials that involve radiologists as well as radiation oncologists and surgeons are needed to get information to potentially identify these patients so that optimum care is delivered to our patients.

Examining the contralateral breast in the staging MR imaging examination

Probably the most compelling reason to perform breast MRI in the patient with known cancer is the assessment of the contralateral breast. It has been well documented that MRI is able to detect occult contralateral breast cancer in approximately 4% to 6% of patients. These cancers are sometimes the more significant lesion and may alter the staging of the patient. Furthermore, knowledge of the extent of disease in both breasts allows optimal treatment options to be discussed at the outset with the patient instead of many years later when the patient develops her contralateral primary. To ignore the opposite breast and assume that the adjuvant chemotherapy will treat unsuspected contralateral disease does not make clinical sense when we expend so much energy, time, and resources to treat the known cancer.

Who should undergo preoperative breast MR imaging?

All patients with a new diagnosis of breast cancer should arguably undergo bilateral MRI examination preoperatively. There are several reasons for this statement. First, the high rate of contralateral carcinoma justifies the use of routine bilateral MRI. Also, for those patients with true multicentric disease the appropriate therapy can be done up front. A conservative recurrence rate of 10% at 10 years certainly justifies the use of a single MRI examination at the time of treatment planning to identify those patients who may benefit from mastectomy. Last, the index lesion is better defined on MRI so that the surgeon may have a better chance at obtaining negative margins at the first attempt of conservation. One study from Stanford [49] demonstrates that bracketing of the lesion by MRI may facilitate complete removal of the lesion if a large DCIS component is not present. Therefore, performing preoperative MRI may increase the chance that the surgeon obtains a negative margin at the initial surgery. More data are needed to address this potential use of MRI to decrease the positive margin rate.

At the very least, perhaps the best patients for preoperative MRI are those who are known to have high rates of positive margins and recurrence. For example, young patients, all patients with dense or moderately dense breasts, and patients with difficult tumor histology such as infiltrating lobular carcinoma [50,51], DCIS, and tumors with extensive intraductal component (EIC), where tumor size assessment is difficult on mammography or ultrasound (Figs. 9 and 10). EIC is when the invasive carcinoma has an associated greater than 25% component of DCIS. EIC is associated with positive margins and high recurrence rates. Interestingly, as MRI is more sensitive to DCIS detection than mammography, it may become the test of choice to evaluate patients preoperatively. Several trials are under way to assess this potential use of MRI.

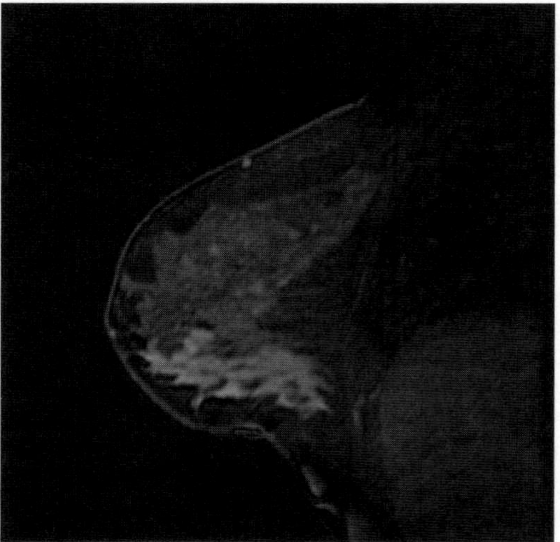

Fig. 9. Infiltrating lobular carcinoma (ILC) extent best shown on MRI. A 43-year-old woman felt a 3-cm area of palpable thickening in the 6 o'clock axis. Mammogram was unrevealing; however, ultrasound demonstrated a vague hypoechoic mass that was biopsied yielding invasive lobular carcinoma. MRI demonstrates a 7-cm area of regional enhancement suspicious for extensive disease. An attempt at conservation was made yielding 4 cm of tumor with positive margins. Further surgery (mastectomy) demonstrated extensive residual DCIS and residual ILC.

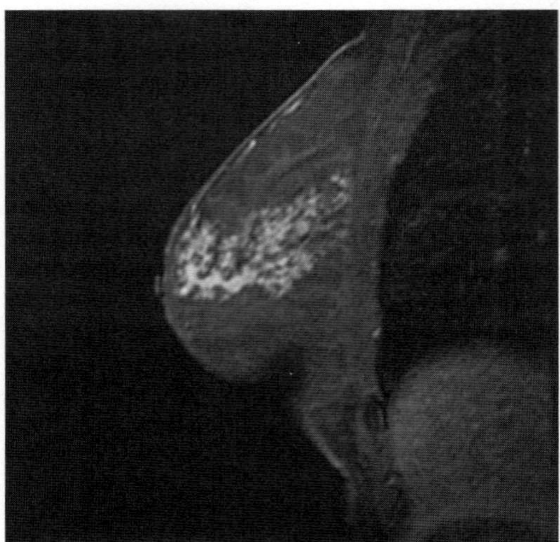

Fig. 10. Unsuspected DCIS in preoperative evaluation. A 57-year-old woman presents with spontaneous bloody nipple discharge. Mammogram was negative. Ductogram on the outside was performed with incomplete opacification of the ducts. MRI was recommended. In the upper outer quadrant of the right breast segmental clumped enhancement was identified. MR biopsy yielded invasive ductal carcinoma and DCIS. Mastectomy yielded extensive DCIS and multifocal invasive ductal carcinoma ranging in size from 0.2 to 0.4 cm with negative sentinel nodes.

Neoadjuvant chemotherapy response

Neoadjuvant chemotherapy is given preoperatively to shrink the tumor before definitive surgery is performed. It is nearly always given in cases of locally advanced breast cancer, yet in recent years it is being used to decrease tumor size in earlier stage cancer as well. The benefit of giving the chemotherapy up front is that one has the ability to determine whether the tumor is going to respond to that particular chosen chemotherapy regimen. A complete pathologic response (elimination of tumor) following neoadjuvant therapy is strongly predictive of excellent long-term survival. Minimal or no response suggests a poor long-term survival regardless of postoperative therapy.

Assessing response to neoadjuvant chemotherapy cancer can be complicated clinically and on mammography. MRI can be useful to overcome the limitations of breast density and fibrosis. MRI may find a role in being able to predict at an earlier time point, perhaps after several cycles of chemotherapy, which patients are responding to neoadjuvant chemotherapy. Early knowledge of suboptimal response may allow switching to alternative treatment regimens earlier rather than later. Unless the response is dramatic, it currently takes longer to predict response, as one must wait to see a volume change in the tumor that is measurable. Volume change may be difficult to assess on the mammogram and physical examination, as fibrosis, a response to chemotherapy, can mimic residual disease. Investigators [14–17] have demonstrated that residual tumor measurements on MRI correlate with the pathologic residual disease following neoadjuvant chemotherapy. Patterns of response are being evaluated in the hope that these findings may predict recurrence and survival. Patterns of response may hold more information because the mere presence or absence of enhancement may be misleading, as fibrosis, a consequence of treatment, may enhance or residual tiny islands of tumor may exist after treatment that are below the detection level of MRI.

Besides volumetric measurements, MRI is able to exploit functional information about the tumor. Kinetic changes occur early in the tumors before volume alterations and another important application that MRI can provide to evaluate response is the use of MR spectroscopy (MRS). MRS evaluates the choline content in the cancer. Several preliminary studies have shown that choline can decrease before a change in the size or morphology of the cancer. It is proposed that choline may be able to predict very early on—perhaps in a day or two—following the first dose of chemotherapy whether or not the patient will have a response [52]. Information that is helpful to the oncologist in deciding the optimal chemotherapy regimen will hopefully give the patient the best chance for response.

Assessment of residual disease

For patients who have not had a preoperative MRI examination and have undergone lumpectomy with positive margins, postoperative MRI can be helpful in the assessment of residual tumor load [13]. Postoperative mammography may be also indicated and is able to detect residual calcifications although it is very limited in the evaluation of residual uncalcified DCIS or residual mass. MRI is able to detect bulky residual disease at the lumpectomy site as well as residual disease in the same quadrant (multifocal) or different quadrant (multicentric). Determination of whether the patient would be best served with directed reexcision (residual disease at the lumpectomy site or multifocal disease) or whether the patient warrants mastectomy (multicentric disease) is where MRI can be helpful. Evaluation for microscopic residual disease directly at the lumpectomy site is not the role of MRI, as the surgeon will perform reexcision based on pathological margins and not based on MRI results.

The role of MRI is to define whether the patient should return to the operating room for a reexcision or would be better served with a mastectomy. Traditionally, a patient can have several trips to the operating room before the decision to perform mastectomy; therefore, MRI may save some patients from these repeated surgical procedures. If multicentric disease is identified on MRI before mastectomy, it is important to sample the lesion to document and verify this impression. A report [13] has shown that MRI identified multifocal or multicentric disease in approximately 35% of patients in whom it was not suspected.

The most appropriate time for scanning a patient to assess for residual disease is as soon as possible after surgery. Immediately after surgery there is a postoperative seroma cavity that is low in signal. Surrounding the cavity there is usually enhancement in the granulation tissue that is formed as a result of the surgical procedure. The enhancement is generally thin and uniform when there is no residual disease or if there is minimal/microscopic residual disease. Bulky residual disease will be easily seen as bulky asymmetrical enhancement around the cavity. More importantly, however, is the assessment of the remainder of the breast for additional disease that would preclude the patient from receiving conservation therapy. The longer one waits following surgery, the more chance there is for the seroma cavity to collapse and cause diagnostic difficulties [53]. Once the seroma cavity collapses the enhancing seroma wall is all that is left and the appearance can mimic a spiculated mass or area of distortion with suspicious morphology and enhancement. When the breast is imaged early following surgery, then these diagnostic dilemmas usually do not arise.

Tumor recurrence at the lumpectomy site

Tumor recurrence after breast conservation occurs at an estimated rate of 1% per year, although with recent improvements in chemotherapy and use of tamoxifen, recurrence at 10 years is under 10%. Recurrence directly at the lumpectomy site occurs earlier than elsewhere in the breast and usually peaks several years following conservation therapy. Early recurrence is generally thought to represent untreated disease that was present at the time of lumpectomy.

Evaluation of the lumpectomy site by mammography may be limited because of postoperative scarring. Physical examination has been reported to have greater sensitivity than mammography in the detection of recurrence. Mammography, however, is still an important tool and should be performed and is able to detect 25% to 45% of recurrences. Mammography is more likely to detect recurrent tumors associated with calcifications than recurrences without calcifications, as the postsurgical distortion limits evaluation for residual masses.

MRI is able to supplement mammography and sonography to detect recurrent disease that may be suspected but not detected by conventional means. All recurrences on MRI in one study enhanced with nodular enhancement in all cases of invasive carcinoma and linear enhancement was observed in the cases of DCIS recurrence. The majority of scars showed no enhancement in this study. Practically, however, active scar can enhance for many years following surgery. Therefore, purely the presence or absence of enhancement alone should not constitute the entire evaluation of whether recurrence is present or not. Morphological analysis and relationship of findings to operative site should factor significantly into the analysis.

Occult primary breast cancer

Patients presenting with axillary metastases suspicious for breast primary and a negative physical examination and negative mammogram must undergo breast MRI. In patients with this rare clinical presentation, MRI has been able to detect cancer in 90% to 100% of cases, if a tumor is indeed present. The tumors are generally small in size, under 2 cm, thus they may evade detection by conventional imaging and physical examination.

The identification of the site of malignancy is important therapeutically. Patients traditionally undergo mastectomy, as the site of malignancy is unknown. Thus, if a site of malignancy can be identified, the patient can be spared mastectomy and offered breast conservation therapy, thereby having a significant impact on patient management. In one study, the results of the MR examination changed therapy in approximately one half of cases, usually allowing conservation in lieu of mastectomy. In our practice, if a site of malignancy is not identified on MRI, the patient receives full breast radiation with careful follow-up with MRI examination.

High-risk screening

An important recent recommendation of breast MRI is in the screening of high-risk patients who have at least a 20% to 25% or greater lifetime risk of developing breast cancer. As mammography has an overall false negative rate of up to 15% in a general population, it is evident that all cancers are not detected by conventional means. The rate of false negative examinations may be even higher in premenopausal women with dense breasts (reaching 50%) and therefore exploration into alternative screening methods such as full breast ultrasound and MRI has occurred. Of the available methods, MRI has proven to have the most promise, mostly due to the high-resolution capabilities, full documentation of the examination, and the potential to detect preinvasive DCIS and small invasive cancers that are usually node negative. Studies that include patients with an overall cumulative lifetime risk of developing breast cancer of approximately 30% show that MRI is able to detect cancer in approximately 1% to 3% of patients.

The use of breast MRI in the high-risk population is limited to those women with documented BRCA 1 or 2 gene or those women with a family member who is a documented carrier but they themselves are untested; any woman with a greater than 20% to 25% lifetime risk (as defined by the BRCAPRO or other models dependent on family history); women with a history of mantle radiation; women with a breast cancer syndrome such as Li-Fraumeni, Cowden, and Bannayan-Riley-Ruvalcaba. There is very little information that exists for screening patients who are at increased risk based on a prior benign biopsy yielding lobular carcinoma in situ (LCIS), atypical ductal hyperplasia (ADH), or atypical lobular hyperplasia (ALH). Furthermore, no information exists for screening "dense, difficult to examine" breasts in patients who are not high risk. There is evidence that women with dense breasts are at increased risk of developing breast cancer and therefore these recommendations may change in the future as more data accumulate. Screening by MRI in this population where the incidence of breast cancer is low would very likely result in too many false positive biopsies to justify its use, although no data exist to support this view.

BRCA 1 and 2 carriers are a group of high-risk patients who have an up to 70% risk of developing breast cancer over their lifetime. The onset of inherited breast cancer is earlier than sporadic cases and the prevalence of bilaterality is higher. Other studies that have included patients at a lower risk than the heterozygote patients [54] have demonstrated that MRI still finds occult breast cancer although at lower rates. It appears that the lower the patient's risk, the lower the prevalence of MRI-detected cancer; however, no screening studies have been performed on the average risk population to determine if this is indeed true. The recommendation to not screen average-risk women with MRI is based solely on expert opinion.

When other reports are inconclusive

When mammography and ultrasound are inconclusive, MRI can sometimes be helpful in the assessment of the breast [55]. By no means should this indication comprise the majority of a breast MRI practice. In fact, the mammographic and sonographic workup should be exhausted before resorting to MRI. MRI should not be used in place of inadequate conventional workup. That said, there are certainly cases where MRI can greatly help. Usually MRI is used in these situations to exclude the presence of disease. Caution should be exercised, however, as a negative MRI in this setting can be over-reassuring and misleading particularly if the conventional workup has been assigned a BI-RADS 0. Use of BI-RADS 0 varies across practices. In our practice we try not to use BI-RADS 0 after a diagnostic workup where MRI is recommended for further evaluation. This is so the entire evaluation does not rest with the MRI results. In the event that the MRI shows nothing, a decision still needs to be rendered regarding the mammographic and sonographic findings. This way the radiologist reading the MRI does not have to reinterpret the entire workup before MRI.

Potential pitfalls in overuse/over-reliance on MR imaging

As with any examination, breast MRI interpretation is dependent on the experience of the reader. A real concern is when inexperienced interpreters generate large numbers of false positive biopsies. Examination of the literature however demonstrates that the positive biopsy rate of MR recommended biopsies is quite high, approaching 45% [4]; however, these numbers come from centers with a lot of experience in MRI interpretation. However, the reputation of MRI as generating too many false positive biopsies is unjustified if one looks at the positive predictive values for biopsy. Indeed, even in a community practice just staring out in their biopsy practice, a positive biopsy rate indicating cancer detection was found in 25% of women recommended for biopsy on the basis of MRI [56]. The biopsy rate is similar to that generated by routine mammography and is certainly better than that generated by ultrasonography [57,58]. What is interesting about the analysis of these biopsy studies is that many of the lesions recommended for biopsy under MRI guidance turn out to be high-risk lesions such as atypical lobular hyperplasia (ALH), atypical ductal hyperplasia (ADH), and lobular carcinoma in situ (LCIS) in 10% to 15% of reported biopsies. Often the presence of a high-risk lesion is an important data point for the patient and referring clinician.

Concern has also been raised about the possibility of inexperienced readers recommending close interval follow-up or biopsies in too many patients. Short-term follow-up recommendation of breast MRI examinations varies in the literature from 5% to 30%. It is clearly apparent that the more experience a radiologist has, the fewer follow-ups are recommended. Additionally, the more comparison MRI examinations a patient has, the lower the recommendation for short-term follow-up. As with mammography, being able to document the stability of a particular finding allows the reader to assign a benign interpretation to the examination in lieu of short-tem follow-up or even biopsy. As patients undergoing breast MRI examination are likely high risk, there may be more of a tendency by the reader to recommend biopsy over short-term follow-up. A minimal number of MRI examinations should be performed by an individual radiologist to gain experience to recognize normal enhancement versus suspicious enhancement. That number has not yet been defined but it is evident that the more examinations a radiologist is responsible for the more comfortable they become with benign enhancement. What these data indicate is that it is important to audit your practice to document the positive biopsy rate as well as the follow-up rate.

Hormonal-related enhancement

As MRI is performed with intravenous contrast, normal fibroglandular parenchyma can demonstrate contrast enhancement [59]. Background enhancement refers to the normal enhancement of the patient's fibroglandular parenchyma. In general, background enhancement is bilateral, symmetrical, and diffuse; however, sometimes it may be focal, regional, and/or asymmetric. Background enhancement may not be directly related to the amount of fibroglandular parenchyma present. Patients with extremely dense breasts may demonstrate little or no background enhancement whereas patients with mildly dense breasts may demonstrate marked background enhancement. In general, younger patients with dense breasts are more likely to demonstrate background enhancement.

In general, background enhancement is progressive over time; however, significant and rapid enhancement can occur on the first post–contrast image even when obtained in the first few minutes following contrast injection. Background enhancement on MRI is analogous to density on mammography in so far as it can "obscure" suspicious possibly malignant enhancing lesions by decreasing conspicuity of enhancing cancers. A description of background enhancement should be included in the breast MRI report because it indicates the likelihood that the interpreting radiologist will be able to discern small or subtle enhancement.

Background enhancement is a combination of both volume of tissue that is enhancing as well as intensity of enhancement. The background enhancement assessed volumetrically is described as MINIMAL (less than 25% of glandular tissue demonstrating enhancement) (Fig. 11), MILD (25% to 50% of glandular tissue demonstrating enhancement) (Fig. 12), MODERATE (50% to 75% of glandular tissue demonstrating enhancement) (Fig. 13), and MARKED (more than 75% of glandular tissue demonstrating enhancement) (Fig. 14). It should be noted that small areas of very intense enhancement may be described as moderate or marked where the volume requirement is not met.

In general, background enhancement is more prominent in the luteal phase of the cycle if the patient is premenopausal. Therefore, for elective examinations (ie, high-risk screening), every effort should be made to schedule the patient in the second week of her cycle (days 7 to 14) to minimize the issue of background enhancement. Despite scheduling the patient at the optimal time of her cycle, enhancement may still occur. Women in whom cancer has been diagnosed and MRI is performed for staging (ie, diagnostic) should be imaged with MRI regardless of the timing of the menstrual cycle or menstrual status.

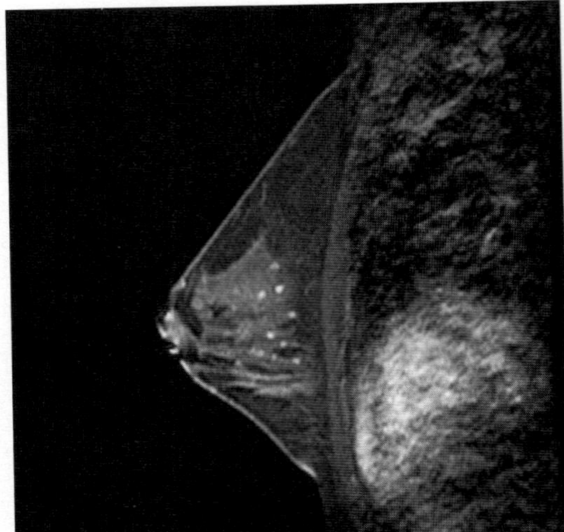

Fig. 12. Mild background enhancement.

Enhancing focus is a tiny, round, pin-point "dot" of enhancement that demonstrates increased signal on postcontrast images (Fig. 15). A corresponding finding is not usually identified on the precontrast image. A focus is distinguished from a mass by a lack of distinguishing features—lack of internal enhancement, lack of assessment by margin analysis, or shape. An enhancing focus may be benign or malignant. Multiple enhancing foci, which are thought to be due in many cases to fibrocystic disease, are more prevalent in premenopausal women and are almost always benign. Foci can be found, however, in women regardless of age and menopausal status.

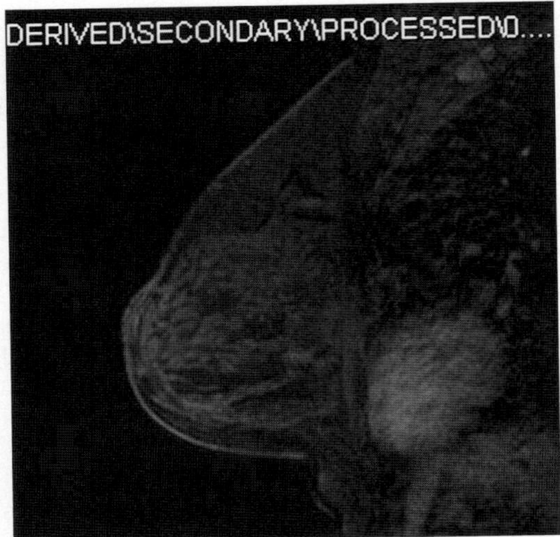

Fig. 11. Minimal background enhancement.

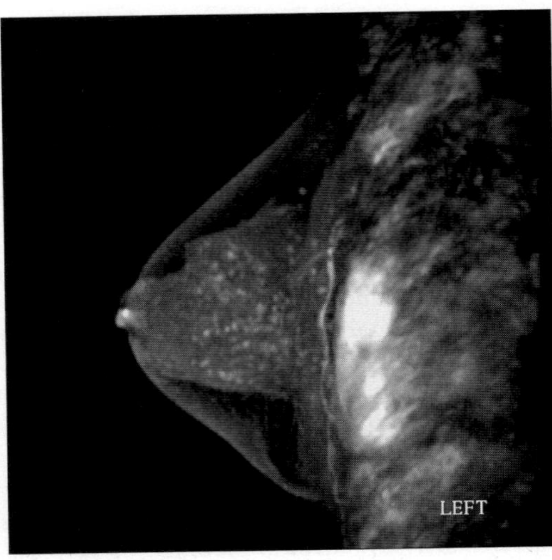

Fig. 13. Moderate background enhancement.

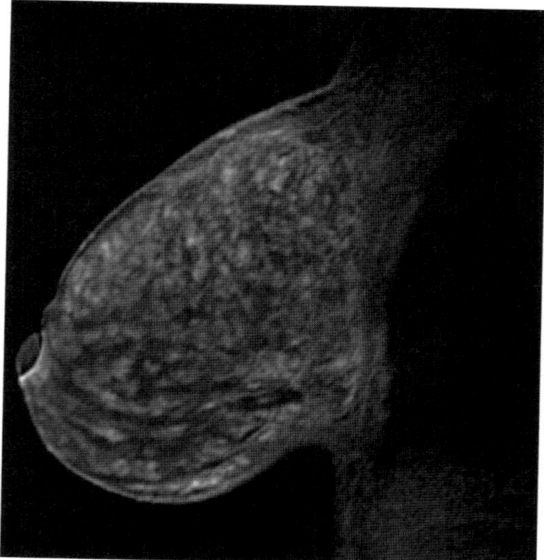

Fig. 14. Marked background enhancement.

In general, foci are less than 5 mm in size; however, applying a strict size criteria is not favored. Size of enhancing lesions can be a helpful in assessing the need for biopsy. A recent study has shown that there is a very low likelihood that lesions under 5 mm represent malignancy [60]. As the size of an MR lesion increases so does the chance of malignancy. Therefore, a helpful guideline that is useful for interpretation of lesions less than 5 mm is as follows: if the lesion is smaller than 5 mm, there should be other suspicious features to warrant biopsy (ie, have rim enhancement, spiculated or irregular margins, clumped appearance). If a lesion is larger than 5 mm, size alone may direct the need for biopsy as a significant proportion of lesions larger than 5 mm prove to be cancer at biopsy. In this situation, the lesion may need to demonstrate benign features to avert biopsy.

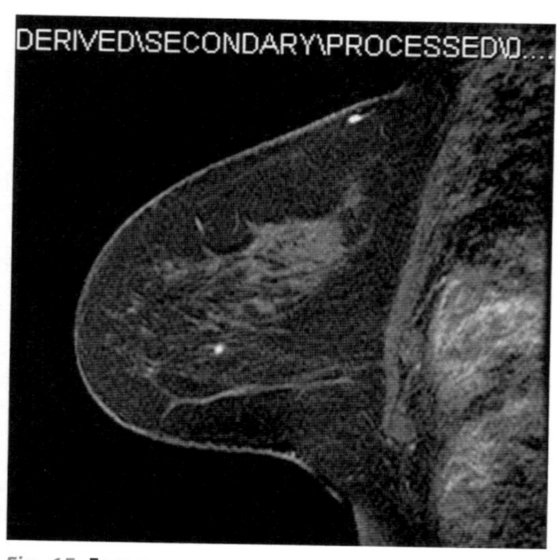

Fig. 15. Focus.

Image acquisition

There is no gold standard technique for performing breast MR imaging. Many techniques are available and widely used depending on hardware and software capabilities and personal preferences. There are however a few minimal technical requirements that should be adhered to when considering your designated protocol. The basic sequence for breast MRI involves a T1-weighted sequence that is obtained within 2 minutes with high resolution ($\sim$1 mm in plane resolution) before and at least 3 times after gadolinium-DTPA administration. High-resolution techniques favor morphologic analysis of lesions and rapid acquisition is used for assessing enhancement profiles. A high-signal fluid sequence (T2-weighted or STIR) is useful for lesion analysis. For example, breast cysts that can be simple or hemorrhagic in addition to myxoid fibroadenomas and lymph nodes that can be very high in signal intensity on this sequence.

Certain minimal technical requirements have been proposed by the International Working Group [3] with the aim of detecting small cancers by assessing lesion morphology and enhancement kinetics. A dedicated breast coil must be used with localization or biopsy capability for MRI-only detected lesions. So far in the literature, only high-field systems have been validated, as these provide adequate high signal to noise and allow fat suppression to be performed.

Parallel imaging applied to breast MRI allows both high spatial and temporal resolution so that neither one needs to be sacrificed. Additionally, these sequences allow simultaneous high-resolution sagittal imaging of both breasts without increasing imaging time. The increased efficiency that parallel imaging affords can be invested in decreasing exam time, improving image quality, and improving spatial and temporal resolution. Parallel imaging is advantageous in that resolution is increased with a concomitant decrease in scan time, artifacts, and acoustic noise. Parallel imaging is a major advantage to those who prefer sagittal small field of view imaging of the breast to axial large field of view imaging. Even for those who prefer axial bilateral imaging, parallel imaging techniques offer advantages and these techniques will likely become the standard techniques in the future.

The suppression of signal from fat is important for increasing conspicuity of breast lesions relative to the breast background tissue that can contain variable amounts of fat. One can suppress signal from fat by performing a fat suppression technique or subtracting the postcontrast image from the precontrast image. For diagnostic purposes, if subtraction is the only method used, misregistration from patient movement between the pre- and the post-contrast images may result, possibly rendering the examination not interpretable.

New developments in MR imaging technology

MRI can provide more information other than vascularity of breast lesions. On MRI, inherent information about the chemical composition of a lesion can be assessed with MRS.

Proton MR Spectroscopy (1H MRS) provides biochemical information about the tissue under investigation [61]. The value of 1H MRS is typically based on the detection of elevated levels of choline compounds, which is a marker of tumor. Proton MRS (1H MRS) is FDA approved and is widely used in the brain and prostate. In vivo 1H MRS studies aimed at improving the discrimination between benign and malignant breast lesions have been done at several centers and have shown to be highly sensitive for all breast cancers, regardless of histology [61–63]. In addition to being used for breast cancer diagnosis, in vivo proton MRS has also been assessed in monitoring breast cancer response to chemotherapies.

A major criticism of breast MRI is that the specificity is relatively low, resulting in benign biopsies. Methods to improve the positive predictive value of MRI biopsy recommendations would improve the acceptability and cost-effectiveness of this imaging technique. MRS has been suggested as an adjunct to breast MRI. Studies performed on 1.5-T MR scanners have reported sensitivities of 70% to 100% and specificities of 67% to 100% for breast MRS. One of these studies suggests that MRS may be a useful supplement to breast MRI, reducing the number of benign biopsies without compromising the diagnosis of breast cancer [63].

Currently breast MRS is available on several vendor MR machines. On 1.5 T, a 1-cm lesion can be analyzed by manually placing an ROI around the lesion and the small area can be interrogated for chemical content. Usually, as lesions on MRI are visualized as enhancement this is done after enhancement. The radiologist, physicist, or technologist must manually perform this task. The acquisition of spectral data takes approximately 10 minutes and the spectral data (in graph form) is later analyzed for chemical content (usually for choline compounds).

Future algorithms for breast conservation therapy

The trend on breast cancer treatment these days to less-invasive therapy needs a reliable modality to map disease. Particularly when partial breast radiation is being tested and used in the clinical setting, exclusion of multicentric disease is imperative as these areas will not be treated with targeted radiation. Additionally, percutaneous treatment options are gaining in interest particularly high-intensity focused ultrasound (HIFUS) where an altrasound bean can thermally ablate tumor without surgical incision [64]. This technology is extremely interesting and may allow more people to have BCT; however, it will rely on meticulous pretreatment planning. The days where all tumor must be surgically removed may be a distant memory in the future.

Summary

Breast MRI has become an integral component in breast imaging. Indications have become clearer and better defined. Guidelines and recommendations are evolving and many are recognized and published. Future applications are exciting and may possibly improve our ability to diagnose breast cancer, improving the patient's treatment options and ultimately patient outcome.

References

[1] Saslow D, Boetes C, Burke W, et al. American Cancer Society guidelines for breast screening with MRI as an adjunct to mammography. CA Cancer J Clin 2007;57:75–89.

[2] American College of Radiology. Breast Imaging Reporting and Data System (BI-RADS). Reston (VA): American College of Radiology; 2003.

[3] Harms SE. Technical report of the international working group on breast MRI. J Magn Reson Imaging 1999;10(6):979.

[4] Lehman CD, Deperi ER, Peacock S, et al. Clinical experience with MRI-guided vacuum-assisted breast biopsy. AJR Am J Roentgenol 2005;184: 1782–7.

[5] Sodickson DK, Griswold MA, Jakob PM. SMASH imaging. Magn Reson Imaging Clin N Am 1999; 7:237–54.

[6] Esserman L, Hylton N, Yassa L, et al. Utility of magnetic resonance imaging in the management of breast cancer: evidence for improved preoperative staging. J Clin Oncol 1999;17:110–9.

[7] Berg WA, Gutierrez L, NessAiver MS, et al. Diagnostic accuracy of mammography, clinical examination, US, and MR imaging in preoperative assessment of breast cancer. Radiology 2004; 233:830–49.

[8] Van Goethem, Shelfout K, Dijckmans, et al. MR mammography in the pre-operative staging of breast cancer in patients with dense breast tissue: comparison with mammography and ultrasound. Eur Radiol 2004;14(5):809–16.

[9] Liberman L. Breast MR imaging in assessing extent of disease. Magn Reson Imaging N Am 2006;14:339–49.

[10] Liberman L, Morris EA, Kim CM, et al. MR imaging findings in the contralateral breast of women with recently diagnosed breast cancer. AJR Am J Roentgenol 2003;180:333–41.

[11] Lee SG, Orel SG, Woo IJ, et al. MR imaging screening of the contralateral breast in patients with newly diagnosed breast cancer: preliminary results. Radiology 2003;226:773–8.

[12] Lehman CD, Gastonis C, Kuhl CK, et al. ACRIN Trial 6667 Investigators Group. MRI evaluation of the contralateral breast in women with recently diagnosed breast cancer. N Engl J Med 2007;356:1295–303.

[13] Orel SG, Reynolds C, Schnall MD, et al. Breast carcinoma: MR imaging before re-excisional biopsy. Radiology 1997;205(2):429–36.

[14] Hylton N. MR imaging for assessment of breast cancer response to neoadjuvant chemotherapy. Magn Reson Imaging N Am 2006;14:383–9.

[15] Partridge SC, Gibbs JE, Lu Y, et al. MRI measurements of breast tumor volume predict response to neoadjuvant chemotherapy and recurrence-free survival. AJR Am J Roentgenol 2005;184: 1774–81.

[16] Schott AF, Roubidoux MA, Helvie MA, et al. Clinical and radiologic assessment to predict breast cancer pathologic complete response to neoadjuvant chemotherapy. Breast Cancer Res Treat 2005;92:231–8.

[17] Yeh E, Slanetz P, Kopans DB, et al. Prospective comparison of mammography, sonography, and MRI in patients undergoing neoadjuvant chemotherapy for palpable breast cancer. AJR Am J Roentgenol 2005;184:868–77.

[18] Preda L, Villa G, Rizzo S, et al. Magnetic resonance mammography in the evaluation of recurrence at the prior lumpectomy site after conservative surgery and radiotherapy. Breast Cancer Res 2006;8:R53.

[19] Morris EA, Schwartz LH, Dershaw DD, et al. MR imaging of the breast in patients with occult primary breast cancer. Radiology 1997;205:437–40.

[20] Orel SG, Weinstein SP, Schnall MD, et al. Breast imaging in patients with axillary node metastases and unknown primary malignancy. Radiology 1999;212:543–9.

[21] Kuhl CK, Schmutzler RK, Leutner CC, et al. Breast MR imaging screening in 192 women proved or suspected to be carriers of a breast cancer susceptibility gene: preliminary results. Radiology 2000;215:267–79.

[22] Warner E, Plewes DB, Shumak RS, et al. Comparison of breast magnetic resonance imaging, mammography, and ultrasound for surveillance of women at high risk for hereditary breast cancer. J Clin Oncol 2001;19:3524–31.

[23] Morris EA, Liberman L, Ballon DJ, et al. MRI of occult breast carcinoma in a high-risk population. AJR Am J Roentgenol 2003;181:619–26.

[24] Podo F, Sardanelli F, Canese R, et al. The Italian multi-centre project on evaluation of MRI and other imaging modalities in early detection of breast cancer in subjects at high genetic risk. J Exp Clin Cancer Res 2002;21:115–24.

[25] Kuhl CK, Schrading S, Leutner CC, et al. Mammography, breast ultrasound, and magnetic resonance imaging for surveillance of women at high familial risk for breast cancer. J Clin Oncol 2005; 23:8469–76.

[26] Leach MO, Boggis CR, Dixon AK, et al. MARIBS study group. Screening with magnetic resonance imaging and mammography of a UK population at high familial risk of breast cancer: a prospective multicentre cohort study (MARIBS). Lancet 2005;365:1769–78.

[27] Kriege M, Brekelmans CT, Boetes C, et al. Magnetic Resonance Imaging Screening Study Group. Efficacy of MRI and mammography for breast-cancer screening in women with a familial or genetic predisposition. N Engl J Med 2004; 351:427–37.

[28] Knopp MV, Weiss E, Sinn HP, et al. Pathophysiologic basis of contrast enhancement in breast tumors. J Magn Reson Imaging 1999;10:260–6.

[29] Boetes C, Strijk SP, Holland R, et al. False-negative MR imaging of malignant breast tumors. Eur Radiol 1997;7:1231–4.

[30] Hwang ES, Kinkel K, Esserman LJ, et al. Magnetic resonance imaging in patients diagnosed with ductal carcinoma-in-situ: value in the diagnosis of residual disease, occult invasion and multicentricity. Ann Surg Oncol 2003;10: 381–8.

[31] Menell JH, Morris EA, Dershaw DD, et al. Determination of the presence and extent of pure ductal carcinoma in situ by mammography and magnetic resonance imaging. Breast J 2005;11: 382–90.

[32] Stomper PC, D'Souza DJ, DiNitto PA, et al. Analysis of parenchymal density on mammograms in 1353 women 25-79 years old. AJR Am J Roentgenol 1996;167:1261–5.

[33] Kerlikowski K, Grady D, Barclay J, et al. Effect of age, breast density, and family history on the sensitivity of first screening mammography. JAMA 1996;276:33–8.

[34] Kolb TM, Lichy J, Newhouse JH. Occult cancer in women with dense breasts: detection with screening US-diagnostic yield and tumor characteristics. Radiology 1998;207:191–9.

[35] Bluemke DA, Gatsonis CA, Chen MH, et al. Magnetic resonance imaging of the breast prior to biopsy. JAMA 2004;292:2735–42.

[36] Achouten van der Velden AP, Boetes C, Bult P, et al. The value of magnetic resonance imaging in diagnosis and size assessment of in situ and

small invasive breast carcinoma. Am J Surg 2006;192:172–8.
[37] Morris EA, Schwartz LH, Drotman MB, et al. Evaluation of pectoralis major muscle in patients with posterior breast tumors on breast MR imaging: preliminary experience. Radiology 2000;214:67–72.
[38] Bedrosian I, Mick R, Orel SG, et al. Changes in the surgical management of patients with breast carcinoma based on preoperative magnetic resonance imaging. Cancer 2003;98:468–73.
[39] Bilimoria KY, Cambic A, Hansen NM, et al. Evaluating the impact of preoperative breast magnetic resonance imaging on the surgical management of newly diagnosed breast cancers. Arch Surg 2007;142:441–5.
[40] Deurloo EE, Klein Zeggelink WF, Teertstra HJ, et al. Contrast-enhanced MRI in breast cancer patients eligible for breast-conserving therapy: complimentary value for subgroups of patients. Eur Radiol 2006;16:692–701.
[41] Schelfout K, Van Goethem M, Kersschot E, et al. Contrast-enhanced MR imaging of breast lesion and effect on treatment. Eur J Surg 2004;30:501–7.
[42] Schnall M. MR imaging evaluation of cancer extent: is there clinical relevance? Magn Reson Imaging N Am 2006;14:379–81.
[43] Holland R, Veling SH, Mravunac M, et al. Histologic multifocality of Tis, T1-2 breast carcinomas. Implications for clinical trials of breast-conserving surgery. Cancer 1985;56:979–90.
[44] Fischer U, Baum F, Luftner-Nagel S. Preopertive MR imaging in patients with breast cancer: preoperative staging, effects on recurrence rates, and outcome analysis. Magn Reson Imaging N Am 2006;14:351–62.
[45] Morrow M. Magnetic resonance imaging in breast cancer: one step forward, two steps back? JAMA 2004;292:2779–80.
[46] Morrow M. Limiting breast surgery to the proper minimum. Breast 2005;14:523–6.
[47] Morrow M, Freedman G. A clinical oncology perspective on the use of breast MR. Magn Reson Imaging N Am 2006;14:363–78.
[48] Freedman G, Fowble B, Hanlon A, et al. Patients with early stage invasive cancer with close or positive margins treated with conservative surgery and radiation have an increased risk of breast recurrence that is delayed by adjuvant systemic therapy. Int J Radiat Oncol Biol Phys 1999;44(5):1005–15.
[49] Wallace AM, Daniel BL, Jeffrey SS, et al. Rates of reexcision for breast cancer after magnetic resonance imaging-guided bracket wire localization. J Am Surg Coll 2005;200:527–37.
[50] Quan ML, Sclafani L, Heerdt AS, et al. Magnetic resonance imaging detects unsuspected disease in patients with invasive lobular cancer. Ann Surg Oncol 2003;10:1048–53.
[51] Kepple J, Layeeque R, Klimberg VS, et al. Correlation of magnetic resonance imaging and pathological size of infiltrating lobular carcinoma of the breast. Am J Surg 2005;190:623–7.
[52] Meisamy S, Bolan PJ, Baker EH, et al. Neoadjuvant chemotherapy of locally advanced breast cancer: predicting response with in vivo (1) H MR spectroscopy—a pilot study at 4T. Radiology 2004;233:424–31.
[53] Frei K, Kinkel K, Bonel HM, et al. MR imaging of the breast in patients with positive margins after lumpectomy: influence of the time interval between lumpectomy and MR imaging. AJR Am J Roentgenol 2000;175:1577–84.
[54] Lehman CD, Blume JD, Weatherall P, et al. International Breast MRI Consortium Working Group. Screening women at high risk for breast cancer with mammography and magnetic resonance imaging. Cancer 2005;203:1898–905.
[55] Lee CH, Smith RC, Levine JA, et al. Clinical usefulness of MR imaging of the breast in the evaluation of the problematic mammogram. AJR Am J Roentgenol 1999;173:1323–9.
[56] Friedman P, Sanders L, Russo J, et al. Detection and localization of occult lesions using breast magnetic resonance imaging: initial experience in a community hospital. Acad Radiol 2005;12:728–38.
[57] Berg WA. Supplemental screening sonography in dense breasts. Radiol Clin North Am 2004;42(5):845–51.
[58] LaTrenta LR, Menell JH, Morris EA, et al. Breast lesions detected with MR imaging: utility and histopathologic importance of identification with US. Radiology 2003;227:856–61.
[59] Kuhl CK, Bieling HB, Gieseke J, et al. Healthy premenopausal breast parenchyma in dynamic contrast-enhanced MR imaging of the breast: normal contrast medium enhancement and cyclical phase dependency. Radiology 1997;203:137–44.
[60] Liberman L, Mason G, Morris EA, et al. Does size matter? Positive predictive value of MRI-detected breast lesions as a function of lesion size. AJR Am J Roentgenol 2006;186:426–30.
[61] Mountford C, Lean C, Malycha P, et al. Proton spectroscopy provides accurate pathology on biopsy and in vivo. J Magn Reson Imaging 2006;24:459–77.
[62] Bolan PJ, Nelson MT, Yee D, et al. Imaging in breast cancer: magnetic resonance spectroscopy. Breast Cancer Res 2005;7:149–52.
[63] Bartella L, Morris EA, Dershaw DD, et al. Proton MR spectroscopy with choline peak as malignancy marker improves positive predictive value for breast cancer diagnosis: preliminary study. Radiology 2006;239:686–92.
[64] Jolesz FA, Hynynen K, McDannold N, et al. MR imaging-controlled focused ultrasound ablation: a noninvasive image-guided surgery. Magn Reson Imaging Clin N Am 2005;13:545–60.

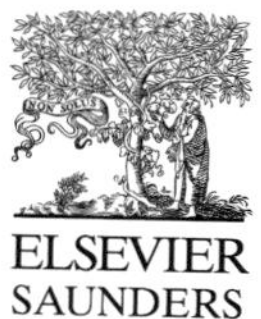

ELSEVIER
SAUNDERS

RADIOLOGIC
CLINICS
OF NORTH AMERICA

Radiol Clin N Am 45 (2007) 881–894

Interventional Breast Imaging: Current Procedures and Assessing for Concordance with Pathology

Lawrence W. Bassett, MD, FACR[a,*], Mary C. Mahoney, MD[b], Sophia K. Apple, MD[c]

The development and now widespread use of minimally invasive breast biopsy has played a major role in expanding the role of breast imaging in the management of breast diseases [1,2]. Most importantly, core-needle biopsy (CNB) has proved to be an acceptable alternative to surgical biopsy [3,4]. The advantages of CNB over surgical biopsy include absence of scarring, no change in future mammograms, lower overall cost, and faster patient recovery [5]. The success of a breast CNB program depends on both the performance of the procedure and the post-CNB management. The article addresses the current procedures for performing breast CNB and the assessment for concordance of imaging and pathology results.

[a] Department of Radiology, David Geffen School of Medicine at the University of California, Los Angeles, 200 UCLA Medical Plaza, Room 165-47, Box 956952, Los Angeles, CA 90095, USA
[b] Department of Radiology, University of Cincinnati Medical Center, Barrett Cancer Center, M.L. 0772, Cincinnati, OH 45267, USA
[c] Department of Pathology and Laboratory Medicine, David Geffen School of Medicine at University of California, Los Angeles, Box 951732, 1P-244 CHS, Los Angeles, CA 90095-17, USA
* Corresponding author.
E-mail address: lawrence.bassett@sbcglobal.net (L.W. Bassett).

radiologic.theclinics.com
doi:10.1016/j.rcl.2007.06.010

Current procedures

The decision to perform an image-guided CNB includes selection of the imaging modality to guide the biopsy and the type of biopsy device to be used. CNB can be performed under stereotactic, ultrasound, or MR imaging guidance. In general, the modality used for imaging guidance should be the one that best demonstrates the lesion. Current CNB devices include the automated large-core (ALC) spring-loaded, rotational, vacuum-assisted (VAD), and total removal devices.

Selecting appropriate imaging guidance

Stereotactically guided core-needle biopsy

Stereotactically guided CNB (SCNB) uses X-ray imaging for localizing and targeting a lesion. Nearly all calcifications and masses identified on mammograms can be biopsied under SCNB with prone or upright tables.

With a prone table, the patient is positioned in a prone or anterior oblique position with the breast extending through an aperture in the table. The breast is compressed and imaged with mammography equipment beneath the table. There is less patient motion and fewer vasovagal reactions than in an upright unit. The compressed position of the breast, extending away from the chest wall, eliminates the risk of pneumothorax.

Upright systems can be added to existing mammography equipment, require less space, and are less expensive than dedicated prone tables. In most cases, the patient sits upright for the procedure. Adaptations in patient positioning allow decubitus or semi-reclining positions for the SCNB. In the upright position, vasovagal reactions are more common.

With either system, the SCNB approach is determined by reviewing the mammograms leading to the biopsy and determining which projection provides the best visualization of the lesion and shortest distance from skin to lesion. Once the patient is positioned, a scout view is obtained to provide information on lesion position in the X- and Y-axes. Stereo images then are obtained 15° from midline in both the positive and negative directions. The depth of the lesion, or the Z-axis coordinate, is determined by calculating the apparent shift of the lesion on the stereotactic images from its location on the scout view.

Once the computer coordinates have been determined, the skin overlying the target lesion is cleansed and anesthetized. A skin incision is made, and the needle is introduced into the breast to the prefire position, just proximal to the target. Stereotactic images are obtained to confirm proper needle positioning (Fig. 1A). The needle then is fired, and postfire stereotactic images are obtained to confirm that the needle is positioned properly (Fig. 1B). SCNB generally is performed with a VAD. A range of needle gauges (7- to 14-gauge) is available, offering large contiguous tissue cores. Although tissue specimens usually are obtained in a circumferential manner around the lesion, the VAD offers the option of selected directional sampling.

When the target is calcifications, a specimen radiograph is performed to ensure that the specimens contain calcifications. At the completion of the procedure, a tissue marker (microclip) can be inserted (Fig. 1C). The needle then is removed, and pressure is held over the biopsy site. The incision is closed with Steri-strips.

Complications are rare and include hematoma or, very rarely, infection. Parker and colleagues [3] reported a 0.2% incidence (6 of 3765 cases) of hematoma in which drainage or antibiotic therapy was required.

Ultrasound-guided breast biopsy

Ultrasound-guided biopsy offers several advantages over stereotactically guided biopsy. Ultrasound biopsy is a real-time procedure, which usually is faster than stereotactically guided biopsy. It requires no breast compression and usually is more comfortable for the patient. Although SCNB is preferable for calcifications, most masses are amenable to ultrasound-guided biopsy [6].

Ultrasound-guided biopsy with a 14-gauge ALC device was first described by Parker and colleagues in 1993 [2]. There was complete concordance in ultrasound-guided CNB and surgical biopsy results in 49 of 181 lesions, including 34 cancers. In the remaining 132 lesions with benign ultrasound-guided biopsy results, no cancers were found at follow-up (range, 12–36 months).

Little preparation is needed for an ultrasound-guided biopsy. The patient lies in the supine or oblique position with the ipsilateral arm raised above the head. Ultrasound scanning is performed with a high-frequency linear array transducer of 7.5 MHz or higher.

Once the lesion is identified, the overlying skin is marked, cleansed, and anesthetized. A skin incision is made to facilitate needle insertion. The operator holds the ultrasound transducer in one hand and the biopsy device in the other hand. The transducer is positioned over the lesion and remains fixed throughout the capture of a specimen. The needle entry site should be adjusted according to the depth of the lesion to enter the lesion without the possibility of pneumothorax. The needle is usually inserted 1 to 2 cm proximal to the edge of the

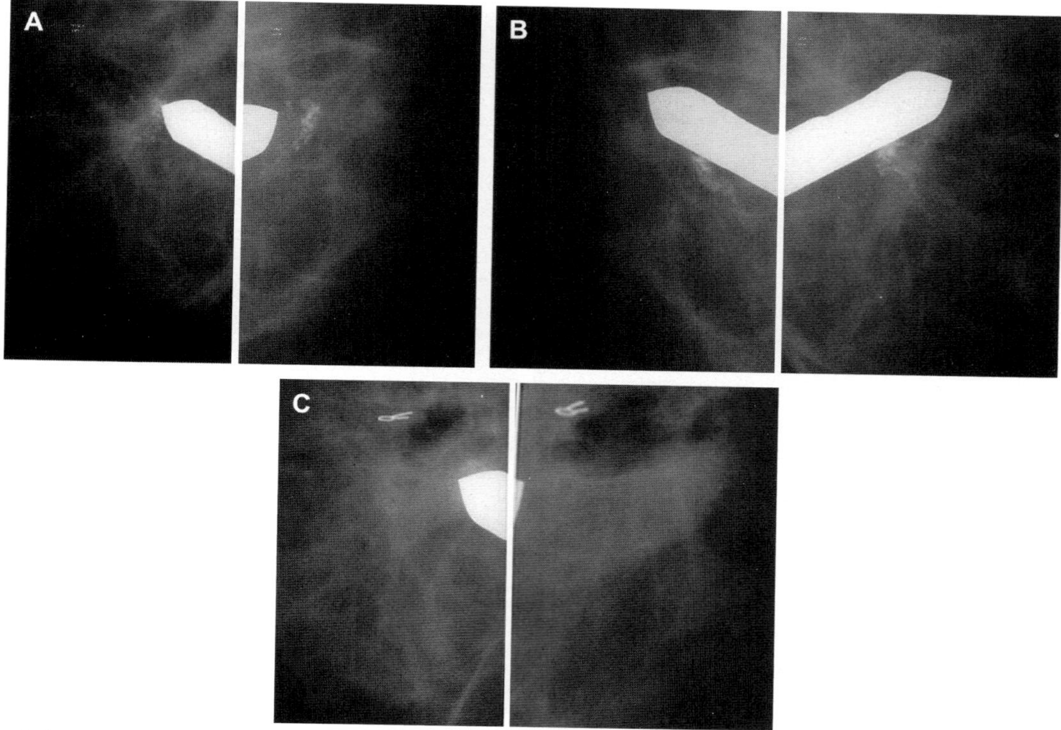

Fig. 1. Stereotactically guided CNB of calcifications. (*A*) Prefire stereotactic images. (*B*) Postfire stereotactic images. (*C*) Postbiopsy stereotactic images. The targeted calcifications have been removed. A tissue marker and gas cavity denote the area of biopsy.

transducer and perpendicular to the plane of the ultrasound beam. The needle is monitored throughout the procedure with real-time ultrasound imaging. The needle is visualized best when parallel to the transducer rather than oriented obliquely to the transducer and ultrasound beam [7,8]. If there is difficulty in visualizing the needle, a sweeping motion is used to identify the needle. The needle then is redirected toward the lesion. In no case should the transducer and the needle be moved simultaneously [8].

When using an ALC device, a 14-gauge needle generally is chosen. The needle tip is advanced to the margin of the lesion, and a prefire image is

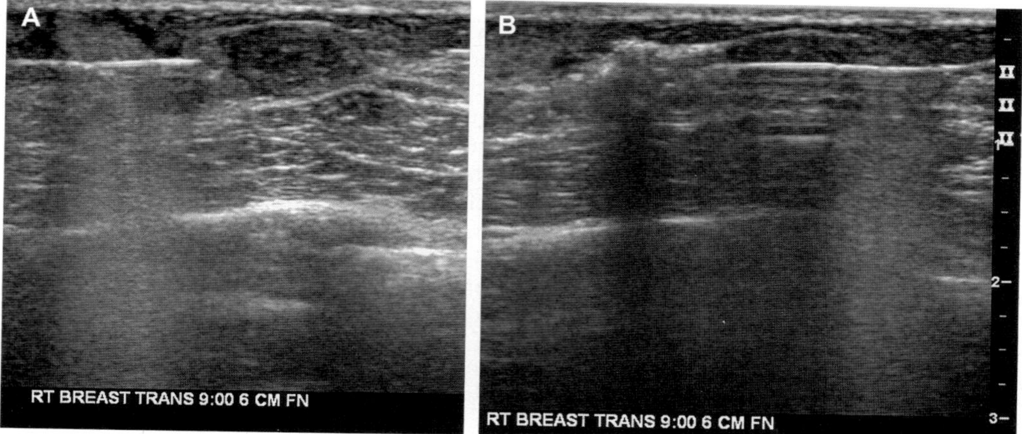

Fig. 2. Ultrasound-guided CNB performed with an ALC device. (*A*) Prefire image with the needle tip at the proximal edge of a solid mass. (*B*) Postfire image demonstrates the needle traversing the mass.

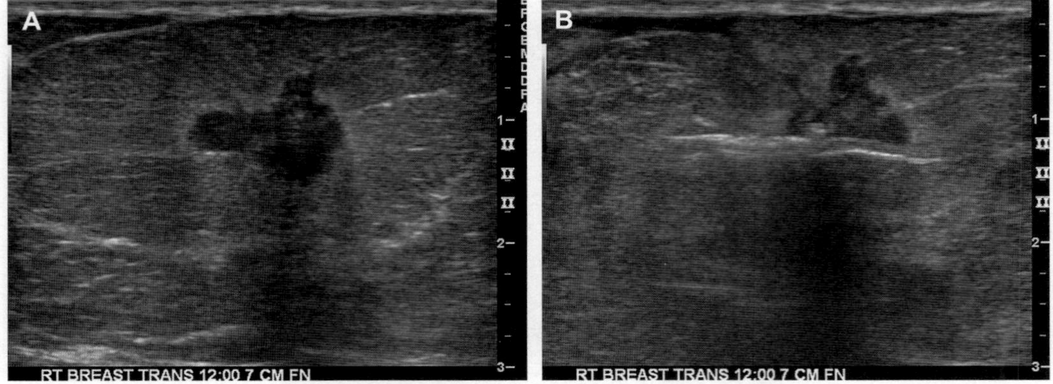

Fig. 3. Ultrasound-guided biopsy performed with a VAD. (*A*) Ultrasound image of an irregularly shaped mass with angular margins. (*B*) Ultrasound image of the VAD positioned inferior to the targeted mass.

obtained (Fig. 2A). Before activating the device, the operator should scan distal to the lesion to the expected postfire position of the needle tip to be certain that no complications will occur. A postfire image documenting the needle traversing the lesion is obtained (Fig. 2B). Usually five tissue core specimens are obtained.

Some breast imagers use a coaxial system in which an introducer (which does not require a skin incision) is inserted proximal to the lesion, and the ALC device is placed through the introducer to take the biopsy. The introducer is left in place when the ALC is removed to place a specimen in the specimen container. Then the ALC again is placed through the introducer, which can be redirected to guide the ALC to a different location in the lesion [9].

A VAD also can be used to perform ultrasound-guided biopsy (Fig. 3). A range of needle gauges (7- to 14-gauge) is available. The needle generally is positioned inferior to the lesion with the sample notch centered under the lesion. Multiple tissue specimens are obtained in an automated fashion. Sampling can be directionally controlled. A marking clip can be inserted into the biopsy cavity at the completion of the procedure.

With both ALC and VAD biopsy devices, direct pressure is applied over the biopsy site after the needle is removed. The skin incision is closed with Steri-strips. As with stereotactic biopsies, potential complications are infrequent and consist primarily of hematoma and rarely infection.

MR imaging-guided breast biopsy

The increasing use of breast MR imaging has necessitated the development of techniques that allow percutaneous sampling of lesions identified only with MR imaging. If the lesion was not identified on mammography or previous ultrasound, targeted or second-look ultrasound usually is performed to determine if an ultrasound correlate allows an ultrasound -guided biopsy. If the MR imaging finding is occult on mammography and ultrasound, MRI-guided biopsy can be used for preoperative wire localization or CNB. VAD biopsies for MRI guidance have improved, and VAD now is the preferred method MR imaging-guided biopsy [10].

MR imaging-guided biopsy requires intravenous injection of gadolinium to localize the lesion (Fig. 4A). Imaging generally is performed in the sagittal and axial planes. As with SCNB, the patient is positioned prone, with the breast dependent in the aperture of a dedicated breast coil. Mild compression is used to stabilize the breast. A fiducial marker is used in conjunction with a biopsy grid, which allows lateral or medial access to the breast in the sagittal projection. After localizing the lesion on sagittal images, the distance from the lesion to the skin is determined by calculating the number of intervening slices. The location of the lesion within the grid is determined, and the overlying skin is cleansed and anesthetized. A skin incision is made, and the needle guide is inserted into the appropriate grid opening. An introducer sheath and trocar are inserted into the breast to the predetermined depth. The trocar then is replaced by the plastic obturator, and imaging is performed to document proper positioning (Fig. 4B, C). The patient then is removed from the magnet bore, and the biopsy needle is inserted into the appropriate location through the introducer sheath. A tissue marker is placed at the completion of the biopsy to document the location of the biopsy site (Fig. 4D). If subsequent surgical intervention is needed, mammography or ultrasound guidance can be used, based on localization of the tissue marker.

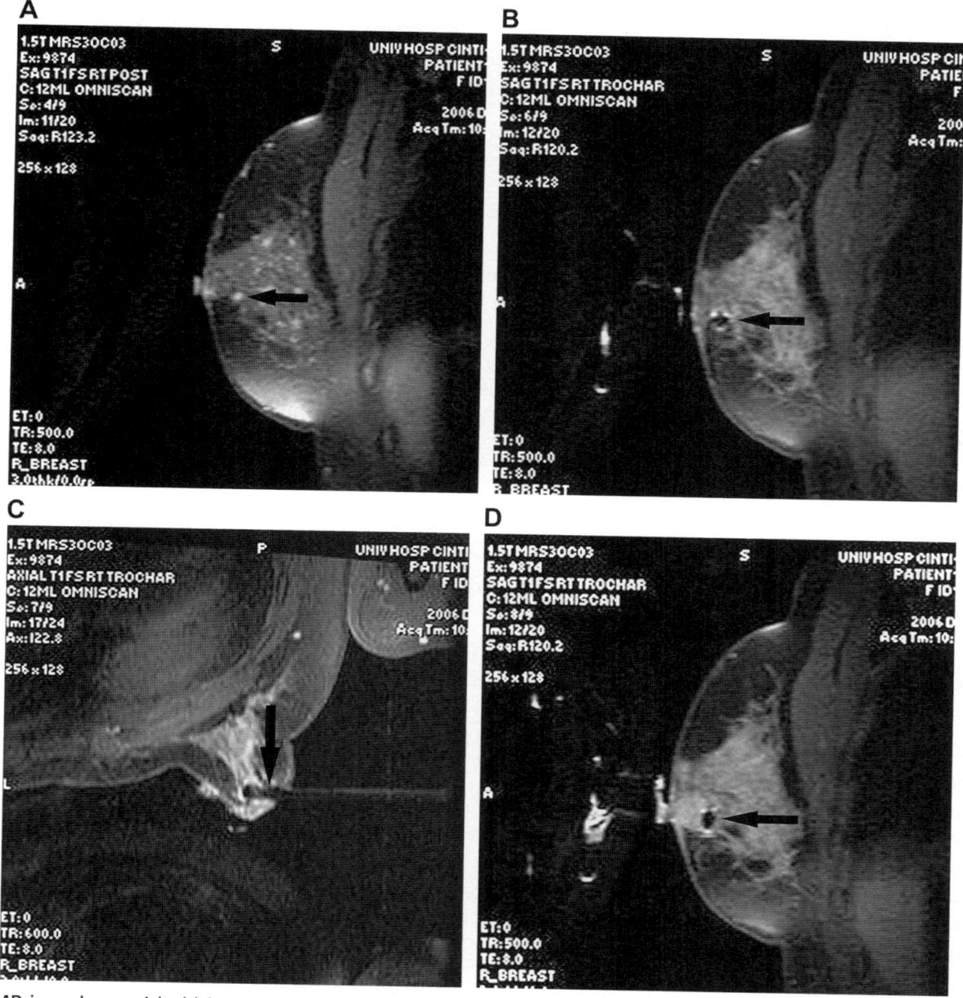

Fig. 4. MR imaging-guided biopsy performed with a VAD. (*A*) T1-weighted contrast-enhanced sagittal image of a focus of enhancement (*arrow*). (*B*) T1-weighted sagittal image demonstrates a signal void (*arrow*) corresponding to the obturator. (*C*) T1-weighted axial image demonstrates the length of the obturator (*arrow*). (*D*) T1-weighted sagittal image at completion of the biopsy. The focus of enhancement is no longer visualized. Signal void (*arrow*) indicates the tissue marker and gas.

Selecting the appropriate acquisition device for breast core-needle biopsy

Automated large-core biopsy

The ALC was introduced in Sweden in 1982. It was adapted by Parker for SCNB in 1990 [1] and for ultrasound-guided biopsies in 1993 [2].

The ALC has a two-step firing mechanism. First the inner stylet is fired into the lesion. Then the outer cutting cannula fires over the stylet to cut the tissue specimen. The needles range is size from 20- to 14-gauge, but usually a 14-gauge needle is used. Today the ALC is used primarily for ultrasound-guided biopsies. The VAD has largely replaced the ALC for stereotactic and MR-guided biopsies.

A new CNB device is the automated rotational core biopsy system. Initially, a 19-gauge needle is fired into the lesion under ultrasound guidance. A carbon dioxide canister in the hand piece is used to freeze, and therefore immobilize, this needle within the lesion. An automated 10-gauge cutting cannula then is rotated over the small needle to obtain tissue samples.

The ALC and rotational devices require a multipass technique with multiple insertions to obtain sufficient tissue samples. Depending on the gauge of the needle used and the number of tissue cores obtained, underestimation of cancer can occur [11].

Vacuum-assisted device

The VAD, developed in the mid-1990s, offers a number of advantages. It allows single insertion of the needle and directional sampling. The primary advantage of the VAD is the larger amount of tissue acquired, resulting in more accurate pathology results and fewer upgrades at the time of surgical excision.

VAD needles range from 14- to 7-gauge. The VAD can be used with stereotactic, ultrasound, or MR imaging guidance. The VAD is positioned in the breast at the site of the lesion. The vacuum is activated, pulling the tissue into the biopsy aperture. A rotating cutter then is advanced through the needle, shearing off the tissue specimen. The cutter is withdrawn to retrieve the tissue specimen, and the needle is rotated to acquire the next specimen in another area of the lesion. Sampling with this technology allows rapid acquisition of multiple large tissue specimens.

Total removal devices

A breast biopsy system that removes a single intact large tissue specimen has been developed recently. This one-pass system that collects the specimen in approximately 10 seconds can be used with stereotactic or ultrasound guidance. The probe is inserted into the breast through an 8-mm skin incision. Radiofrequency is used to advance the device through the breast to the lesion. Five struts then open to form a basket that circumscribes the lesion. The specimen is withdrawn through the entry channel, which collapses after the specimen is withdrawn. Specimens range in weight from 1 to 3 g and are 10 to 20 mm in diameter, depending on the size of the device.

The advantage of this system is that it retrieves an intact specimen, preserving the architecture of the lesion. In theory, histologic analysis of this sample should be simpler than evaluating multiple core specimens taken throughout the lesion. Furthermore, retrieving an intact specimen could improve the ability to assess the margins of a lesion. Clinical studies currently are evaluating these potential advantages. Two studies have demonstrated that underestimation rates for ductal carcinoma in situ (DCIS) and atypical ductal hyperplasia (ADH) at subsequent surgery are lower for a total removal system (3%–20%) than for a VAD (11%–16%) [12,13]. There are potential therapeutic applications for this system, but greater experience with this new device is required.

Assessing for concordance with pathology

The imaging–pathology team

A successful imaging-guided CNB program requires a strong working relationship between the radiologist and pathologist. The pathologist must be aware of sampling limitations and problem lesions and must have adequate clinical information when evaluating CNB specimens. To assist the pathologist, the authors have devised a modified pathology requisition for breast CNB (Fig. 5). The information provided includes location of the lesion (crucial if there is more than one biopsy site), relevant imaging findings, and the likelihood of malignancy. To communicate the likelihood of malignancy, the authors use an option in the most recent American College of Radiology Breast Imaging Reporting and Data System (ACR BI-RADS) [14]. Using this option, the final assessment category 4 (suspicious), to which the majority of recommended biopsies are assigned and in which the likelihood of malignancy ranges from 2% to 95%, is divided into three subcategories: 4A, low suspicion for malignancy (< 10%); 4B, moderate suspicion (10%–50%); and 4C, high suspicion (50%–95%). Because these subcategories have not yet been incorporated into the Mammography Quality Standards Act, the imaging report final assessment should be category 4, suspicious, with an added comment that the findings suggest category 4A (low suspicion), category 4B (moderate suspicion), or category 4C (high suspicion).

Normal anatomy

In assessing for concordance, it is important to understand certain aspects of normal breast anatomy. Most breast lesions arise in the ductal system. There are 10 to 12 duct systems (lobes), each beginning as a lactiferous duct with an orifice at the nipple. Within the breast the lactiferous ducts divide into the excretory ducts, which divide and subdivide, finally ending in the terminal duct lobular unit (Fig. 6). The majority of breast cancers arise at the terminal duct lobular unit.

Assessing for concordance

Assessment for concordance of imaging and pathology findings is based on the "triple test," first developed for breast fine-needle aspiration biopsy and standardized under the auspices of the National Cancer Institute in 1996 [15]. Based on the triple test, an excisional biopsy should be performed if there is any discordance between clinical, imaging, or pathology findings.

Because most CNBs are performed for nonpalpable lesions, assessment for concordance usually

Breast CNB Pathology Requisition

Patient ID number: *201-68-22* **Name:** *Jones, Mary J*

Ordering physician: *L Bassett* **ID #:** *04203*

Referring physician: *D.Smith* **ID #:** *01868*

Phone: *310-825-7106*

Location of lesion: *R 11:00, middle 1/3 depth*

Abnormality: Mass ___ Calcifications √ Other ___

Most likely diagnosis: Benign ___ Malignant √

BI-RADS Final Assessment: 2 __ 3__ 4A __ 4B __ 4C √ 5 __

Biopsy specimen contains calcifications: Yes √ No ___

Calcs in teabag in specimen container: Yes √ No ___

Comments:

Suspect DCIS. Patient has a family history of breast cancer.

She has had several benign biopsies but theses calcifications are more worrisome.

Fig. 5. Breast CNB pathology requisition designed to provide the pathologist the essential information needed to optimize interpretation of CNB specimens.

involves comparing imaging and pathology findings. If these are discordant, excisional biopsy should be performed. The assessment for concordance can be performed by several methods:

1. A case-by-case or scheduled meeting with the pathologist
2. Reviewing imaging findings alongside the pathology report

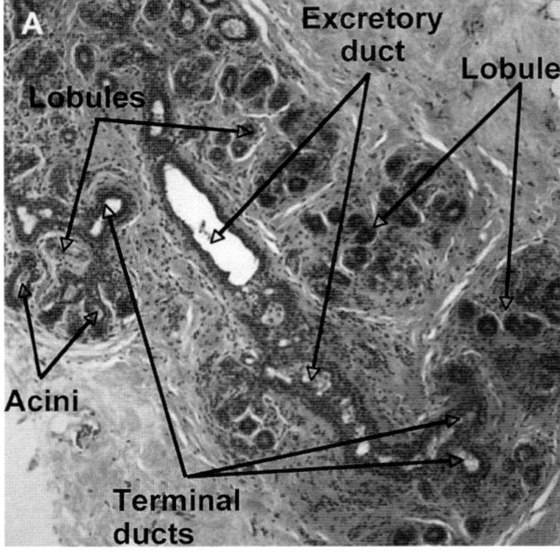

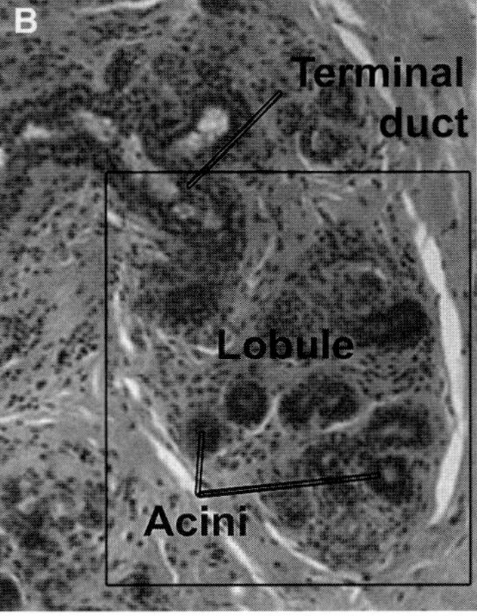

Fig. 6. Normal anatomy of an excretory duct ending at the terminal duct lobular unit (TDLU). (*A*) Hematoxylin and eosin stain (original magnification × 200). The branching excretory ducts end as terminal ducts that enter the lobules. In the lobule the terminal ducts divide into small ductules that enter the acini (where fluid, or milk during lactation, is produced). (*B*) Hematoxylin and eosin stain (original magnification × 400). The TDLU includes the terminal duct and its branches ending in the acini. The lobule is surrounded by a loose connective tissue that allows expansion of the lobule when fluid or milk is produced in the acini. Greater than 90% of cancers arise in the TDLU.

3. Comparing imaging reports and pathology reports for concordance

Images documented during the imaging-guided CNB can be reviewed to verify that the lesion was targeted accurately (eg, for ultrasound-guided CNB, documentation that the ALC device traversed the lesion or that the VAD was properly placed) and that post-CNB images verify that the lesion was sampled. For SCNB of calcifications, specimen radiographs and the pathology findings should document the presence of calcifications.

After the assessment for concordance has been completed, a management plan is devised. Concordant malignant cases are referred to a surgeon for definitive treatment. Concordant benign cases are placed in a follow-up imaging protocol, because CNB has a 2% false-negative rate [16]. One-year follow-up is an alternative interval for "definite benign" results (eg, imaging indicated typical fibroadenoma, and pathology showed fibroadenoma).

Limitations of core-needle biopsy

The major limitation of CNB is sampling error. If pathology results do not explain imaging findings adequately (discordance), excisional biopsy should be performed. In addition, several benign and high-risk CNB pathology findings have been linked to potential underestimation of disease. In other words, some benign pathology findings have been shown to coexist with carcinoma, and a cancer might be missed because of sampling error. Discordance between imaging and pathology or potential underestimation of disease requires excisional biopsy.

Underestimation of disease

Which CNB benign histology diagnoses justify an excisional biopsy to rule out coexistent malignancy leading to potential underestimation of disease? It is well established that a CNB revealing ADH requires excisional biopsy. The need for excisional biopsy for some other CNB diagnoses, including lobular neoplasia, radial scar, papillary lesions, and columnar cell lesions, has been controversial [17,18]. Underestimation of disease also occurs when a CNB diagnosis is DCIS but subsequent surgery reveals invasive cancer.

Atypical ductal hyperplasia

ADH is a proven high-risk lesion with potential for CNB underestimation of disease. On mammography ADH presents as calcifications, sometimes identical to DCIS. On histology, ADH shows features that lie midway between usual ductal hyperplasia and DCIS. There are several reasons surgical excision should be performed after a CNB diagnosis of ADH. First, distinguishing advanced ADH from low-grade DCIS can be difficult for the most experienced pathologists [19,20]. Secondly, DCIS may lie at the periphery of ADH [21,22]. Underestimation rates for a CNB showing ADH, range from 15% to 50%. VADs reduce the incidence of underestimation [23], but even with the use of an 11-gauge VAD, underestimation of DCIS or invasive carcinoma has been reported in 20% to 25% of CNB diagnoses of ADH. Therefore, there is consensus that ADH on CNB mandates excisional biopsy [11].

Lobular neoplasia

Lobular neoplasia is a spectrum of lesions including lobular carcinoma in situ (LCIS), atypical lobular hyperplasia (ALH), and ductal involvement with cells of ALH. On histology, LCIS is characterized by distention of the lobules with proliferating small, uniform cells; if the proliferating cells do not distend the lobule, the diagnosis is ALH (Fig. 7). Lobular neoplasia typically does not have clinical or imaging findings and is an incidental finding at biopsy [24].

Traditional teaching was that lobular neoplasia is not a direct precursor of malignancy but rather is a marker that identifies women who have an increased risk of developing breast cancer in the future (a three times greater risk for ADH and a ten times greater risk for LCIS); the increased risk is equal for either breast and at any location. Thus, it would be reasonable to recommend excisional biopsy after a CNB with lobular neoplasia [25].

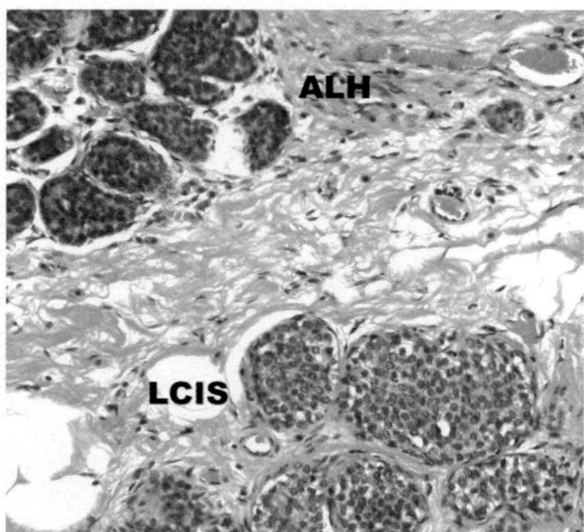

Fig. 7. Hematoxylin and eosin stain (original magnification × 400). Lobular neoplasia. Atypical lobular hyperplasia (ALH) characterized by proliferation of small uniform cells within the lobule and adjacent lobular carcinoma in situ (LCIS) characterized by increased proliferation of small uniform cells resulting in distention of the acini.

A report of 14 cases of LCIS or ALH on CNB, however, revealed that 3 (21%) of 14 patients who had a CNB diagnosis of LCIS had DCIS or invasive carcinoma at excisional biopsy [26]. Among six CNBs with ALH, one had infiltrating lobular carcinoma. The conclusion was that excisional biopsy should be considered after CNB diagnosis of LCIS and discordant ALH.

Traditional teaching about lobular neoplasia has been challenged. A retrospective study by Page and colleagues [27] found that the distribution of cancers that developed after a CNB showing lobular neoplasia was not bilaterally equal. If lobular neoplasia was diagnosed on biopsy, subsequent cancers were three times more likely to develop in the ipsilateral breast. This report suggests that lobular neoplasia is intermediate between a local precursor and a generalized risk factor for breast cancer.

A review of 6081 consecutive patients who underwent CNB identified 35 (0.58%) who had LCIS or ALH [28]. In 15 patients who had LCIS at CNB, 4 (27%) were upgraded to DCIS or invasive cancer at excisional biopsy. In 20 patients who had ALH, 2 (10%) were upgraded to DCIS at surgical excision. The CNB underestimation of lobular neoplasia after excisional biopsy (17%) was not significantly different from that for ADH. Excisional biopsy was recommended when CNB showed LCIS or ADH.

A recent review of 27 patients who had lobular neoplasia as the most severe pathology at SCNB (with an 11-gauge VAD and a mean of 13 specimens) showed carcinoma at surgical excision in 5 cases (19%) [29]. No mammography features allowed distinction between the patients whose lesions were upgraded at the time of surgery and those whose lesions were not upgraded.

Furthermore, histologic features of LCIS and DCIS can overlap. Usual "bland" LCIS has small, uniform cells, but in some cases the cells may have cytologic pleomorphism suggesting DCIS. In addition, "cancerization of the lobules" can occur when DCIS extends retrograde from nearby ducts into the lobules. If the CNB diagnosis of LCIS versus DCIS is uncertain, an E-cadherin stain can be applied [30]. E-cadherin stain, taken up by DCIS but not by LCIS, can be used to differentiate ductal from lobular phenotypes (Fig. 8).

Radial scar

A radial scar is a nonpalpable, proliferative lesion identified on mammography as an architectural distortion that cannot be differentiated from invasive carcinoma (Fig. 9A) [31]. At pathology, radial scars harbor an array of proliferative elements. The center of the lesion undergoes fibrosis and elastosis, with resultant retraction of the periphery. As a result, fibrous strands with distorted entrapped ducts arranged in a radiating pattern are seen (Fig. 9B).

At one time it was believed that radial scars were high-risk lesions that could evolve to tubular carcinoma. Although experts no longer believe that a radial scar is a precursor of tubular carcinoma, it does increase the risk of developing breast cancer, and the risk increases with a larger size of the radial scar [32–34]. Some experts recommend excisional biopsy for all radial scars diagnosed on CNB [35].

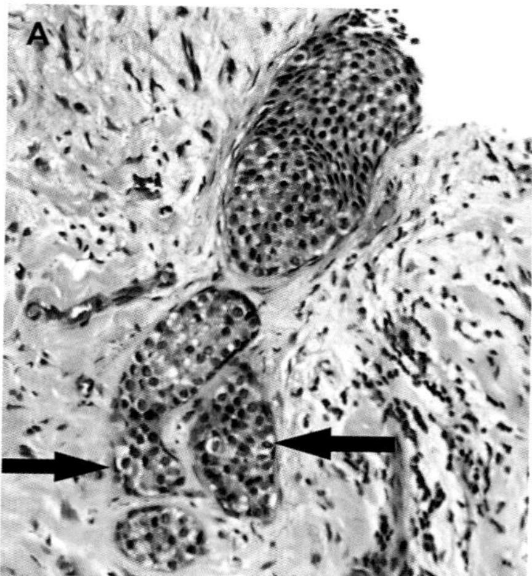

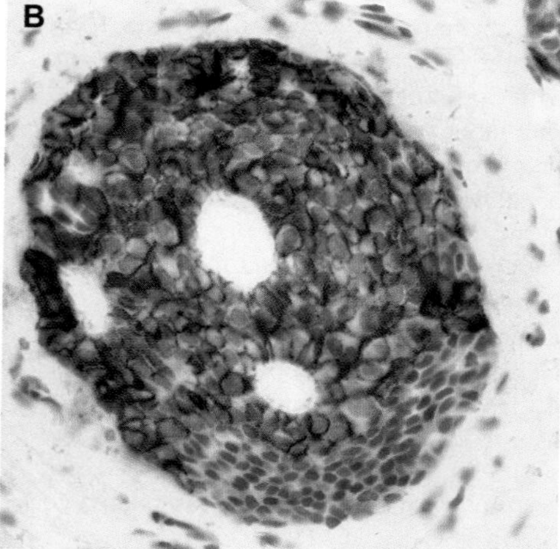

Fig. 8. Lobular carcinoma in situ (LCIS) versus ductal carcinoma in situ (DCIS). (*A*) Hematoxylin and eosin stain (original magnification × 400). This CNB specimen was diagnosed as LCIS, but atypical cells (*arrows*) rather than the usual uniform small cells characteristic of bland or usual LCIS were present. (*B*) E-cadherin stain shows uptake of the brown stain, indicating the correct diagnosis is DCIS, not LCIS.

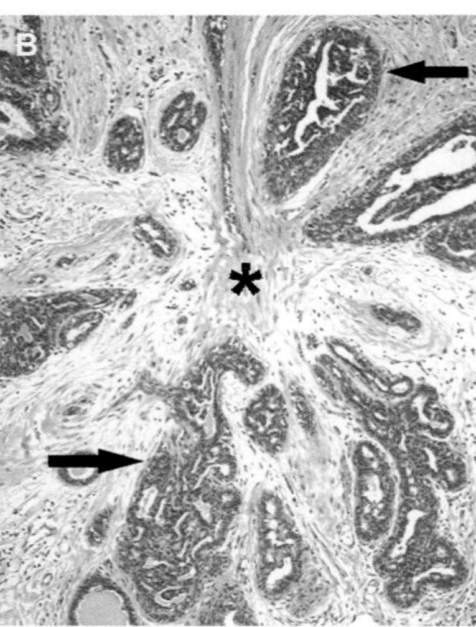

Fig. 9. Radial scar. (*A*) Mammogram. Close-up shows an area of architectural distortion (*arrow*) with long spicules and calcifications. (*B*) Pathology (hematoxylin and eosin stain; original magnification × 100). The center of the lesion (*) shows fibrosis and elastosis with retraction of the peripheral fibrous strands and distorted entrapped ducts (*arrows*) arranged in a radiating pattern with an array of proliferative elements.

A recent multi-institutional study of 157 cases of radial scar diagnosed at CNB found carcinoma in 8% at excision [36]. This percentage increased to 28% if the radial scar was associated with atypia (ADH, ALH, LCIS) and fell to 4% if there was no atypia. Coexisting malignancy was missed in 9% of lesions biopsied with an ALC device but in none of those biopsied with a VAD. The rate of missed cancer fell from 8% to zero when 12 or more specimens were obtained. Thus, diagnosis of benign radial scar by CNB was reliable when there was no atypia and at least 12 VAD specimens.

Papilloma

Papillomas include solitary, large central duct papillomas and multiple peripheral papillomas. A papilloma is composed of arborescent fronds of fibrovascular stroma with a stalk that arises from the duct lumen (Fig. 10). The fronds usually are covered with a benign two-cell epithelial layer; however, the large volume of the epithelial lining may undergo hyperplasia at any location and evolve to ADH, DCIS, or invasive papillary carcinoma.

Mammographically, a papilloma may present as a small, circumscribed mass or a small group of calcifications. On ultrasound it may present as a complex mass. Central large duct papillomas may cause bloody or clear nipple discharge, but peripheral papillomas are asymptomatic. A study by Page and colleagues [37] concluded that increased risk of breast cancer from a papilloma was related to the presence or absence of ADH.

Evaluation of the epithelial lining determines whether a papilloma is benign, high risk, or malignant. There are concerns when papillary lesions are diagnosed on CNB. First, there is difficulty in differentiating atypical from malignant papillary lesions on limited, fragmented material. Secondly, it is uncertain if the CNB specimens represent the most worrisome areas of the papilloma.

One study of 26 papillary lesions diagnosed on CNB and managed with either surgical excision or 2 years' follow-up included 7 papillary lesions without atypia and with concordant imaging findings

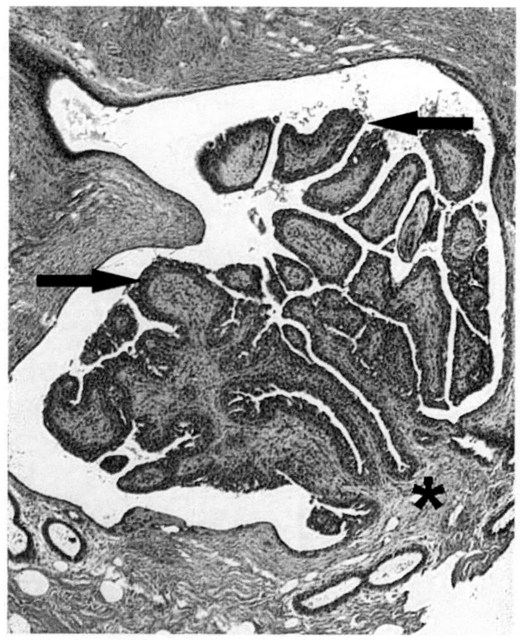

Fig. 10. Papilloma arising from the duct lining as a fibrovascular stalk (*) and extending into the lumen with numerous arborescent fronds, each with a fibrovascular stalk and epithelial lining (*arrow*). Hematoxylin and stain (original magnification × 200).

identified at CNB [38]. Of these seven cases, no cancers were found at surgical excision or follow-up unless atypia was identified or there was imaging–histologic discordance. In a retrospective review, Mercado and colleagues [39] reported on 12 benign papillomas (1.6% of all CNBs), of which 6 had surgical excision. One of these six revealed DCIS adjacent to a papilloma with atypia, but this case had discordant imaging–pathology findings, with the mammogram showing calcifications in a linear distribution. In another study of 46 papillomas identified at CNB (4% of all CNBs), the authors concluded that, when the histologic diagnosis was benign and there was no atypia (26 cases), the papillary lesions could be managed safely with imaging follow-up (for at least 2 years) rather than with surgical excision [40]. In summary, atypical papillary lesions diagnosed at CNB require surgical excision because the frequency of histologic underestimation is similar to that in other atypical lesions.

Columnar cell lesions

Advances in mammography and the increasing use of CNB for microcalcifications have increased the diagnosis of a columnar cell lesion [41]. This entity includes a wide range of pathologic findings distinguished by columnar (ovoid, elongated) epithelial cells lining the terminal duct lobular unit. Columnar cell lesions have been described variably as columnar cell hyperplasia, blunt duct adenosis, hyperplastic terminal groupings, columnar metaplasia, and columnar alteration with prominent apical snouts and secretions [42]. Columnar cell lesions can be placed into two categories: columnar cell change and columnar cell hyperplasia (Fig. 11). Columnar cell change is defined as a terminal duct lobular unit with variably dilated acini lined by one or two layers of columnar epithelial cells. Flocculent secretions and apical snouts often are present. Columnar cell hyperplasia is defined as cellular stratification of more than two cell layers of columnar epithelial cells and otherwise sharing many of the features of columnar cell change. Calcifications are reported to be present in 75% of columnar cell lesions. The calcifications are usually psammomatous, nonblanching, and round on mammography.

CNB of a columnar cell lesion with atypia (Fig. 12) shows DCIS or invasive cancer at excisional biopsy in up to 30% of cases [17,18]. The cancer risk associated with columnar cell lesions that do not fulfill the criteria for ADH or DCIS is unknown and requires follow-up studies. Based on current literature, excisional biopsy should be performed if CNB demonstrates a columnar cell lesion with atypia.

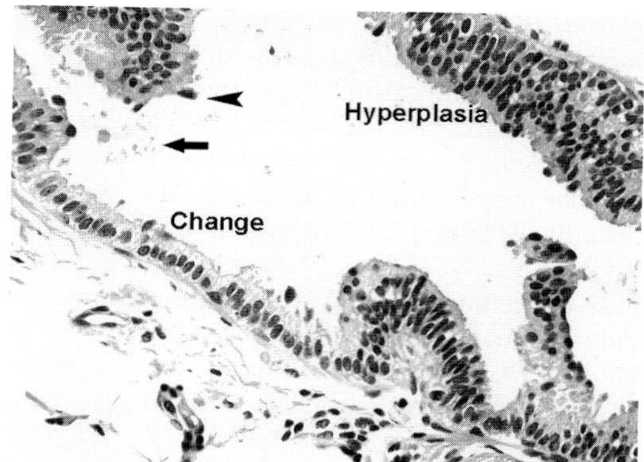

Fig. 11. This columnar cell lesion in the terminal duct lobular unit shows features of both columnar cell change (one or two cell layers of ovoid, elongated lining cells) and columnar cell hyperplasia (more than two layers of columnar cells) lining dilated acini with flocculent secretions (*arrow*) and prominent apical snouts (*arrowhead*). Hematoxylin and eosin stain (original magnification × 400).

Underestimation of ductal carcinoma in situ

Underestimation of DCIS occurs when a CNB of calcifications reveals DCIS but invasive carcinoma is identified at surgery. In one study, 305 consecutive cases of breast carcinoma manifested only by calcifications were evaluated in a prospective manner and then correlated with pathology [43].

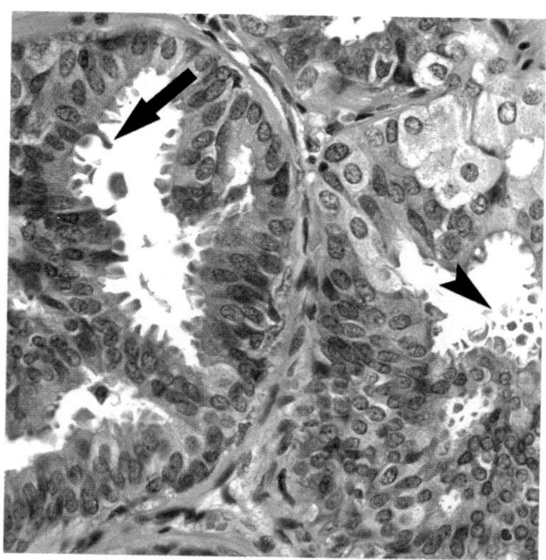

Fig. 12. Columnar cell lesion with atypia. These dilated acini in the terminal duct lobular unit show atypical cells rather than the typical ovoid, elongated cells of a columnar cell lesion. Other features of columnar cell lesions, such as prominent apical snouts (*arrow*) and flocculent secretions with calcifications (*arrowhead*), are present. Hematoxylin and eosin stain (original magnification × 600).

Invasive foci were more likely to be associated with calcifications extending 11 mm or more (40% of cases) than with calcifications extending 1 to 10 mm (26%). Invasive foci were more likely to be associated with linear calcifications (44%) than with granular calcifications (29%). An ALC device is more likely than a VAD to underestimate invasive carcinoma as DCIS [44]. The consequence of CNB underestimation of DCIS is that the patient must undergo a two-stage surgical procedure: one for excision of DCIS and another for axillary node evaluation when invasive cancer is identified at surgery.

False-positive core-needle biopsy

If a false-positive CNB is suspected because surgical excision did not identify malignancy, several courses of action should be taken:

1. The entire surgery specimen is processed for evaluation by the pathologist. The pathologist should see the prior CNB site (fat necrosis, hemorrhage, and/or a microclip) to verify the correct site was removed at surgery.
2. The original CNB specimens should be reviewed. If this review determines the specimens actually were benign, the CNB was a false positive.
3. If the CNB review confirms malignancy, repeat imaging should be performed to verify that the suspicious imaging finding was removed at surgery.
4. If the CNB review confirmed malignancy, and postsurgical imaging is negative, it is likely that a small suspicious lesion was removed entirely at CNB. Complete removal is more likely with sampling devices such as an 8- or 11-gauge VAD.

Sclerosing adenosis: a potential false-positive core-needle biopsy

Sclerosing adenosis is a benign lesion characterized by proliferation of lobules and fibrous tissue. Occasionally the fibrosis is so severe that the acini of the lobules are distorted enough to mimic invasive tubular carcinoma [45]. On mammograms, sclerosing adenosis is characterized by calcifications that can range from uniform and round to pleomorphic or linear (Fig. 13A).

On high-power magnification, sclerosing adenosis has a two-cell-layer epithelium, identified by the presence of myoepithelial cells; but tubular carcinoma has a one-cell-layer epithelial lining with no myoepithelial cells. On low-power magnification, sclerosing adenosis has a lobular configuration, but carcinoma has a haphazard pattern (Fig. 13B). If there is any doubt, smooth muscle myosin heavy chain and p63 stains should be performed to identify the presence of myoepithelial cells, which are present in sclerosing adenosis but not in invasive carcinoma [46].

Potential false negatives and follow-up for benign core-needle biopsy

A false-negative CNB is defined as one diagnosed as benign on pathology but with cancer detected within 2 years in the same quadrant of the ipsilateral breast. A false-negative CNB does not include cases with discordance or underestimation of disease if excisional biopsy is performed and a cancer is identified with no significant delay in diagnosis. The false-negative rate for CNB is approximately 2%, which is not higher than that of excisional biopsy [16]. Imaging follow-up is recommended to

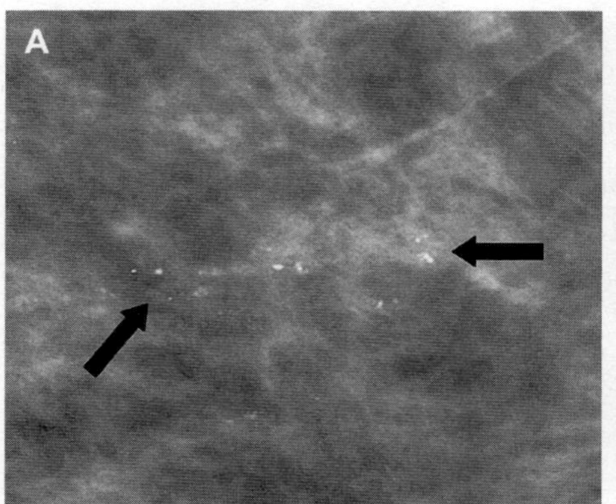

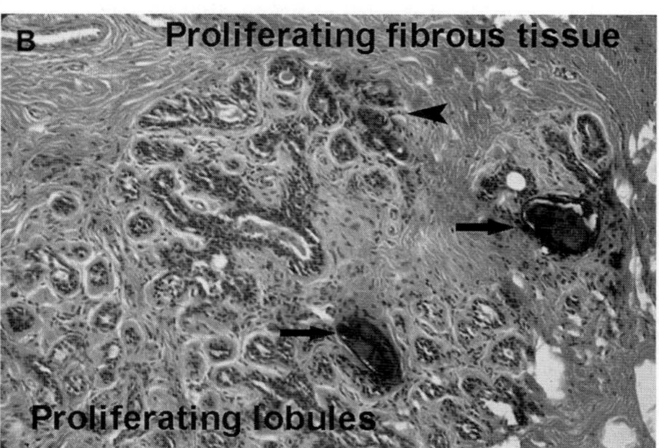

Fig. 13. Sclerosing adenosis. (*A*) Mammograms revealed pleomorphic calcifications in a linear distribution (*arrows*). CNB was recommended. (*B*) Pathology specimens revealed proliferation of fibrous tissue and lobules (hematoxylin and eosin stain; original magnification × 100). Calcifications (*arrows*) were identified in distorted lobules. The pathologist identified a lobular organization (*arrowhead*) in the distorted tissue indicating sclerosing adenosis, which was confirmed by a smooth muscle myosin heavy chain stain, which was taken up by myoepithelial cells throughout the CNB specimens.

avoid delay in diagnosis of a possible false-negative CNB. For most benign concordant CNB biopsy results, a 6-month follow-up is recommended. A 1-year follow-up is adequate for "definite benign" cases, such as a typical fibroadenoma at imaging with a concordant pathology diagnosis of fibroadenoma [16]. The follow-up imaging modality should be the one that best demonstrates the lesion.

It is important to be aware of potential noncompliance with follow-up recommendations. One study reported that only 74% of patients complied with recommendations for excisional biopsy, and only 54% complied with short-term follow-up imaging studies [47]. A quality assurance program that monitors recommended follow-up imaging is recommended.

Communicating results

Patients have unusually high anxiety related to a breast biopsy [48]. Therefore, results should be obtained and communicated to patients within a reasonable time. Usually results can be obtained in 2 to 3 days without compromising accuracy. The authors avoid communicating "preliminary" pathology readings because changing a diagnosis from a benign to a malignant final interpretation can be devastating for the patient. The CNB results and recommended management plan can be communicated to the patient by either the referring health care provider or the radiologist.

Summary

Minimally invasive breast biopsy procedures for suspicious imaging findings have played a major role in expanding the role of breast imaging in the management of breast diseases. This article has reviewed the current procedures and devices for performing CNB under stereotactic, ultrasound, or MR imaging guidance. In addition, post-CNB management protocols have been presented, including the assessment for concordance of radiology and pathology findings and the potential underestimation of disease. Based on the post-CNB evaluation, the patient is managed with imaging follow-up or referred for breast surgery.

References

[1] Parker SH, Lovin JD, Jobe WE, et al. Stereotactic breast biopsy with a biopsy gun. Radiology 1990; 176(3):741–7.

[2] Parker SH, Jobe WE, Dennis MA, et al. US-guided automated large-core breast biopsy. Radiology 1993;187(2):507–11.

[3] Parker SH, Burbank F, Jackman RJ. Percutaneous large-core breast biopsy: a multi-institutional study. Radiology 1994;193(2):359–64.

[4] Brenner RJ, Bassett LW, Fajardo LL, et al. Stereotactic core-needle breast biopsy: a multiinstitutional prospective trial. Radiology 2001;218(3):866–72.

[5] March DE, Raslavicus A, Coughlin BF, et al. Use of core biopsy in the United States. AJR Am J Roentgenol 1997;169(3):697–701.

[6] Parker SH, Burbank F. A practical approach to minimally invasive breast biopsy. Radiology 1996;2000(1):11–20.

[7] Harvey JA, Moran RE. US-guided core needle biopsy of the breast: technique and pitfalls. Radiographics 1998;18(4):867–77.

[8] Georgian-Smith D, Shiels WE 2nd. Freehand interventional sonography in the breast: basic principles and clinical applications. Radiographics 1996;16(1):149–61.

[9] Kaplan SS, Racenstein MJ, Wong WS, et al. US-guided core biopsy of the breast with a coaxial system. Radiology 1995;194(2):573–5.

[10] Eby PR, Lehman C. MRI-guided breast interventions. Semin Ultrasound CT MR 2006;27(4): 339–50.

[11] Bassett L, Winchester DP, Caplan RB, et al. Stereotactic core-needle biopsy of the breast: a report of the Joint Task Force of the American College of Radiology, American College of Surgeons, and College of American Pathologists. CA Cancer J Clin 1997;47(3):171–90.

[12] Sie A, Bryan DC, Gaines V, et al. Multicenter evaluation of the breast lesion excision system, a percutaneous, vacuum-assisted, intact specimen breast biopsy device. Cancer 2006;107(5):945–9.

[13] Killebrew LK, Oneson RH. Comparison of the diagnostic accuracy of a vacuum-assisted percutaneous intact specimen sampling device to a vacuum-assisted core needle sampling device for breast biopsy: initial experience. Breast J 2006; 12(4):302–8.

[14] American College of Radiology breast imaging reporting and data system, breast imaging atlas. Reston, (VA): American College of Radiology; 2003.

[15] The uniform approach to breast fine needle aspiration biopsy: a synopsis. Developed and approved at the NCI Sponsored Conference, Bethesda, Maryland, September 9–10, 1996. Breast J 1996;2(6):357–63.

[16] Lee CH, Philpotts LE, Horvath LJ, et al. Follow-up of breast lesions diagnosed as benign with stereotactic core needle biopsy: frequency of mammographic change and false-negative rate. Radiology 1999;212(1):189–94.

[17] Reynolds HE. Core needle biopsy of challenging benign breast conditions. AJR Am J Roengenol 2000;174(5):1245–50.

[18] Jacobs TW, Connolly JL, Schnitt SJ. Nonmalignant lesions in breast core needle biopsies: to excise or not to excise? Am J Surg Pathol 2002; 26(9):1095–110.

[19] Rosai J. Borderline epithelial lesions of the breast. Am J Surg Pathol 1991;15(3):209–21.
[20] Schnitt SJ, Connolly JL, Tavassoli FA, et al. Interobserver reproducibility in the diagnosis of ductal proliferative breast lesions using standard criteria. Am J Surg pathol 1992;16(12):1133–43.
[21] Lennington WJ, Jensen RA, Dalton LW, et al. Ductal carcinoma in situ of the breast: heterogeneity of individual lesions. Cancer 1994;73(1):118–24.
[22] Brem RF, Behrndt VS, Sanow L, et al. Atypical ductal hyperplasia: histologic underestimation of carcinoma in tissue harvested from impalpable breast lesions using 11-gauge stereotactically guided directional vacuum-assisted biopsy. AJR Am J Roentgenol 1999;172(5):1405–7.
[23] Philpotts LE, Shaheen NA, Carter D, et al. Comparison of rebiopsy rates after stereotactic core-needle biopsy of the breast with 11-gauge vacuum suction probe versus 14-gauge needle and automatic gun. AJR Am J Roentgenol 1999;172(3):683–7.
[24] Pope TL Jr, Fechner RE, Wilhelm MC, et al. Lobular carcinoma in situ of the breast: mammographic features. Radiology 1988;168(1):63–6.
[25] Andersen JA. Lobular carcinoma in situ of the breast. An approach to rational treatment. Cancer 1977;39(5):2597–602.
[26] Shin SJ, Rosen PP. Excisional biopsy should be performed if lobular carcinoma in situ is seen on needle core biopsy. Arch Pathol Lab Med 2002;126(6):697–701.
[27] Page DL, Schuyler PA, Dupont WD, et al. Atypical lobular hyperplasia as a unilateral predictor of breast cancer risk: a retrospective cohort study. Lancet 2003;361(5):125–9.
[28] Foster MC, Helvie MA, Gregory NE, et al. Lobular carcinoma in situ or atypical lobular hyperplasia: is excisional biopsy necessary? Radiology 2004;231:813–9.
[29] Mahoney MC, Robinson-Smith TM, Shaughnessy EA. Lobular neoplasia at 11-gauge vacuum-assisted stereotactic biopsy: correlation with surgical excision and mammographic follow-up. AJR Am J Roentgenol 2006;187(4):949–54.
[30] Jacobs TW, Pliss N, Kouria G, et al. Carcinoma in situ of the breast with intermediate features: role of E-cadherin staining in categorization. Am J Surg Pathol 2001;25(2):229–36.
[31] Frouge C, Tristant H, Guinebretiere JM, et al. Mammographic lesions suggestive of radial scars: microscopic findings in 40 cases. Radiology 1994;195(3):623–5.
[32] Jacobs TW, Byrne C, Colditz G, et al. Radial scars in benign breast-biopsy specimens and the risk of breast cancer. N Engl J Med 1999;340(3):340–6.
[33] Alvarado-Cabrero I, Tavassoli FA. Neoplastic and malignant lesions involving or arising in a radial scar: a clinicopathologic analysis of 17 cases. Breast J 2000;6(2):96–102.
[34] Sloane JP, Mayers MM. Carcinoma and atypical hyperplasia in radial scars and complex sclerosing lesions: importance of lesion size and patient age. Histopathology 1993;23(3):225–31.
[35] Patterson JA, Scott M, Anderson N, et al. Radial scar, complex sclerosing lesion and risk of breast cancer. Analysis of 175 cases in Northern Ireland. Eur J Surg Oncol 2004;30(10):1065–8.
[36] Brenner RJ, Jackman RJ, Parker SH, et al. Percutaneous core needle biopsy of radial scars of the breast: when is excision necessary? AJR Am J Roentgenol 2002;179(5):1179–84.
[37] Page DL, Salhany KE, Jensen RA, et al. Subsequent breast carcinoma risk after biopsy with atypia in a breast papilloma. Cancer 1996;78(2):258–66.
[38] Liberman L, Bracero N, Vuolo MA, et al. Percutaneous large-core biopsy of papillary breast lesions. AJR Am J Roentgenol 1999;172(2):331–7.
[39] Mercado CL, Hamele-Bena D, Singer C, et al. Papillary lesions of the breast: evaluation with stereotactic directional vacuum-assisted biopsy. Radiology 2001;221(3):650–5.
[40] Rosen EL, Bentley RC, Baker JA, et al. Imaging-guided core needle biopsy of papillary lesions of the breast. AJR Am J Roentgenol 2002;179(5):1185–92.
[41] Schnitt SJ, Vincent-Salomon A. Columnar cell lesions of the breast. Adv Anat Pathol 2003;10(3):113–24.
[42] Fraser JL, Raza S, Chorny K, et al. Columnar alteration with prominent apical snouts and secretions: a spectrum of changes frequently present in breast biopsies performed for microcalcifications. Am J Surg Pathol 1998;22(12):1521–7.
[43] Stomper PC, Geradts J, Edge SB, et al. Mammographic predictors of the presence and size of invasive carcinomas associated with malignant microcalcification lesions without a mass. AJR Am J Roentgenol 2003;181(6):1679–84.
[44] Jackman RJ, Burbank F, Parker SH, et al. Stereotactic breast biopsy of nonpalpable lesions: determinants of ductal carcinoma in situ underestimation rates. Radiology 2001;218(2):497–502.
[45] Jao W, Recant W, Swerdlow MA. Comparative ultrastructure of tubular carcinoma and sclerosing adenosis of the breast. Cancer 1976;38(1):180–6.
[46] Bose S, Derosa CM, Ozzello L. Immunostaining of type IV collagen and smooth muscle actin as an aid in the diagnosis of breast lesions. Breast J 1999;5(3):194–201.
[47] Goodman KA, Birdwell RL, Ikeda DM. Compliance with recommended follow-up after percutaneous breast core biopsy. AJR Am J Roentgenol 1998;170(1):89–92.
[48] Maxwell JR, Bugbee ME, Wellisch D, et al. Imaging-guided core needle biopsy of the breast: study of psychological outcomes. Breast J 2000;6:53–61.

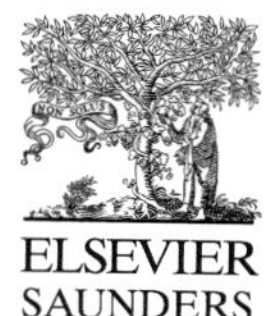

ELSEVIER
SAUNDERS

RADIOLOGIC
CLINICS
OF NORTH AMERICA

Radiol Clin N Am 45 (2007) 895–906

Beyond Standard Mammographic Screening: Mammography at Age Extremes, Ultrasound, and MR Imaging

Wendie A. Berg, MD, PhD, FACR

The basic principles of screening are as follows: (1) earlier detection of disease will reduce mortality; (2) healthy individuals who are screened will not be harmed; (3) the screening test must be widely available and well tolerated; and (4) screening should be cost effective. Randomized, controlled trials have proven mammographic screening to be effective by each of these criteria. Across seven randomized, controlled trials, in women aged 50 to 69 years, a 22% reduction in mortality was observed among women screened at 14 years of observation (95% confidence interval [CI], 13%–30%) [1]. Among women aged 40 to 49 years, the summary risk reduction was 15% (95% CI, 1%–27%). Among women aged 40 to 69 who actually were screened by service screening from 1988 through 1996 in the Swedish Two County trial, a 63% reduction in mortality was observed, which represented a 50% reduction in mortality compared with the period between 1968 and 1977 when no mammographic screening was available [2]. Improved treatment can be credited with a 12% to 13% reduction in mortality during the same period [2].

Randomized, controlled trials of mammographic screening have not included women younger than 40 years of age or older than 69 years, nor have they analyzed outcomes specifically in women at increased risk of developing breast cancer. This article explores the status of screening in such women and, in particular, the use of supplemental screening with ultrasound (US) and/or MR imaging for screening high-risk women.

Policy decisions to begin screening at age 40 or 50 years are derived largely from the prevalence of disease, which is less than 40 cases per 100,000 population below age 35 years across all ethnic groups and increases moderately beginning in the forties [3]. One in 2500 women without any known risk factors will develop breast cancer by age 30 years, one in 200 by age 40 years, and one in 50 by age 50 years. Rates peak from ages 75 to 79 years and decrease after age 80 years; one in eight women who live to age 85 will develop breast cancer [3].

WAB is supported by grants from The Avon Foundation and the National Cancer Institute (CA89008) through the American College of Radiology Imaging Network.

American Radiology Services, Johns Hopkins Green Spring, 301 Merrie Hunt Dr., Lutherville, MD 21093, USA
E-mail address: wendieberg@gmail.com

radiologic.theclinics.com

doi:10.1016/j.rcl.2007.06.001

High risk

Definitions of "high risk" vary. Generally, women with the risk factor who are at least three times more likely to develop breast cancer than those without the risk factor (ie, relative risk $\geq$ 3.0) are considered at "high risk." High risk often is defined by use of models that incorporate family history and prior biopsies. A lifetime risk of breast cancer of 20% or 25% by the models of Gail and colleagues [4,5] or Claus and colleagues [6] or at least a 1.7% 5-year risk of breast cancer by the Gail model [7] is considered high risk. Fibrocystic changes, even when proliferative, confer only minimal increased risk of 1.5 to 2.0, as do early menarche (< age 13) or late menopause (> age 55).

The age at which to begin screening women who are at increased risk would reasonably derive from the age at which the risk is equal to that for an average woman of age 40 or 50 years, depending on national policy. Table 1 summarizes risk factor data. A family history of male breast cancer and/or a relative who had both breast and ovarian cancer increases the likelihood of a *BRCA* mutation, and many high-risk screening programs enroll women who have either or both of these criteria [8,9]. The BRCAPRO model calculates the risk of carrying a *BRCA* gene mutation as well as the subsequent risk of breast or ovarian cancer for individuals in families with known or suspected carriers [10]. It has been estimated that 2% of Ashkenazi Jewish women are *BRCA*-mutation carriers, and genetic testing should be considered [11]. For women who have a known or suspected *BRCA* mutation, most studies begin screening at age 25 years. For women who have an intermediate family history of breast cancer (see Table 1), screening usually begins 10 years before the age of diagnosis of the first-degree relative who had breast cancer or at least by age 40 years [12].

Earlier studies of women who had mantle radiation therapy to the breasts (eg, for Hodgkin's disease) after age 18 years and before age 30 years showed a very high risk of breast cancer beginning 8 years after treatment and peaking at 15 years after treatment [13]. When treatment began after 1974 and used lower doses of radiation and more limited fields, no such increased risk has been found [14].

No studies have addressed specifically the reduction in mortality from screening high-risk women. Therefore this article considers surrogate end points.

Surrogate end points and mortality

Lymph node status is the single most important prognostic factor for predicting disease-free and overall survival in breast cancer [15,16]. The decrease in mortality from randomized, controlled trials of mammographic screening is almost entirely attributable to earlier detection. The decrease in mortality parallels the reduction in size distribution of cancers depicted [17] and closely parallels the reduction in rates of node-positive breast cancer [18]. Many screening programs have performed only biannual screening in women 40 to 49 years of age, and there has been relatively little reduction in the size distribution or rates of node-positive cancers compared with women aged 50 to 69 years who were screened annually [19]. The single most important predictor of the success of a screening program, independent of the type of intervention or imaging, is likely to be the reduction in node-positive cancers. Absent a control group, this article considers the percentage of cancers that are node positive at diagnosis as a surrogate measure of the efficacy of various screening strategies.

Although mortality is not considered specifically in most of this discussion, it is important to recognize that the benefit from mammographic screening in terms of reduction in mortality is not seen until 5 to 7 years after the onset of screening. As such, a woman who has a life expectancy of less than 5 years is not expected to benefit from screening. The cost effectiveness of screening usually is measured in cost per year of life saved. There is a higher cost to screening younger women, especially women younger than 40 years of age, due to lower prevalence of disease. This may be justifiable because of the increased number of years of life that can be saved. In young women at high risk for breast cancer, it may even be cost effective to screen with more expensive technologies, such as MRI. For women older than 69 years, life expectancy is relatively shorter, and comorbidities are frequent, but the yield of screening is higher because of the higher prevalence of disease. In women older than 69 years, the cost effectiveness of screening needs to be considered in terms of potential years of life saved based on the individual woman's life expectancy.

Digital mammography and dense breasts

Dense breast tissue itself is a risk factor for breast cancer. The risk is four- to sixfold higher in women who have extremely dense breasts than in matched controls who have fatty breasts [20–23], and breast cancer is more likely to develop in denser areas of the breast [24]. Extremely dense (> 75% dense) or heterogeneously dense (51%–75% dense) parenchyma [25] is present in more than half of women younger than age 50 years and in one third of women age 50 years and older [26].

Mammography has reduced sensitivity in dense breast tissue, with sensitivity as low as 30% to 48% in extremely dense parenchyma [27,28]. There is a correspondingly high rate of interval cancers (cancers coming to clinical attention between screening intervals) among women who have dense breasts, and more than half of interval cancers have a poor prognosis [29]. The multicenter Digital Mammographic Imaging Screening Trial showed improved performance of digital mammography in women who had dense breasts, with 70% sensitivity compared with 55% sensitivity for film-screen mammography [30]. False negatives were identified by a single annual mammographic follow-up or by cancers coming to clinical attention although no systematic clinical breast examination program was included [30]. The true sensitivity of digital mammography in dense breasts may be far lower than 70%, but digital mammography, when available, is recommended in such women. A similar detection benefit was observed for digital mammography in screening women younger than 50 years and in pre- or perimenopausal women, with substantial overlap among the groups attributable largely to denser parenchyma in younger women.

Screening ultrasound

Supplemental screening with US and MR imaging is being studied in women who are at increased risk of breast cancer because of increased breast density, family or personal history, or both. Across seven published series of whole-breast US screening, using only film-screen mammography for comparison, 178 cancers were identified only sonographically in 49,586 women, for a yield of 0.36% (Table 2). In all but one series [28], only a single prevalence screen was performed; an estimate of the yield from annual screening sonography is not available. Women who have fatty breast tissue were excluded from screening US, and more than 90% of cancers seen only sonographically have been in heterogeneously dense or extremely dense parenchyma (hereafter collectively termed "dense" breast tissue) [31]. Ductal carcinoma in situ (DCIS) is difficult to visualize on US; 94% of cancers seen only on US were invasive [31]. More than 70% of cancers seen only on US were 1 cm in size or smaller [31], and, when reported, 63 of 73 (86%) of cancers seen only on US were node negative [28,32–34] (with update by S. Ciatto, personal communication, 2006). In the recently published Italian multicenter study, screening US more than doubled the rate of breast cancer detection in women who had dense breasts, with 34 cancers seen in 7615 women on mammography and 36 seen only on US [34] (update by S. Ciatto, personal communication, 2006). Eighteen of 36 (50%) cancers seen only on US were visible in retrospect on mammography [34] (update by S. Ciatto, personal communication, 2006).

On average, 3% of patients who have screening breast US have been recommended for an US-guided biopsy (see Table 2). In some of the series, additional patients were recommended for US-guided cyst aspiration, but the numbers of such patients are not always identified easily from the reports. Although the positive predictive value of biopsy has been low for lesions seen only on US (averaging 11%, see Table 2), US-guided biopsy is not considered particularly onerous by patients (M. Schleinitz, MD, personal communication and American College of Radiology Imaging Network [ACRIN] 6666, unpublished data, 2006) or practitioners. Recall for additional work-up from screening US is not specifically reported in the studies to date, because most screening US has been physician performed (see Table 2), with results given to the patient at the time of the examination; this practice may change with use of automated devices and potential resulting batch reading. Short-interval follow-up has been recommended in another 3% to 10% (averaging 6%) of women screened with US [28,32,35,36].

Although screening US seems to allow detection of cancers that are clinically significant at an early stage, an important but heretofore missing piece of information is the rate of interval cancers and number of such cancers that are node positive: even combined US and mammography on an annual basis may not detect the cancers that clinically are most significant. The ongoing ACRIN 6666 protocol [37,38] is a prospective, multicenter study of three rounds of annual screening US and mammography. The rate of interval cancers and the node status of both interval and screen-detected cancers will be important outcomes.

Screening US is well tolerated by patients and is inexpensive. If results of the studies in Table 2 are maintained, and three cancers are found per 1000 women screened with US, at the age of 45 years, preliminary cost effectiveness analysis shows a $50,000 to $70,000 cost per year of life saved (MD Schleinitz, MD, personal communication, 2003). This cost is within the accepted range for seat belts, mammography, and other public health interventions [39]. As of a 2005 report from survey of Fellows of the Society of Breast Imaging, supplemental screening sonography was offered at approximately 35% of United States facilities [40]. Current reimbursement (used to calculate costs) probably does not cover the true costs of this examination if performed by a physician. Automated whole-breast US may

Table 1: **Summary of relative risk and absolute risk of breast cancer by family history and other high-risk factors**

Risk factor	Relative risk (95% CI)	Absolute risk (95% CI)	References
No known risk factors	1	12% by age 80 years 0.04% in next 10 years if age 20 years 0.4% in next 10 years if age 30 years 1.4% in next 10 years if age 40 years 1.9% in next 10 years if age 50 years 2.3% in next 10 years if age 60 years 2.5% in next 10 years if age 70 years	[66]
BRCA-1 or *-2* mutation	—	33% by age 50 years 56% by age 70 years	[11]
BRCA-1 mutation	—	18% by age 39 years 59% by age 49 years 65% (44–78%) by age 70 years	[67]
BRCA-2 mutation	—	15% by age 39 years 34% by age 49 years 45% (31–56%) by age 70 years	[67]
Li-Fraumeni syndrome (*TP53* mutation)	—	90% lifetime risk	[68]
CHEK2 mutation	—	<20% lifetime risk	[69]
First-degree relative with breast cancer before age 40 years	5.7 (2.7–11.8) for a woman < age 40 years; 3.0 (1.8–4.9) for a woman aged 40–49 years	—	[66]
Mother diagnosed before age 50 years	2.4 (1.86–3.12)	—	[70]
Sister diagnosed before age 50 years	3.18 (2.15–4.72)	—	[70]

Two family members with breast cancer, at least one diagnosed before age 40 years	13.5 (3.4–53.9) for a woman < age 50 years 3.9 (1.8–8.6) for a woman ≥ age 50 years	—	[66]
Two or more family members with breast cancer	2.9 (2.4–3.6)	2% in next 10 years if age 30 years 5.2%–5.7% in next 10 years if age 40–70 years	[66]
Three or more family members with breast cancer	3.9 (2.0–7.5)	—	[66,70]
Personal history of breast cancer[a]	8–10 overall; 3–4 for second primary	10% risk of recurrence within 12 years if radiation given; 14% risk of recurrence within 20 years	[71–73]
Personal history of lobular carcinoma in situ	8–12	18–37% lifetime risk	[74]
Personal history of atypical ductal hyperplasia[a]	4–5	—	[75]
Personal history of atypical lobular hyperplasia	3	—	[76]
Age greater than 60 years	—	> 1.7% 5-year risk	Gail model [4]
Extremely dense breast tissue[b]	4–6	—	[20–24]

Relative risk is the risk of developing breast cancer for women with the risk factor compared with risk of developing breast cancer for women without any known risk factors (95% confidence interval). Note: "High risk" is usually defined as an absolute risk which is ≥three-fold that of an average woman in her 40s (ie, ≥4.2% in the next 10 years) or 50s (ie, ≥5.7% in the next 10 years), depending on national policy for the age to begin routine screening. In women who are at high risk, supplemental screening with ultrasound or MR imaging may be considered in addition to routine mammography. In general, risks from various risk factors are multiplicative [70].

[a] Chemoprevention with tamoxifen or aromatase inhibitors decreases relative risk by 0.47–0.74.

[b] For women who have known *BRCA* mutations, the effect of increasing breast density is similar in magnitude to the effect in controls without known mutations [77]. Relative risks associated with other risk factors, such as nulliparity, alcohol use, early menarche, late menopause, and hormone use are similar in women who have a family history of breast cancer and women without a family history [66].

Table 2: Results with screening breast ultrasound

Author	# in Study	# Biopsies (%)	# Cancers (% of biopsies)	Details
Gordon and Goldenberg 1995 [35]	12,706	279 (2.2)	44 (16)	Screening and diagnostic patients, physician performed
Buchberger et al 2000 [36]	8103[a]	362 (4.5)[b]	32 (8.8)	Screening, physician performed
Kaplan 2001 [32]	1862	102 (5.5)	6 (6.6)	Screening, technologist performed
Kolb et al 2002 [28]	13,547[c]	358 (2.6)[b]	37 (10)	Screening over several years, physician performed
Crystal et al 2003 [33]	1517	38 (2.5)	7 (18)	Screening, physician performed
Leconte et al 2003 [78]	4236	NS	16	Screening, physician performed
Corsetti et al 2006 [34], with update by S. Ciatto, personal communication, 2006	7615	NS[d]	36	Multicenter, screening, physician performed
Total	49,586	1139/37,735 (3.0)	178	

Abbreviation: NS, not stated.
[a] Not included are another eight cancers found in another 867 examinations performed in the diagnostic setting.
[b] Biopsies as stated do not include cyst aspirations.
[c] Number of examinations performed in 5418 women; in all other series, the number of women evaluated is the same as the number of examinations.
[d] In the published series [34], 15 core biopsies, 66 surgical biopsies, and 405 aspirations were performed in 6449 women examined with screening US.

improve the practical implementation of screening US.

MR imaging

MR imaging is limited as a screening test because of its high cost and requirement for intravenous contrast injection. Claustrophobia further reduces patient tolerance of MR imaging. As of the 2005 survey previously mentioned, 51% of United States facilities offered diagnostic breast MR imaging, and 12% offered screening MR imaging [40]. As a result of these limitations, MR imaging is being considered only for screening women at high risk of breast cancer. MR imaging screening of the contralateral breast in women who have newly diagnosed cancer has been shown to depict mammographically and clinically occult cancer in 3–6% of women but is not discussed further in this article [41–45].

Tables 3 and 4 summarize results from five studies of screening of women at high risk using MR imaging. Series in which patients were selected for MR imaging on the basis of negative mammography have been excluded from this analysis [46], and insufficient data are available on use of MR imaging to screen women at increased risk because of lobular carcinoma in situ or atypical hyperplasias [47]. With normalizing for the number of MR imaging screening rounds, on average 8.3 cancers were depicted only on MR imaging for every 1000 examinations performed (70 cancers per 8426 examinations, 0.83%, Table 4). The higher yield observed in these studies than reported for screening US is explained, at least in part, by differences in the patient populations studied. In four of the MR imaging series [8,48–50], women were enrolled because they were known or suspected carriers of *BRCA-1* or *-2* mutations, and rates of cancers detected only on MR imaging (normalized per screening round) were 1.0% to 1.5% [8,48–50]. In the series of Kriege and colleagues [51,52], 358 women were proven mutation carriers, and the other 1551 enrolled women had a risk of breast cancer as low as 15% or greater by the Claus model [6]; the rate of cancer detected only on MR imaging (normalized per screening round) was 0.48%. In the US series, where reported, the rate of breast cancer detected only on US in the subset of women at higher risk because

Table 3: Detection of cancers with mammography, ultrasound, MR imaging, or a combination of mammography with ultrasound or MR imaging across five series of high-risk women

Study	# Women[a]	# Cancers	# cancers Seen on Mammography (% of cancers)	# Cancers Seen on Ultrasound (%)	# Cancers Seen on Ultrasound Plus Mammography (%)	# Cancers Seen on MR Imaging (%)	# Cancers Seen on Mammography Plus MR Imaging (%)
Warner et al 2004 [48]	236	22	8 (36)	7 (32)	12 (55)	17 (77)	20 (91)
Kriege et al 2004 [51]	1909	45[b]	15 (33)	ND	ND	29 (64)	40 (89)
Kuhl et al 2005 [8]	529	43	14 (33)	17 (40)	21 (49)	39 (91)	40 (93)
Leach et al 2005 [49]	649	35	14 (40)	ND	ND	27 (77)	33 (94)
Sardanelli et al 2007 [50]	278	14[c]	8 (57)	8 (57)	9 (64)	13 (93)	14 (100)
Total	3601	159	59 (37)	32/79 (41)	42/79 (53)	125 (79)	147 (92)

Abbreviation: ND, not determined.
[a] Women were screened annually for multiple rounds in each of these studies.
[b] A total of 50 cancers were found in this study, with results summarized for the 45 cancers found in women who had been imaged by both mammography and MR imaging.
[c] A total of 18 cancers were found in this study, with results summarized for the 14 cancers found in women who had been imaged by all screening modalities.

Table 4: Results of high-risk screening with MR imaging across five series

Study	# Patients	# Cancers	# Invasive Cancers (%)	# Node-Positive Cancers (%)[a]	Cancers Seen Only on MR Imaging (% Of Cancers)	MR Imaging Recalls/# MR Imaging Examinations (%)	PPV MR Imaging Recall (%)	# Interval Cancers (%)
Warner 2004 [48]	236	22	16 (73)	2 (13)	7 (32)	37/457 (8.1)	17 (46)	1 (4.5)
Kriege 2004 [51]	1909	50	44 (88)	9 (20)	20 (40)	177/4169 (4.2)	29 (16)	4 (8.0)
Kuhl 2005 [8]	529	43	34 (79)	5 (15)	19 (44)	78/1542 (5.1)	39 (50)	1 (2.3)
Leach 2005 [49]	649	35	29 (83)	5 (17)	19 (54)	344/1881 (18.3)	27 (7.8)	2 (5.7)
Sardanelli 2007 [50][b]	278	14	10 (71)	1 (10)	5 (36)	24/377 (6.4)	15 (63)	0 (0)
Total	3601	164	133 (81)	22 (16)	70 (43)	660/8426 (7.8)	127 (19)	8 (4.9)

Abbreviation: PPV, positive predictive value.
[a] % = Percentage of invasive cancers that are node positive.
[b] A total of 18 cancers were found in this study, with results summarized for the 14 cancers found in women who had been imaged by all screening modalities.

of personal or family history of breast cancer, was 0.48% to 1.3%, versus 0.18% to 0.26% in women at average risk [28,33,36].

On average, 7.8% of women who had screening by MR imaging were recalled for additional evaluation or biopsy (see Table 4). Of those recalled, 19% proved to have cancer (see Table 4). In several series [8,51], a relatively high proportion of cancers detected on MR imaging were classified initially as Breast Imaging Reporting and Data System category 3, probably benign [53]. Only 16% of cancers were node positive at detection, and only 8 of 164 cancers (4.9%) were interval cancers (see Table 4). DCIS is readily depicted on MR imaging; 11 of 70 (17%) of cancers seen only on MR imaging were DCIS [8,48–51]. The relatively low specificity of MR imaging improved with subsequent rounds of screening, although the rate of cancer detection by annual MR imaging remained relatively constant [8,48,52]. Both the low observed interval cancer rate and the relatively constant rate of detection with annual MR imaging screening suggest that the annual interval is appropriate.

In three of these series [8,48,50], mammography, US, and MR imaging were performed and interpreted independently. Across those three series [8,48,50], only 2 of 81 (2.5%) of cancers were seen only on US, compared with 31 of 81 (38%) seen only on MR imaging. Screening with US seems to have little value after combined mammography and MR imaging, although targeted US often is successful in guiding biopsy of suspicious findings seen on MR imaging even when the initial survey US is negative [43]. Even after combined mammography and US, across these series, only 53% of cancers were depicted, whereas combined mammography and MR imaging depicted 92% of cancers (see Table 3). Thus it would seem that even the combination of mammography and US is inadequate in screening women at high risk. This assumption may not be true, however. It may be that cancers seen only on MR imaging would be detected at the next annual screening with combined mammography and US and would still be node negative at detection. The ACRIN 6666 protocol will provide the rate of interval cancers and node-positive cancers at each round of combined mammography and US screening, and at 24 months a subset of patients will undergo screening with MR imaging [38]. The difference in rates of node-positive cancers at 36 months in the subgroup of ACRIN 6666 participants who have had MR imaging and the group that has not will be important information. In the series of Kriege and colleagues [51], 21% of cases of invasive cancer were node positive in the group screened with MR imaging, compared with 52% to 56% in two control groups. These findings suggest that, compared with mammography alone, supplemental screening with MR imaging should reduce mortality caused by breast cancer in high-risk women.

Based on Medicare reimbursement, breast MR imaging costs about 10 times as much as film-screen mammography. The cost effectiveness of screening with MR imaging has been studied in *BRCA-1* and *-2* carriers and varies substantially with patient age at screening [54]. Addition of annual screening with MR imaging after mammography between the ages of 35 and 54 years yielded a cost per quality-adjusted year of life saved of $55,420 for all *BRCA-1* carriers and of $98,454 for the subset of *BRCA-2* carriers who had dense breasts [54]. Based on cost effectiveness estimates from the United Kingdom study [55], MR imaging screening will be offered to women aged 30 to 39 years at familial risk who have a 10-year risk greater than 8% and to women aged 40 to 49 years who have at a 10-year risk greater than 20% or greater than 12% if the breast parenchyma is dense [56].

The latest guidelines from the American Cancer Society [56] endorse annual screening with both MR imaging and mammography of all women with who have a *BRCA* mutation, Li-Fraumeni, Cowden, or Bannayan-Riley-Ruvalcaba syndromes, of untested first-degree (mother, sister, daughter) relatives of a *BRCA* carrier or those who have the listed syndromes, and of those who have lifetime risk of 20% to 25% or greater by validated risk-assessment models. The American Cancer Society recommends against MR imaging screening in women who have less than a 15% lifetime risk of breast cancer [56]. For women at intermediate risk, including those for whom dense breast tissue is the only risk factor, the American Cancer Society states payment should not be a barrier and that further study is warranted [56].

Screening in women older than age 69 years

Because of the high prevalence of breast cancer in this population, all women over age 69 years are considered to be at high risk and to have a 5-year risk of developing breast cancer of at least 1.7% (see Table 1). Mammographic sensitivity is as high as 98% in fatty breasts [57], and fatty replacement increases with age (in the absence of hormone replacement therapy). Thus, there is reason to expect success with mammographic screening in older women.

As stated, the mortality benefit to screening mammography begins to be seen from 5 to 7 years after the onset of screening [1]. Therefore patients who have life expectancies of less than 5 years are unlikely to benefit from screening. Further, there may be harm from detecting cancers that would never have become clinically important. The risk of detecting nonprogressive cancer is estimated at 37% of DCIS on the prevalence (first) screen and only 4% on subsequent incidence screens [58], although it may take 7 to 10 years for most DCIS to become clinically significant. The average life expectancy of a woman reaching age 80 years is 8.6 years and of a woman reaching age 85 years is 5.9 years [59]. The upper quartile of women reaching age 90 years still has a life expectancy of 6.8 years [59]. Smith-Bindman and colleagues [60] showed a reduced risk of metastatic breast cancer among California Medicare beneficiaries aged 66 to 79 years who underwent screening mammography (relative risk, 0.57; 95% CI, 0.45–0.72) and a corresponding increase of in situ, local, and regional breast cancer among those screened. McPherson and colleagues [61] analyzed the relative risk of all-cause mortality among women diagnosed as having invasive breast cancer from the Upper Midwest Tumor Registry System as a function of age and comorbidities. Patients who had mammographically detected tumors had a significantly lower risk of death among all age groups over age 69 years, even when mild-to-moderate comorbidities were present. They found that only women over age 74 years who had severe or multiple comorbidities were unlikely to benefit from screening [61].

Currently the American Cancer Society does not set an upper age limit in guidelines for mammographic screening, with the caveats that a woman should be in reasonably good health and would be a candidate for treatment should cancer be detected [62]. Nonetheless, most organized screening programs throughout the world currently restrict screening to women younger than 70 years, or 75 years at most [63].

Summary

The reduction in mortality achieved by mammographic screening is proven for women between the ages of 40 and 69 years, and more limited data suggest a benefit in women older than 69 years. At the same time, there is increasing awareness of the limitations of mammography, particularly in women who have dense breast tissue. Indeed, dense breast tissue itself has been validated increasingly as a marker of a high risk of developing breast cancer. In women who have dense breast tissue, several steps should be considered. When available, digital mammography has better performance in dense breast tissue. Having the mammogram interpreted by a radiologist who specializes in breast imaging improves the likelihood of cancer detection [64] and diagnosis [65]. Substantial data have shown improved detection of breast cancer with a single screening US examination. Data are needed to support the use of supplemental US in annual screening, and results from the ongoing ACRIN 6666 protocol will help inform such a policy. At present, there is a lack of trained personnel to offer widespread US screening. There is a need for whole-breast automated devices and their validation.

Because of its high cost, limited availability, and reduced patient tolerance, supplemental screening using MR imaging probably will remain more selective, on a case-by-case basis, for the foreseeable future. In women known or suspected to be carriers of a known mutation in *BRCA-1* or *-2*, it seems appropriate to consider screening beginning as early as age 25 years with both mammography and MR imaging. Although data support using supplemental MR imaging in other women at high risk, specific performance characteristics of MR imaging in many subgroups merits further evaluation.

References

[1] Humphrey LL, Helfand M, Chan BK, et al. Breast cancer screening: a summary of the evidence for the U.S. Preventive Services Task Force. Ann Intern Med 2002;137:347–60.

[2] Tabar L, Vitak B, Tony HH, et al. Beyond randomized controlled trials: organized mammographic screening substantially reduces breast carcinoma mortality. Cancer 2001;91:1724–31.

[3] National Cancer Institute. Surveillance, Epidemiology, and End Results. Available at: www.seer.gov/. Accessed July 4, 2007.

[4] Gail MH, Brinton LA, Byar DP, et al. Projecting individualized probabilities of developing breast cancer for white females who are being examined annually. J Natl Cancer Inst 1989;81:1879–86.

[5] Gail MH, Costantino JP. Validating and improving models for projecting the absolute risk of breast cancer. J Natl Cancer Inst 2001;93:334–5.

[6] Claus EB, Risch N, Thompson WD. Autosomal dominant inheritance of early-onset breast cancer. Implications for risk prediction. Cancer 1994;73:643–51.

[7] National Cancer Institute. Available at: http://www.cancer.gov/bcrisktool/. Accessed on July 4, 2007.

[8] Kuhl CK, Schrading S, Leutner CC, et al. Mammography, breast ultrasound, and magnetic resonance imaging for surveillance of women at high familial risk for breast cancer. J Clin Oncol 2005;23:8469–76.

[9] Cortesi L, Turchetti D, Marchi I, et al. Breast cancer screening in women at increased risk according to different family histories: an update of the

Modena Study Group experience. BMC Cancer 2006;6:210.

[10] Berry DA, Iversen ES Jr, Gudbjartsson DF, et al. BRCAPRO validation, sensitivity of genetic testing of BRCA1/BRCA2, and prevalence of other breast cancer susceptibility genes. J Clin Oncol 2002;20:2701–12.

[11] Struewing JP, Hartge P, Wacholder S, et al. The risk of cancer associated with specific mutations of BRCA1 and BRCA2 among Ashkenazi Jews. N Engl J Med 1997;336:1401–8.

[12] Dershaw DD. Are there any indications for routine breast cancer screening of asymptomatic women who are less than 40 years old? AJR Am J Roentgenol 1999;172:1136–7.

[13] Aisenberg AC, Finkelstein DM, Doppke KP, et al. High risk of breast carcinoma after irradiation of young women with Hodgkin's disease. Cancer 1997;79:1203–10.

[14] Tinger A, Wasserman TH, Klein EE, et al. The incidence of breast cancer following mantle field radiation therapy as a function of dose and technique. Int J Radiat Oncol Biol Phys 1997;37: 865–70.

[15] Russo J, Frederick J, Ownby HE, et al. Predictors of recurrence and survival of patients with breast cancer. Am J Clin Pathol 1987;88:123–31.

[16] Fisher ER, Anderson S, Redmond C, et al. Pathologic findings from the National Surgical Adjuvant Breast Project protocol B-06. 10-year pathologic and clinical prognostic discriminants. Cancer 1993;71:2507–14.

[17] Michaelson JS, Silverstein M, Sgroi D, et al. The effect of tumor size and lymph node status on breast carcinoma lethality. Cancer 2003;98:2133–43.

[18] Smith RA, Duffy SW, Gabe R, et al. The randomized trials of breast cancer screening: what have we learned? Radiol Clin North Am 2004;42: 793–806, v.

[19] Zabicki K, Colbert JA, Dominguez FJ, et al. Breast cancer diagnosis in women < or = 40 versus 50 to 60 years: increasing size and stage disparity compared with older women over time. Ann Surg Oncol 2006;13:1072–7.

[20] Wolfe JN, Saftlas AF, Salane M. Mammographic parenchymal patterns and quantitative evaluation of mammographic densities: a case-control study. AJR Am J Roentgenol 1987;148: 1087–92.

[21] Boyd NF, Byng JW, Jong RA, et al. Quantitative classification of mammographic densities and breast cancer risk: results from the Canadian National Breast Screening Study. J Natl Cancer Inst 1995;87:670–5.

[22] Harvey JA, Bovbjerg VE. Quantitative assessment of mammographic breast density: relationship with breast cancer risk. Radiology 2004;230: 29–41.

[23] McCormack VA, dos Santos Silva I. Breast density and parenchymal patterns as markers of breast cancer risk: a meta-analysis. Cancer Epidemiol Biomarkers Prev 2006;15:1159–69.

[24] Boyd NF, Guo H, Martin LJ, et al. Mammographic density and the risk and detection of breast cancer. N Engl J Med 2007;356:227–36.

[25] D'Orsi CJ, Bassett LW, Berg WA, et al. Breast imaging reporting and data system, BI-RADS: mammography. 4th edition. Reston (VA): American College of Radiology; 2003.

[26] Stomper PC, D'Souza DJ, DiNitto PA, et al. Analysis of parenchymal density on mammograms in 1353 women 25-79 years old. AJR Am J Roentgenol 1996;167:1261–5.

[27] Mandelson MT, Oestreicher N, Porter PL, et al. Breast density as a predictor of mammographic detection: comparison of interval- and screen-detected cancers. J Natl Cancer Inst 2000;92: 1081–7.

[28] Kolb TM, Lichy J, Newhouse JH. Comparison of the performance of screening mammography, physical examination, and breast US and evaluation of factors that influence them: an analysis of 27,825 patient evaluations. Radiology 2002;225: 165–75.

[29] Tabar L, Vitak B, Chen HH, et al. The Swedish Two-County Trial twenty years later. Updated mortality results and new insights from long-term follow-up. Radiol Clin North Am 2000; 38:625–51.

[30] Pisano ED, Gatsonis C, Hendrick E, et al. Diagnostic performance of digital versus film mammography for breast-cancer screening. N Engl J Med 2005;353:1773–83.

[31] Berg WA. Supplemental screening sonography in dense breasts. Radiol Clin North Am 2004;42: 845–51, vi.

[32] Kaplan SS. Clinical utility of bilateral whole-breast US in the evaluation of women with dense breast tissue. Radiology 2001;221: 641–9.

[33] Crystal P, Strano SD, Shcharynski S, et al. Using sonography to screen women with mammographically dense breasts. AJR Am J Roentgenol 2003;181:177–82.

[34] Corsetti V, Ferrari A, Ghirardi M, et al. Role of ultrasonography in detecting mammographically occult breast carcinoma in women with dense breasts. Radiol Med (Torino) 2006;111:440–8.

[35] Gordon PB, Goldenberg SL. Malignant breast masses detected only by ultrasound. A retrospective review. [see comments]. Cancer 1995;76: 626–30.

[36] Buchberger W, Niehoff A, Obrist P, et al. Clinically and mammographically occult breast lesions: detection and classification with high-resolution sonography. Semin Ultrasound CT MR 2000;21:325–36.

[37] Berg WA. Rationale for a trial of screening breast ultrasound: American College of Radiology Imaging Network (ACRIN) 6666. AJR Am J Roentgenol 2003;180:1225–8.

[38] American College of Radiology Imaging Network. Available at: http://www.acrin.org/6666_protocol.html. Accessed July 4, 2007.

[39] Farria D, Feig SA. An introduction to economic issues in breast imaging. Radiol Clin North Am 2000;38:825–42.

[40] Farria DM, Schmidt ME, Monsees BS, et al. Professional and economic factors affecting access to mammography: a crisis today, or tomorrow? Cancer 2005;104:491–8.

[41] Liberman L, Morris EA, Kim CM, et al. MR imaging findings in the contralateral breast of women with recently diagnosed breast cancer. AJR Am J Roentgenol 2003;180:333–41.

[42] Lee SG, Orel SG, Woo IJ, et al. MR imaging screening of the contralateral breast in patients with newly diagnosed breast cancer: preliminary results. Radiology 2003;226:773–8.

[43] Berg WA, Gutierrez L, Nessaiver MS, et al. Diagnostic accuracy of mammography, clinical examination, US, and MR imaging in preoperative assessment of breast cancer. Radiology 2004; 233:830–49.

[44] Lehman CD, Blume JD, Thickman D, et al. Added cancer yield of MRI in screening the contralateral breast of women recently diagnosed with breast cancer: results from the International Breast Magnetic Resonance Consortium (IBMC) trial. J Surg Oncol 2005;92:9–15 [discussion: 15–6].

[45] Lehman CD, Gatsonis C, Kuhl CK, et al. MRI evaluation of the contralateral breast in women with recently diagnosed breast cancer. N Engl J Med 2007;356:1295–303.

[46] Morris EA, Liberman L, Ballon DJ, et al. MRI of occult breast carcinoma in a high-risk population. AJR Am J Roentgenol 2003;181:619–26.

[47] Port ER, Park A, Borgen PI, et al. Results of MRI screening for breast cancer in high-risk patients with LCIS and atypical hyperplasia. Ann Surg Oncol 2007;14:1051–7.

[48] Warner E, Plewes DB, Hill KA, et al. Surveillance of BRCA1 and BRCA2 mutation carriers with magnetic resonance imaging, ultrasound, mammography, and clinical breast examination. JAMA 2004;292:1317–25.

[49] Leach MO, Boggis CR, Dixon AK, et al. Screening with magnetic resonance imaging and mammography of a UK population at high familial risk of breast cancer: a prospective multicentre cohort study (MARIBS). Lancet 2005;365:1769–78.

[50] Sardanelli F, Podo F, D'Agnolo G, et al. Multicenter comparative multimodality surveillance of women at genetic-familial high risk for breast cancer (HIBCRIT study): interim results. Radiology 2007;242:698–715.

[51] Kriege M, Brekelmans CT, Boetes C, et al. Efficacy of MRI and mammography for breast-cancer screening in women with a familial or genetic predisposition. N Engl J Med 2004; 351:427–37.

[52] Kriege M, Brekelmans CT, Boetes C, et al. Differences between first and subsequent rounds of the MRISC breast cancer screening program for women with a familial or genetic predisposition. Cancer 2006;106:2318–26.

[53] Ikeda DM, Hylton NM, Kuhl CK, et al. Breast Imaging Reporting and Data System, BI-RADS: magnetic resonance imaging. Reston (VA): American College of Radiology; 2003.

[54] Plevritis SK, Kurian AW, Sigal BM, et al. Cost-effectiveness of screening BRCA1/2 mutation carriers with breast magnetic resonance imaging. JAMA 2006;295:2374–84.

[55] Griebsch I, Brown J, Boggis C, et al. Cost-effectiveness of screening with contrast enhanced magnetic resonance imaging vs X-ray mammography of women at a high familial risk of breast cancer. Br J Cancer 2006;95:801–10.

[56] Saslow D, Boetes C, Burke W, et al. American Cancer Society guidelines for breast screening with MRI as an adjunct to mammography. CA Cancer J Clin 2007;57:75–89.

[57] Kerlikowske K, Grady D, Barclay J, et al. Effect of age, breast density, and family history on the sensitivity of first screening mammography. [see comments]. JAMA 1996;276:33–8.

[58] Yen MF, Tabar L, Vitak B, et al. Quantifying the potential problem of overdiagnosis of ductal carcinoma in situ in breast cancer screening. Eur J Cancer 2003;39:1746–54.

[59] Walter LC, Covinsky KE. Cancer screening in elderly patients: a framework for individualized decision making. JAMA 2001;285:2750–6.

[60] Smith-Bindman R, Kerlikowske K, Gebretsadik T, et al. Is screening mammography effective in elderly women? Am J Med 2000;108:112–9.

[61] McPherson CP, Swenson KK, Lee MW. The effects of mammographic detection and comorbidity on the survival of older women with breast cancer. J Am Geriatr Soc 2002;50:1061–8.

[62] Smith RA, Saslow D, Sawyer KA, et al. American Cancer Society guidelines for breast cancer screening: update 2003. CA Cancer J Clin 2003;53:141–69.

[63] Ballard-Barbash R, Klabunde C, Paci E, et al. Breast cancer screening in 21 countries: delivery of services, notification of results and outcomes ascertainment. Eur J Cancer Prev 1999;8: 417–26.

[64] Sickles EA, Wolverton DE, Dee KE. Performance parameters for screening and diagnostic mammography: specialist and general radiologists. Radiology 2002;224:861–9.

[65] Leung JW, Margolin FR, Dee KE, et al. Performance parameters for screening and diagnostic mammography in a community practice: are there differences between specialists and general radiologists? AJR Am J Roentgenol 2007;188: 236–41.

[66] Collaborative Group on Hormonal Factors in Breast Cancer Familial breast cancer. Collaborative reanalysis of individual data from 52 epidemiological studies including 58,209 women with breast cancer and 101,986 women without the disease. Lancet 2001;358:1389–99.

[67] Easton DF, Ford D, Bishop DT. Breast and ovarian cancer incidence in BRCA1-mutation

carriers. Breast cancer linkage consortium. Am J Hum Genet 1995;56:265–71.
[68] Lux MP, Fasching PA, Beckmann MW. Hereditary breast and ovarian cancer: review and future perspectives. J Mol Med 2006;84:16–28.
[69] Wooster R, Weber BL. Breast and ovarian cancer. N Engl J Med 2003;348:2339–47.
[70] Easton DF. Familial risks of breast cancer. Breast Cancer Res 2002;4:179–81.
[71] Fisher B, Anderson S, Redmond CK, et al. Reanalysis and results after 12 years of follow-up in a randomized clinical trial comparing total mastectomy with lumpectomy with or without irradiation in the treatment of breast cancer. N Engl J Med 1995;333:1456–61.
[72] Fisher B, Anderson S, Bryant J, et al. Twenty-year follow-up of a randomized trial comparing total mastectomy, lumpectomy, and lumpectomy plus irradiation for the treatment of invasive breast cancer. N Engl J Med 2002;347:1233–41.
[73] American Chemical Society. 2007. Available at: www.acs.org. Accessed July 18, 2007.
[74] Frykberg ER. Lobular carcinoma in situ of the breast. Breast J 1999;5:296–303.
[75] Dupont WD, Parl FF, Hartmann WH, et al. Breast cancer risk associated with proliferative breast disease and atypical hyperplasia. Cancer 1993;71:1258–65.
[76] Page DL, Schuyler PA, Dupont WD, et al. Atypical lobular hyperplasia as a unilateral predictor of breast cancer risk: a retrospective cohort study. Lancet 2003;361:125–9.
[77] Mitchell G, Antoniou AC, Warren R, et al. Mammographic density and breast cancer risk in BRCA1 and BRCA2 mutation carriers. Cancer Res 2006;66:1866–72.
[78] Leconte I, Feger C, Galant C, et al. Mammography and subsequent whole-breast sonography of nonpalpable breast cancers: the importance of radiologic breast density. AJR Am J Roentgenol 2003;180:1675–9.

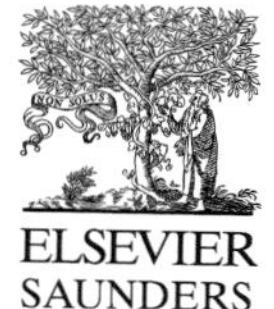

ELSEVIER
SAUNDERS

RADIOLOGIC
CLINICS
OF NORTH AMERICA

Radiol Clin N Am 45 (2007) 907–923

Alternative Breast-Imaging Approaches

R. James Brenner, MD, FACR[a,*], Yuri Parisky, MD[b]

In 1992, the National Cancer Institute convened a group of imaging investigators to assess the current feasibility and future directions related to clinical research for imaging with the use of positron emission tomography (PET) in oncology. The four areas of clinical potential with this method were identified as depicting and characterizing masses; depicting regional metastatic disease involving lymph nodes; depicting systemic metastases of cancer; and helping to assess the response of cancers to a variety of therapies [1].

The history and current status of breast-imaging strategies have incorporated similar rationales. From the first mammographic image reported in 1930 by Warren [2] to the present frontiers of noninvasive spectroscopic analysis of disease, several techniques have been proposed and studied. Because breast imaging often is distinguished—although lung and colon imaging are now entering a similar venue—by its dual goals of screening and diagnosis, the field has always required the additional parameter that efficacy and outcomes must be related to size of lesions detected. Appropriating a new technology that adds little to the current evaluation and management of small lesions is of questionable value. For example, if a proposed test has comparable accuracy in diagnosing cancer of a palpable lesion, for which conventional mammography and ultrasound are highly suspicious, but lesser accuracy for smaller nonpalpable lesions, its added value is questionable.

Most of the current clinical methods for breast cancer evaluation are based in the depiction of abnormal anatomy. This approach is an indirect method for detection and diagnosis. It is the abnormal (patho) physiology that is producing anatomic changes that are observed in mammography, ultrasound, CT, and MR imaging. The latter two studies are influenced by abnormal physiology; MR imaging or CT contrast studies reflect perfusion abnormalities surrounding pathologic lesions. Even this measure, however, is a secondary phenomenon, based on the primary development of tumor vessels and various growth factors; the observation of

[a] Breast Imaging Section, University of California, UCSF-Mt. Zion Hospital, Radiology H2804, 1600 Divisadero Street, San Francisco, CA 94115-1667, USA
[b] Mammoth Hospital, PO Box 660, 85 Sierra Park Road, Mammoth Lakes, CA 93546, USA.
* Corresponding author.
E-mail address: james.brenner@radiology.ucsf.edu (R.J. Brenner).

radiologic.theclinics.com
doi:10.1016/j.rcl.2007.06.006

contrast enhancement and washout is a product of increased vessel density and the absence of vascular endothelial "tight junctions" which are responses to, but not primary events in, the development of cancer.

More physiologic approaches have been advocated in an attempt to provide noninvasive methods to image breast cancer and distinguish it from benign changes in the breast. Perhaps most prominent of these are nuclear medicine studies that depend on the incorporation of a radioactive tracer into a tumor to provide the basis for imaging of a primary event or abnormality. Because alterations in physiology usually precede anatomic changes, the aim of this approach is to provide earlier diagnoses. Nuclear imaging is dependent upon the development of specific tracers to answer clinical problems and technology that is capable of distinguishing focal accumulation of the tracer from background normal tissue uptake or "noise." Protocols are developed that balance sufficient "count" rates and "target to background" features with patient throughput. For example, the injection of certain tracers to identify sentinel nodes requires a sufficient dose and proper timing of the imaging or target detection. Too little material may not be imaged or detected, and too much or too long a time between injection and detection may obscure the distinction between sentinel and nonsentinel axillary lymph nodes. This challenge has been especially severe in the development of monoclonal antibodies, where the advantages of specificity for cancer accumulation are compromised by difficulties in having the agent reach the target with sufficient imaging parameters for diagnosis.

Other approaches have received attention during the past decade, many attempting to exploit other portions of the electromagnetic (EM) spectrum beyond ultrasound and x-ray energies. Most of these have used computerized models and software previously unavailable in either revisiting older concepts with newer image processing or developing new areas yet unexplored. Many of these techniques, sometimes referred to as "physiologic" imaging, rely on basic biochemical perturbations in normal physiology that signal disease. The logistics of this approach have been applied to many fields. For example, some of the earliest work in PET imaging in the early 1980s explored differential blood flow and oxygen consumption associated with pathologic conditions [3].

The regulatory environment, especially in the United States, often conditions the manner in which new technology is introduced. Because mammography has been so established as a current standard for breast cancer screening, most technologies under investigation are proposed as ancillary studies for lesions already detected during screening and, thus, are aimed at improving the specificity of diagnosis. In performing such examinations, however, the identification of unsuspected abnormalities that are pursued to a diagnosis of cancer provides a basis for suggesting improved sensitivity. Continued clinical investigation helps to better define the potentials and limitations of such claims, even providing a basis for advocating a potential role for screening.

This article explores many proposed techniques—imaging and otherwise—that are predicated more on abnormal physiologic alterations than anatomic ones. Many of these approaches are being better defined in terms of their clinical applicability or are early "works in progress," where theoretic notions that are based in science are being tested for their clinically applicability.

Diagnostic nuclear medicine studies

Technetium-based agents

Much of the history of breast imaging with radionuclear agents reflects the serendipitous observation of tracer accumulation in the breast during studies performed for other reasons. Thus, for example, gallium and phosphonates have been detected in lesions subsequently demonstrated to represent breast adenocarcinoma; however, studies showing their efficacy in regular clinical practice have been lacking.

In this context, agents used for cardiac function evaluation have been noted to accumulate in tumors. Cox and colleagues [4], in The Netherlands, first reported in 1976 focal uptake in a lung cancer for a patient being evaluated for heart disease with Tl-201. More dedicated evaluation of this agent initially was described by Hisada and colleagues [5] 2 years later. Palpable carcinomas of the breast subsequently were reported to have a high likelihood of uptake (96%), a conclusion that could not necessarily be applied to smaller, nonpalpable cancers [6].

Given the superior imaging characteristics of 99mTechnetium (a scintillation camera is more sensitive to the 140 photon energy of this agent than the 80 photon energy of Tl) and its general replacement as the radionuclide of choice in cardiac imaging, similar observation patterns with respect to lung cancer were reported first by Hassan and colleagues [7] in 1989 using 99mTc-sestamibi. The precise mechanism for 99mTc-sestamibi is unknown. Much of the tracer activity is concentrated in the mitochondria [8] and its accumulation in primary malignant or metastatic lesions have been described for thyroid, lung, bronchial, and breast [9]. Various techniques have been advocated to improve depiction of breast tumors with this agent, including the use of prone positioning (to separate the breast from the chest wall), increased counts, and delayed images.

In the mid-1990s, many single-institutional reports using Tc-99m sestamibi were optimistic, but frequently did not specify the size of the tumor in the studied population or selected a population likely to represent larger cancers. For example, a Canadian study suggested sensitivity and specificity for primary tumors in a population of 65 women with palpable or highly suspicious mammograms of 91.5% and 94.4% respectively. In advancing the efficacy of the technique, the investigators also reported metastatic lymph node sensitivity and specificity of 84.2% and 90.9%, respectively [10]. Herein the issue of lesion size can be inferred, even if not reported. Nearly 90% of the studied population had metastatic lymph nodes, indicating a cohort with advanced disease. Similarly, an American study of 147 women reported sensitivity of 92.2% and specificity of 89.2%, but two thirds of the lesions were palpable, with a mean size on mammogram of 2.82 cm [11]. Other studies that more critically evaluated the results of sestamibi imaging with respect to size were less encouraging. Sensitivity for lesions less than 1 cm in size was 50% [12]. Perhaps the best profile of the use of sestamibi can be viewed from a multi-institutional trial [13]. For palpable lesions, sensitivity and specificity were 87% and 76%, respectively; however, for nonpalpable lesions, the sensitivity and specificity were 61% and 87%, respectively. Given these results, screening for small breast cancers is unlikely to be validated with this agent.

Others have advocated the role of Tc-sestamibi in helping to develop a management plan for cases that are problematic based on conventional imaging. One private practice group reported sensitivities and specificities of 90% and 93%, respectively [14], prompting commentary even by an enthusiast of this technique that such numbers were "unique!" [15]. One important problem with this approach, especially for nonpalpable lesions, is that the negative predictive value of sestamibi studies, as evidenced in the above mentioned multi-institutional trial, is insufficiently high to validate a decision to avoid biopsy based on the nuclear medicine study results. Difficult though decisions may be for complex conventional imaging cases, reliance on a negative sestamibi study may not be justified.

The role of Tc-sestamibi has been revisited, however. Early reports regarding the use of Tc-99m tetrofosmin scintimammography suggested its possible role in diagnostic imaging, although little has been published to indicate significantly improved results when compared with sestamibi [16]. More recently, however, new approaches and, especially new technology, have been suggested that might improve results [17]. By looking more critically at dose, compression (how far the lesion is from the detector, decreased attenuation), acquisition time, field of view, and especially semi-conductor electronics or other modifications in instrumentation, improved results have been demonstrated under limited circumstances [17–22]. For example, using a small multicrystal sodium iodide–based system, the sensitivity for detection of tumors 1 cm or less was increased from 47% to 67% [17]. Whether such improvements will encourage the use of such agents is difficult to predict. Dual detectors may improve sensitivity. Conversely, added value will need to be shown over current techniques. For example, studies reporting on the accuracy of sestamibi with the more expensive use of MR imaging showed comparable specificities but lower sensitivities, suggesting a possible role for the postoperative breast [22].

Another proposed use of technetium-based radionuclear agents has been as a noninvasive method to assess response to treatment, such as neoadjuvant therapy with limited, but encouraging, results [23]. This rationale applies to other imaging techniques, such as MR imaging for local disease assessment and PET for systemic determinations. Because PET scanning is less accessible, by requiring special equipment beyond the more widely available gamma cameras, technetium-based compounds might have wider applicability. An important role might be to assess early response to neoadjuvant therapy, an approach that is gaining popularity. A recent report on the use of 99mTc-depreotide scintigraphy suggested that success in selecting patients for endocrine therapy in advanced breast cancer, based on down-regulation of somatostatin receptors, could be accomplished and assessed at 3 weeks following initial therapy [24]. If better instrumentation and electronics can be applied to hand-held probes, then lesions identified only by sestamibi might be identified more easily for operative excision [9].

Positron emission tomography

Obtaining sufficient uptake of a radionuclide at anatomic sites of disease and registering such sites properly can be challenging. Elements that undergo radioactive decay by means of emitting positrons lend themselves, with proper instrumentation, to more sophisticated methods of anatomic delineation. When the positron encounters an electron, the two particles undergo an annihilation reaction, such that two residual photons with energy of 512 keV each attempt travel at 180° angles from one another. Thus, penetration through the body is improved, and the coincident events can be recorded (recall technetium decay photons have an energy of 140 keV). Special equipment is necessary to capture such information, and computers are used to coregister such events and assign anatomic placement. The slight timing differences that can be registered by detectors at 180° from each other permit a more closely approximated anatomic location for such events. Thus, where tracer accumulates, the location can be better defined and imaged.

PET imaging attempts to achieve such goals. Because there is some variation as to the detected event—the positron may travel up to 3 mm before encountering an electron that triggers the annihilation reaction—resolution can approximate 5 mm, depending on how concentrated the tracer is at an anatomic focus and where such a focus is located. This registration can be delineated further when coupled to a CT scan in what often is termed PET-CT or fusion studies. The physics of both studies is beyond the scope of this discussion but has been well described [25]. Because dedicated PET equipment is expensive and less accessible than standard nuclear imaging hardware, investigations have been conducted on modified standard equipment using a single photon emission CT (SPECT) approach. Reporting on phantoms and 24 patients with known or suspected cancer, hypermetabolic lesions were seen by PET in 46 foci and by SPECT in 36 cases in one study [26]. Other investigators indicated that, given the more uniform attenuation issues in the lung, SPECT was useful only in this organ when compared with PET [27]. In this context, it should be noted that for whole-body PET scanning, only about 5% of the photons reach the detector.

Early PET investigations used C-11– or O-15–labeled tracers to determine blood flow to tumors or to analyze oxygen extraction and use by tumors [3]. Most oncologic use of PET, however, has used 2-[fluorine-18] fluoro-2-deoxy-D-glucose (FDG). The half-life of F-18, which is cyclotron produced, is long enough (109 minutes) to permit transport to imaging facilities. This glucose analog is taken into the cell and phosphorylated by hexokinase, like glucose; however, the phosphorylated compound cannot undergo further metabolism and, following the action of hexokinase, cannot escape the cell. Thus, the basic biochemistry and physiology of the compound, unlike sestamibi, is understood to a large extent. FDG is one of most studied tracers, which portend a new era for molecular imaging. Although some tumors (eg, bronchial carcinoid) do not accumulate this tracer, most metabolically active tumors do to some extent. Furthermore, breast cancer has demonstrated overexpression of the glucose transport molecule GLUT1, which may contribute to the target imaging [28]. The exact mechanisms of cell membrane transport have not been elucidated, however; thus, the empiric observation that some breast carcinomas (sometimes even advanced ones) do not accumulate FDG cannot be reconciled.

FDG can be taken up under normal physiologic conditions in skeletal muscle, myocardium, bone marrow, the genito-urinary tract, healing bone, lymph nodes, infection, and any type of inflammation [29,30]. The latter is especially problematic during imaging surveillance following treatment for breast cancer because fat necrosis often appears similar to carcinoma, and the distinction between recurrence and inflammation cannot be made. This is complicated by MR imaging studies that often are unable to resolve the issue because of intense contrast uptake that often is associated with fat necrosis. In addition, there may be unexplained uptake at the nipple areolar complex and variable uptake due to breast proliferative changes, especially in younger women, limiting the role of PET. Activity in normal thymus, thyroid, and pelvic structures also has been observed. With proper preprocedure fasting and limited body motion, most of these background physiologic accumulations can be minimized.

PET scanners often have a limited axial field of view of less than 15 cm. The ability to detect sufficient tracer accumulation over background is subject to all of the conditions described above for all nuclear medicine studies. Attempts to quantitate such uptake as a standardized uptake value have met with limited success [31]. Because of the inherent resolution of PET, its role in primary breast cancer detection has not been validated, although sporadic cases of small lesions have been seen, most likely secondary to inexplicable intense uptake (favorable target/background ratio). A meta-analysis of 13 studies showed an overall sensitivity of 89% (range, 79%–100%), but the mean size of studied tumors ranged from 2 to 4 cm [32]. Prototype dedicated PET units for breast were reported first in 2000 [33], although the feasibility of this approach was considered in 1994 [34]. More recently, with a different prototype, 23 patients with highly suspicious abnormalities by mammography or ultrasound were studied with the unit conforming to a conventional mammography machine [35]. Of 23 lesions seen by FDG-PET, 18 were malignant, with a mean size of 1.9 cm (range, 0–6 cm). For malignant lesions not seen by PET images that were reconstructed in transverse, craniocaudal, and coronal planes, the mean size was 1.3 cm. Actual histology of such lesions were larger by a mean of 4 mm in diameter. Therefore, the sensitivity was 86% (95% confidence interval [CI]: 65%–95%) and specificity was 33% (95% CI: 2%–79%). False positives included a calcific lesion that was fibrocystic and two masses that represented fat necrosis. PET identified an 8-mm mass representing papillary ductal carcinoma in situ (DCIS) that was not seen initially by ultrasound but was identified at a "second-look" examination. In like manner and with a similar population providing a validation study for a commercially available unit, 39 of 44 (89%) index lesions were seen [36]. Using a different protocol unit, 14 of 16 patients were imaged successfully, demonstrating 10 cancers and 4 benign lesions [37]. Claims regarding the promise of PET imaging for DCIS remain unsubstantiated [30].

The most important and possibly unequaled impact of FDG-PET imaging has been in its whole-body application, which can be performed in about 1 hour. Initial staging and surveillance reassessment lend themselves well to whole-body imaging modalities, such as PET. Its correlation to other imaging studies has been promoted, but often without a tissue diagnosis [38]. In a British Columbia study of 165 patients, axillary metastases were identified with a sensitivity of 28% and a specificity of 86% [39]. The impact of the study, however, is illustrated by the observation that, of the 5% of patients who had distant metastases, nearly one third of them were believed to have only local-regional disease by clinical and conventional imaging. Thus, staging and management were altered substantively by the results. For cases in this study with suspected recurrence, the sensitivity was 89% and the specificity was 88%.

The impact of FDG-PET on management was reported recently from a cancer center [40]. Studying 125 consecutive patients and comparing results with conventional imaging, the extent of disease was increased in 43% (n = 54), unchanged in 33% (n = 41), and decreased in 24% (n = 30). Therapeutic plans were altered in 32% of cases (n = 40), validated in 27% of cases (n = 34), and not considered affected in 41% of cases (n = 51). As in the previously mentioned study, the major impact of initial PET scanning caused the treating physician to change the assessment from local-regional disease to systemic disease, as well as helping to evaluate treatment response. Findings at PET were confirmed with a tissue diagnosis, however, in just less than half of the cases.

PET has been used with some success to identify unknown primary carcinomas. One study reported 7 of 29 such primary carcinomas detected by PET, including 2 breast cancers, 4 oral cavity cancers, and 1 colon cancer [41]. The current authors have seen positive results in such a context for PET, but all have been demonstrated on MR imaging, with many cases detected by MR imaging and not PET. MR imaging likely remains the modality of choice for an unknown primary carcinoma presenting with axillary metastasis [42].

Like sestamibi, PET scanning with FDG also has been suggested for evaluation of response to neoadjuvant therapy. Although the results are encouraging, the expense and availability of this technique, combined with results that do not seem to be better than MR imaging, may limit its application in this regard [43].

Like with sestamibi, improvement in PET imaging has been proposed. Other positron emitters coupled to amino acids with known physiologic mechanisms have been proposed, including C-11 methionine and F-18 tyrosine, but have met with limited success [44]. For reasons advocated in the imaging of sestamibi, prone table imaging for PET has been suggested, also with limited enthusiasm [45]. The use of estrogen receptors for those tumors demonstrating receptor positivity has been advocated, with one trial indicating a 93% sensitivity for primary tumor and axillary node disease; however, these results have not been embraced for several technical reasons [46]. PET-FDG is likely to remain a benchmark for whole-body surveillance, against which all other imaging modalities likely will be compared. As a primary breast cancer imaging study, better instrumentation and accessibility may be required to validate its use, especially in situations where MR imaging is available and fulfills a similar role at less cost.

Radionuclear tracers for identification of sentinel node in staging breast cancer

The proper staging of breast cancer is fundamental to establishing a prognosis and determining appropriate treatment. Because most carcinomas (not necessarily applicable to breast sarcomas, which constitute a small percentage of breast malignancies) demonstrate early spread by means of the lymphatic system, proper assessment of nodal status is essential in this determination. Regardless of tumor anatomic location, the embryologic basis for lymphatic development provides a basis for careful evaluation of the axillary lymph nodes, because 97% of all tumors, if they spread beyond the breast, involve such structures [47].

Full axillary lymph node dissection (ALND) is associated with a 2% false negative rate and is considered the standard by which the axillary nodal chain is evaluated [1,48]. The procedure incurs consequential morbidity [49], a particular problem for the large number of cases that have no axillary involvement. Conversely, about one third of patients in whom the axillary nodal examination is normal demonstrate sites of tumor involvement at microscopy [50]. The concept of identifying sentinel nodes—whereby the first node associated with primary lymphatic drainage can be specified—began in 1977 for penile carcinoma and was popularized in the evaluation of melanoma in 1992 [51,52]. The approach was applied subsequently to breast cancer, initially with isosulfan blue dye and later with technetium-based compounds [53,54]. Various techniques have been investigated with this nuclear medicine approach, all using technetium-99m tracers that can be imaged in terms of their pattern of spread or simply detected manually by gamma-probes in the axilla. Injection into the peritumoral site, the subdermis, or the subareolar complex produces satisfactory results, consequent to the development of the lymphatic system [55]. In addition, different tracers have been studied with variable success, including sulfur colloid (filtered and ultrafiltered), human serum albumin colloid, dextran 40, microlite, and cardiolite, as well as combinations of isosulfan blue and technetium radiotracers. One important advantage of radionuclear techniques over blue dye, but only when accompanied by imaging scintigraphy, is the ability to detect the unusual case of primary and exclusive drainage to internal mammary nodes with no axillary drainage, as well as the rare instances of contralateral drainage. Under such situations, the absence of axillary sentinel node metastases at dissection is of no, and perhaps even misleading, value.

Results of sentinel node scintigraphy have been variable, often depending on the technique used. A multicenter validation study of probe-directed sentinel node biopsy followed by ALND provided standardized training for surgeons at 11 centers [56]. Sentinel nodes were identified successfully in 405 of 443 (91%) enrolled patients. The accuracy of predicting axillary involvement was reported as 97% (392/405), with a false negative rate of 11%. An attempt to evaluate the impact of imaging—"sentinel node mapping"—combined three protocols in reporting a success rate of 94%, with 105 of 466 patients showing positive disease. False negative rates could not be determined because not all patients underwent completion ALND.

Issues impacting the results of this technique include patient selection, tracer selection, operator experience and expertise, and definitions of positive nodes. Patients with large tumors of greater than 5 cm may have drainage to multiple nodes. Patients with prior axillary surgery or large biopsy cavities (>6 cm) and distorted lymphatics may be candidates for radionuclear tracer studies, but results will be compromised. Determining a "hot" sentinel node often is dependent on the operator determining the rate of gamma-detected counts as a factor of background, so that a learning curve and clinical judgment are part of the assessment. Finally, with the advent of immunohistochemical stains that more easily detect epithelial cells within the lymph node, the significance of standard hematoxylin and eosin–negative, and, for example, cytokeratin-positive, disease (and its quantitative extent) influences reported results.

Current techniques operate with a benchmark that the sentinel node should be identified in at least 95% of cases. Injection sites, with or without imaging guidance (eg, ultrasound guidance of biopsy cavity walls—the actual cavity should not be injected), and different types of tracers have success, with false negative rates reported at 0% to 15% and correlation to axillary nodal status reported as 95% or better [49].

CT with radiography

Early trials in the late 1970s with CT prompted the generation of three dedicated CT units for breast cancer evaluation. Whether with whole-body scanners or dedicated units, the attempt to image lesions and assess malignant potential was based on lesion morphology and contrast enhancement characteristics. Because contrast enhancement as demonstrated on CT is a secondary phenomenon of breast tumors related to perfusion, the likelihood of discriminating benign from malignant lesions without morphologic criteria would be proven by empiric observations. In fact, this did not happen. CT enhancement was not sufficiently discriminatory to significantly improve accuracy [57,58]. Given the nonionizing use of MR imaging with a similar basis for lesion detection (ie, differential perfusion), there may not be a compelling need to demonstrate improved results, especially if some of the same issues of sensitivity and specificity apply to both approaches, which is likely. If comparable sensitivity is achieved with improved specificity, however, there may yet be a role for CT in this context, especially if dose considerations are reconciled, as will be discussed infra.

CT, like MR imaging, is a cross-sectional imaging modality. Thus, certain lesions that escape mammographic orthogonal geometry projection may be visualized on CT. Although MR imaging has the same capability, preoperative localization of lesions using a CT scanner can be facilitated with less time, fewer resources, and comparable accuracy compared with MR-guided techniques. Percutaneous biopsy using CT has not been developed to the extent as for MR imaging, however, so the advantages of preoperative localization with CT remain the only tissue sampling application.

CT can detect abnormalities in silicone implant integrity, demonstrating the same features ("linguine sign, inverted loop sign") of implant failure as described for MR imaging; however, there is no advantage to the former, with the disadvantage of ionizing radiation. Nonetheless, CT performed for other reasons related to the thoracic structures can detect such abnormalities, even if incidental to the primary purpose of the intended examination.

Staging of breast cancer has been an important role for CT. As in any staging modality, evaluation of lung parenchyma as well as axillary, hilar, and mediastinal nodal chains frequently are depicted well on CT scanning. In addition, the relationship of the breast to the chest wall and the ability to demonstrate enlarged internal mammary lymph nodes and lymph nodes associated with the clavicular region permit deliberate planning for adjuvant radiation therapy.

Recent interest has been developing in revisiting the issue of dedicated breast CT for detection and diagnosis. Following the enthusiasm generated for potential applications of digital mammography—specifically, tomosynthesis—the feasibility of providing direct tomographic depiction of cancer and other lesions has been explored. Unlike earlier versions of CT (see supra), where little benefit was found for a high dose of radiation from scanners developed before helical or multichannel instruments, new approaches seek to exploit current technologic improvements with scan time and radiation dose. Of particular note is the use of a flat panel detector specifically suited to the breast [59,60]. (Recall discussion regarding instrumentation modifications designed to improve the accuracy of Tc99mSestamibi studies). Preliminary results suggest that a full breast scan may be attended by a radiation dose comparable to a two-view mammographic study, with sufficiently better spatial and contrast resolution as to provide all of the benefits—if not more—of digital tomosynthesis. One issue that current prototype units face is that the scans are done in the prone position, even though scan time may be less than 5 minutes. Such hardware and patient positioning considerations compromise this approach, when considering its application to wide-scale screening. Although useful in an adjunctive sense, the most powerful benefit of a tomographic examination of the breast likely would be in the screening environment, where cancer that is detected poorly by conventional mammography may be identified and overlapping tissue summation artifacts of conventional radiography may be resolved easily without recalling the patient for additional imaging [61,62].

Nonconventional techniques

Given the elusive balance between sensitivity and specificity of current breast-imaging techniques, there remains interest in nonconventional imaging of the breast. The authors chose the descriptor "nonconventional" to avoid unintentional bias sometimes associated with these modalities. Many of these nonconventional imaging modalities are founded in physical science; measurement of heat, electrical conductivity, or impedance to light are physical properties that can be altered by disease states and provide a basis for suggesting certain pathologic entities.

Numerous factors seem to influence the continued pursuit of exploiting such modalities. These include the limitations of mammography (lack of sensitivity in dense breasts), patient apprehension because of painful examination or perceived dangers of radiation exposure, and low specificity resulting in too many biopsies. Most of the nonconventional modalities purport nondestructive or pain-free imaging, imply harm from radiation or ultrasound, or attempt to find a justifiable clinical practice, such as helping to reduce the overall cost of "unnecessary biopsies."

Nonconventional imaging techniques are being studied, from basic in vitro experimentation to multicenter clinical trials. The history and description of many of these techniques have been reviewed in textbooks dedicated to the subject [63,64]. Several physical properties related to the breast, observed or induced, can be measured in an attempt to define unique and early identifiable breast cancer characteristics. To simplify and categorize the vast spectrum of potential imaging modalities related to this discussion, one can divide them into imaging involving emission or transmission properties. Within these two categories, we examine certain types of nonconventional breast imaging: thermal, electrical impedance, ultrasound CT, and transillumination, as well as other techniques that do not conform easily to categorization. The purpose of this discussion is to identify different methods to use energies of the EM spectrum to better identify breast cancer and to evaluate recurring rationales that provide a basis for continued and potentially revealing investigations (Fig. 1).

Emission imaging

Two thousand years ago, the Roman physician Celsus – Aulus (Aurelius) Cornelius, described the clinical features of disease or inflammation as rubor (redness), calor (warmth), tumor (swelling), and dolor (pain). Hippocrates is credited with first observing differential body temperature. He described covering an ill patient's thorax with an earth-soaked cloth. Warmer areas dried faster, resulting in a temperature distribution thermogram. Of the four original observations of inflammation, only calor or warmth can be quantitatively measured and correlated to the degree of disease.

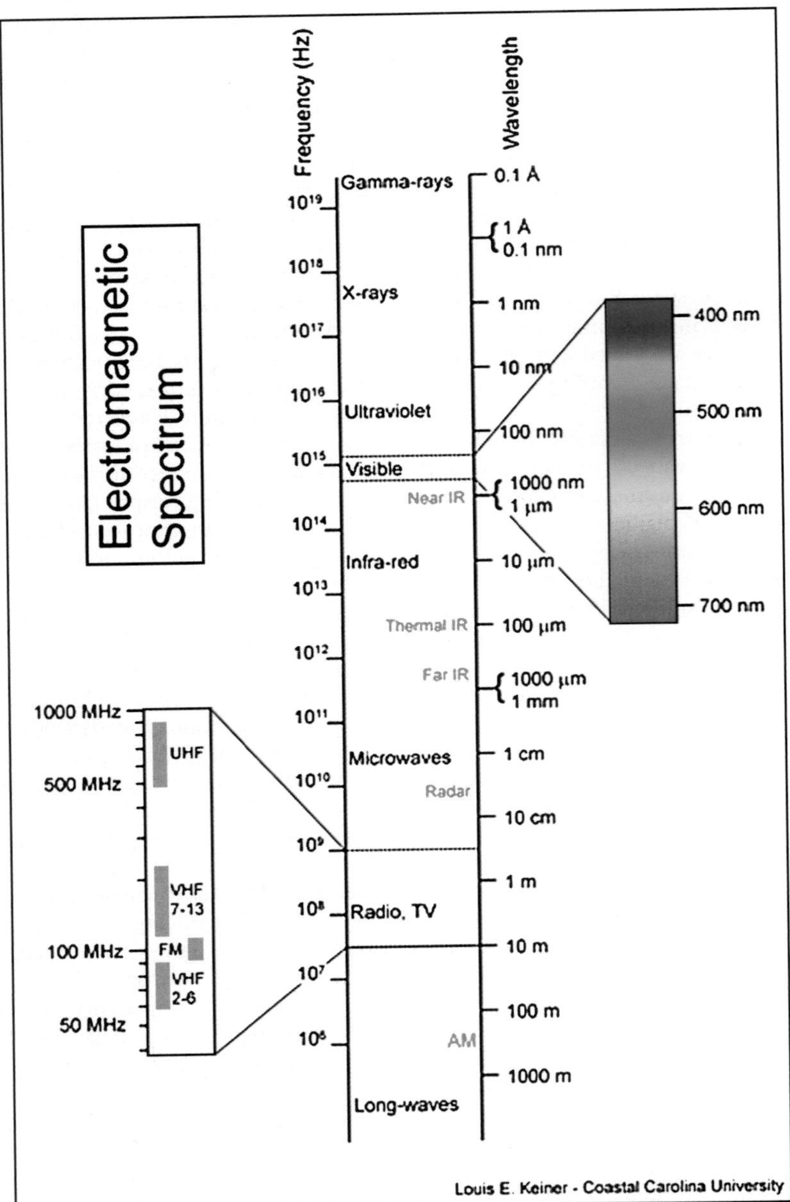

Fig. 1. The electromagnetic spectrum. (*Courtesy of* L. Keiner, PhD, Conway, SC.)

Heat can be transmitted by three means: convection, conduction, and radiation. Investigations using heat radiation use a narrow wavelength on the EM spectrum. Emission of infrared radiation, at a particular wavelength, is related to temperature; the warmer the source, the shorter the wavelength. Microwave thermal emission also can be used, a subject that has been studied less clinically than infrared radiation. Microwave emission is believed to represent deeper tissue heat emission, whereas infrared emission is considered to be a result of more superficial processes. Infrared emission can be measured accurately to fractions of a degree by a specialized infrared camera (millimeter resolution topographically) and displayed as a spectrum on a color or gray scale, representing temperature: a "thermogram." Lawson [65] showed the first breast thermogram in 1956. Numerous investigators have observed that patients who have breast cancer demonstrate an elevation of focal ipsilateral breast skin temperature of 1°C to 3°C [66,67]. Early investigations proposed that thermographic imaging of the breast could increase diagnostic accuracy when coupled with mammography and identify occult early breast cancer or presumably patients who are at risk for developing cancer [68].

The interest in thermal imaging as a tool to identify breast cancer prompted investigation of this technology in the Breast Cancer Detection Demonstration Project (BCDDP), a multicenter study conducted in the 1970s, where it performed with unsatisfactory results. As an independent imaging modality for asymptomatic women, the false positive rate was 25%, and the false negative rate exceeded 60%. When results were coupled with physical examination and mammography, the false positive rate increased, and the false negative rate decreased minimally [69]. Despite the untoward results from the BCDDP, there continued research into thermal imaging. Favorable results from small trials and anecdotal cases of improved efficacy were reported in the 1980s and 1990s. Scientific debate regarding the source of the thermal signal as cell division and increased metabolism eventually were discarded in favor of increased vascularity. Based on work in breast cancer angiogenesis [70], thermal imagery was proposed as a predictor of primary aggressiveness, and the potential for metastasis was postulated by Head and colleagues [71]. Despite the lack of sufficient data, a relationship between the tumor, vascularity, and generated heat relative to adjacent normal breast tissue activity has generated new inquiries [72]. Retrospective analysis of a subgroup of BCDDP patients suggested a possible merit to thermographic findings. A scoring system was applied, and patients with poor thermographic prognostic factors at initial screening were observed to have shorter survival [73].

Interest in this technology continues, notwithstanding the absence of data to support an established clinical role. In the late 1990s, a public company approached the US Food and Drug Administration (FDA) and received guidance for a prospective blinded multicenter trial for evaluating thermometric features in an adjunctive setting, Computerized Thermal Imaging. The trial enrolled patients with mammographically suspicious lesions scheduled for biopsy. The dynamic infrared imaging was performed with a challenge of cooled circulating air to increase the conspicuity of abnormal (tumoral) vascularity, which presumably lacked normal physiologic vasoconstrictive response. A proprietary algorithm was applied to the data. For all breast lesions recommended for biopsy and eventually biopsied, the "index of suspicion" suggested a 97% sensitivity, a 14% specificity, a 95% negative predictive value, and a 24% positive predictive value [74]. Because of methodologic concerns, the FDA panel did not approve the application for clinical use.

Another device, the Sentinel Breastscan (Infrared Sciences Corp., Stony Brook, New York) system, received FDA approval in 2004, predicated on prior approval of infrared imaging technology with respect to safety but not necessarily efficacy. The device purports to enhance the awareness of the clinician and radiologist to "those sites where a cancer is most likely to be found." Data published in biomedical conference proceedings, from nonblinded trials involving screening and diagnostic patients, suggested a false negative rate of less than 1%, a true positive rate greater than 99%, but marginal specificity. Half of the normal screening population was deemed at risk for possibly developing breast cancer, a number that is of limited value to patients and clinicians and is about threefold greater than the actual population who will develop breast cancer [75]. Thus, thermal imaging, although reflecting physiologic parameters related to cancer, has been found insufficiently discriminatory to be accepted into routine clinical use. Further investigations into a simple method to assess response to neoadjuvant therapy have been proposed so that interest in thermal features of breast cancer remains.

Transmission imaging

A multitude of energy sources along the EM spectrum may be directed into the breast in a nondestructive manner and the consequences subsequently measured. These types of radiation, with wavelengths equal to or longer than that of visible and infrared light, are considered nondestructive because they do not appear to interact harmfully with molecular structures during the short imaging acquisition periods. The forms of radiation can be altered by physical properties of tumor and diseased tissue and differentiated from those energies, which traverse normal breast tissue. Ultrasound is a form of such imaging, as is visible light transillumination, the first recorded transmission imaging of the breast, performed in the 1920s. Simple transillumination or visible light diaphanography was unsuccessful in distinguishing benign from malignant disease during clinical trials that were conducted in the 1980s [76].

Optical imaging

The general term "optical imaging" encompasses a wide spectrum of light-transmission imaging modalities. Nonvisible light, ranging in wavelength from 700 to 1200 nm, transmitted into the breast can interact with the physical and absorptive properties of normal and abnormal tissue. The light can be absorbed, reflected, refracted, or scattered.

Measurement of the detected changes in the transmitted light is the subject of much research, most of which is preliminary. Although the use of this technology has been studied in determining water or lipid concentration in breast tissue and lesions, most of the work has focused on the imaging of angiogenesis, specifically the light absorption by hemoglobin in various oxygenated states. The absorption of light, like magnetic properties exploited with MR imaging, differs in oxygenated or deoxygenated hemoglobin. Normal tissue is differentiated from cancerous tissue by the density of microvessels, with higher concentrations of deoxyhemoglobin found within the higher density of microvessels of tumors. Selection of appropriate wavelengths for imaging is dependent on the "target" absorptive properties [77]. Hemoglobin is best imaged at the narrow wavelength of the near infrared spectrum, 650 to 850 nm [78]. A small clinical trial using such infrared imaging characteristics as an adjunct to sonography, in differentiating benign from malignant lesions based on relative concentrations of deoxyhemoglobin, was conducted. The trial suggested a potential to distinguish prebiopsy benign from malignant lesions based on relative deoxyhemoglobin concentrations [79]. Current investigations are being conducted to permit fusing or coregistrating mammography with optical imaging, to create a hybrid optical and x-ray mammography system [80].

The manufacturers of the DOBI Medical ComfortScan (Mahwah, New Jersey) conducted a multicenter trial to evaluate their optical technology—an array of near-infrared light-emitting diodes—as an adjunctive imaging modality to mammography and physical examination.

Examination of each breast takes less than 1 minute, in a specifically designed cushioned imaging apparatus. A charge-coupled device camera is placed opposite the diode source to measure the transmitted near-infrared light. Near-infrared light is absorbed differently by blood, depending on the oxygenated state of the hemoglobin. The examination requires gentle compression of the breast at approximately 10 to 15 mm Hg, which presumably traps blood in abnormal "neo-angiogenesis" tumoral vasculature. The process is dynamic and subject to computerized differentiation of the transmitted signal to produce an interpretable image.

Preliminary data provided by the company from four clinical trial sites, which were interpreted by a single blinded reader (n = 68) indicating benign or malignant results, yielded a sensitivity of between 92% and 98%, dependent on the manner of data presentation, and an average specificity of 63% [81]. (Unfortunately, the company has experienced financial difficulties while supporting the clinical trials, and validation of this technology has fallen victim to finances rather than science.)

Another company, Imaging Diagnostics Systems (Plantation, Florida), is evaluating Computed Tomography Laser Mammography (CTLM) and is seeking FDA approval. The technology is dependent on the differential absorption of the transmitted 808-nm wavelength laser light by the relative concentrations of oxy- and deoxyhemoglobin. The selected wavelength, according to company literature, maximally detects the hemoglobin (Fig. 2). Case studies suggest the physical area of increased absorption is several fold greater than the tumor itself. Imaging is performed supine, with the uncompressed breast suspended. Images are collected in a manner similar to CT, with laser beam source diameter of 3 mm. Object detectability in vitro has been reported at 2.0 mm. Processed images are reconstructed into two- or three-dimensional displays onto a workstation and can be compared directly with mammography or fused with MR imaging.

Much of the published clinical work evaluating CTML has been conducted in Europe. A blinded study, involving 100 female patients with 105 lesions categorized as Breast Imaging and Reporting Data System (BI-RADS) 4 or 5 based on mammography, yielded a significant increase in laser absorption by malignant lesions (70.0% versus 32.7%, $P = .028$). Also observed was an increased absorption in larger volumes (85.7% of malignant and 77.8% of benign lesions) and in lesions with round shapes (78.1% of malignant and 73.3% of benign lesions), although these features were less useful [82].

Both of these technologies await FDA clinical evaluation. Both seek approval as adjunctive breast-imaging technologies, which may be used to determine the likelihood of malignancy following conventional image–detected abnormalities. This approach, as opposed to a screening device, is the usual method to obtain approval for new technology in assessing the likelihood of breast cancer in clinical practice.

Ultrasound CT

Conventional diagnostic breast ultrasound uses reflected sound waves detected by a transducer to create an image. Technology used by the UltraSound CT device (Techniscan Medical Systems, Salt Lake City, Utah) characterizes lesions within the breast by determining characteristics of speed and attenuation of sound using transmission, rather than reflection, ultrasound. The device incorporates two opposing transducers in a water bath to obtain the data and provides two separate image sets for analysis. This transmitter and receiver pair rotates about the immersed suspended breast in a manner

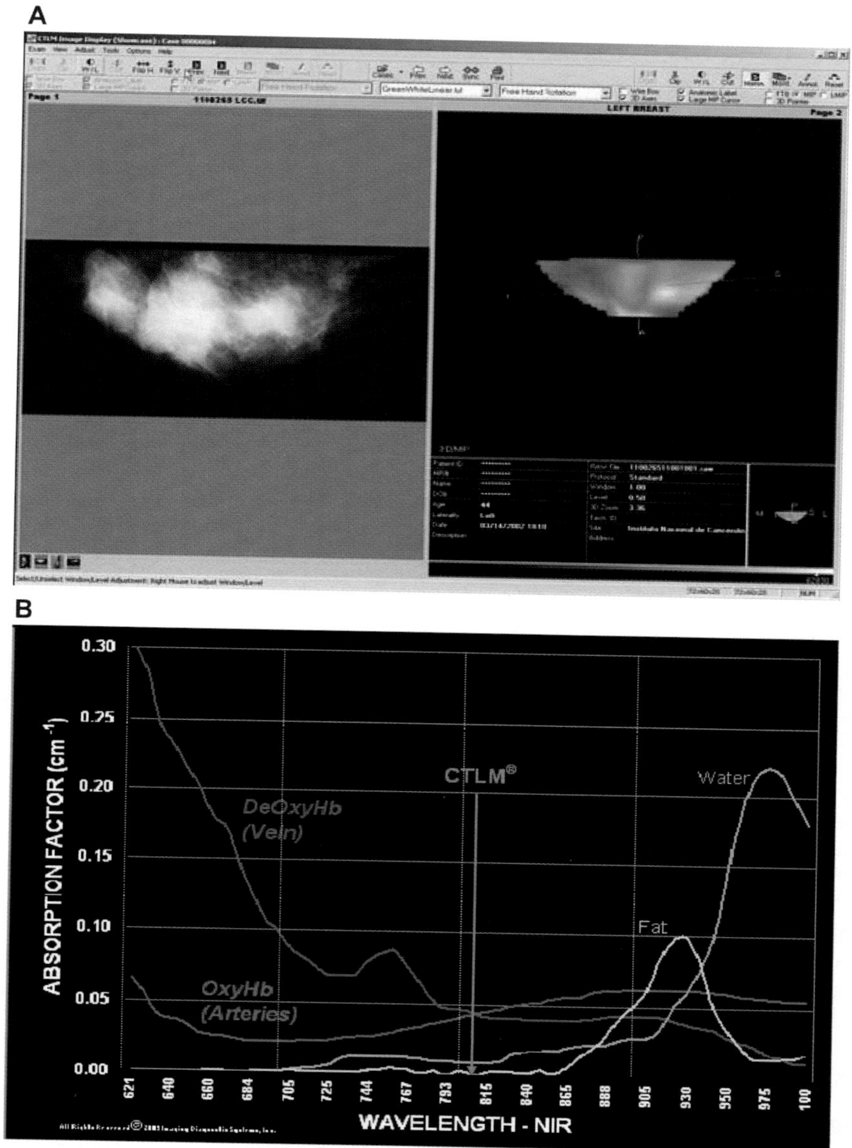

Fig. 2. CTLM. (*A*) Cranial caudal mammogram (*left*) with correlative CTLM image (*right*). Increased absorption of light in the lateral aspect correlates to an area of increased hemoglobin, suggesting angiogenesis in an area that is nonspecific on mammogram. (*B*) Absorption of light (wavelength by various structures within the breast). At a wavelength of 808 nm, there is optimal absorption of near-infrared (NIR) light by oxyhemoglobin (OxyHb) and deoxyhemoglobin (DeOxyHb), with minimum absorption by water or fat.

similar to CT. Each slice is 2 mm in thickness, and the transducer pair scans every 2° in 180 locations. The receiving transducer is a 960-element multirow detector that receives direct and scattered sound waves from the source as the sound travels through the breast. Once a slice is completed, the transducer pair moves up or down the breast in 2-mm increments. The data are interpreted based on the mathematics of inverse scattering, which allows calculation of waveform information from these signals, as they interact with numerous physical interfaces within the breast. Thus, for each thickness plane a two-dimensional image is created, and when stacked together, a three-dimensional image is formed, for speed and sound attenuation (Fig. 3). The manipulations of such data are proprietary, so that only empiric results can be evaluated.

Early data analysis suggests little overlap between benign and malignant lesions, with attenuation values having a much greater predictive value than

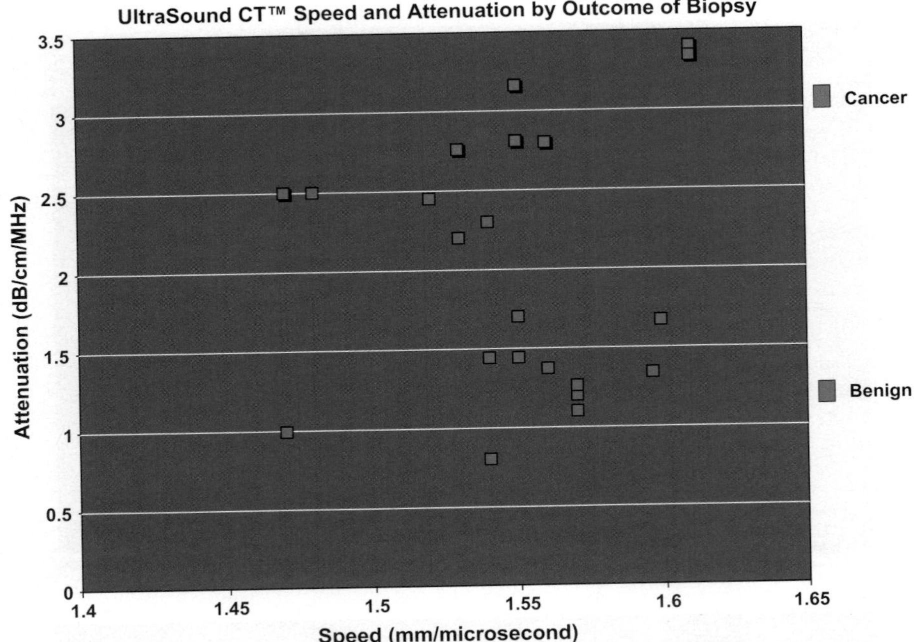

Fig. 3. Ultrasound CT—relationship of transmission speed and attenuation values to lesion outcome. (*Adapted from* Johnson SA, Abbott T, Bell R, et al. Non-invasive breast tissue characterization using ultrasound speed and attenuation: in vivo validation. In: Andre MP, editor. Acoustical imaging. Vol 28. The Netherlands: Springer Netherlands; 2007. p. 147–54; with permission.)

speed of sound transmission. Mean comparisons indicated higher average attenuation values for the malignant lesions (3.05 dB/cm/MHz, standard deviation [SD]: 0.290 dB/cm/MHz) than for the benign abnormalities (1.50 dB/cm/MHz, SD: 0.474 dB/cm/MHz). Sound speed–derived data provide images with greater visual detail and resolution. The ability to routinely acquire data to provide such distinguishing values remains an area of ongoing investigations (Fig. 4) [83].

Electrical impedance imaging

The local milieu surrounding a cancer is altered in several ways: increased vascularity, fibrosis, altered cellular and extracellular contents, electrolyte balances, and altered cellular membrane properties of the tumor cells. These alterations can affect the transmission of low voltage current through tissue. This is the principle upon which electrical impedance imaging is based. The changes that occur within and adjacent to cancerous tissue alter capacitance, and conductivity decreases its impedance. TransScan Medical (Ramsey, New Jersey) received premarket approval for adjunctive breast imaging of its device TS2000 in 1999.

The introduction of this technology had limited acceptance by the clinical community. The company and product went through several changes, resulting in relocation (Mirabel Medical, Inc., Austin Texas), a new product (T-scan 2000ED), and new clinical trials in search of acceptable indications.

Electrical imaging impedance is accomplished with transmission of a 1-V electrical signal generated through the breast by means of an electrode placed on the arm or held by the patient on the side contralateral to the breast being imaged. Electrodes or a hand-held scanner measures the breast's internal electrical impedance. A real-time computer display of local impedance is obtained, with a predetermined threshold indicating an abnormality. Low impedance in tissue is displayed as bright signals on a topographic computer screen display. At its FDA PMA hearing, the manufacturer claimed, on the basis of combined results from pre-PMA trials, that the adjunctive use of this technology improved the diagnostic sensitivity of mammography by 15.6% and the diagnostic specificity by 20.2% over those of mammography alone [84].

More recently, this technology has been studied in terms of risk stratification and adjunctive use for mammography results. Proposed identification of women at higher risk yielded a relative probability of a woman with a positive electrical impedance spectroscopy (EIS) examination as 7.68, whereas sensitivity was poor, 38%, in a cancer-enriched cohort. In an asymptomatic arm of the study, specificity was 95% [85]. Another study, using a different strategy, imaged patients with BI-RADS 4

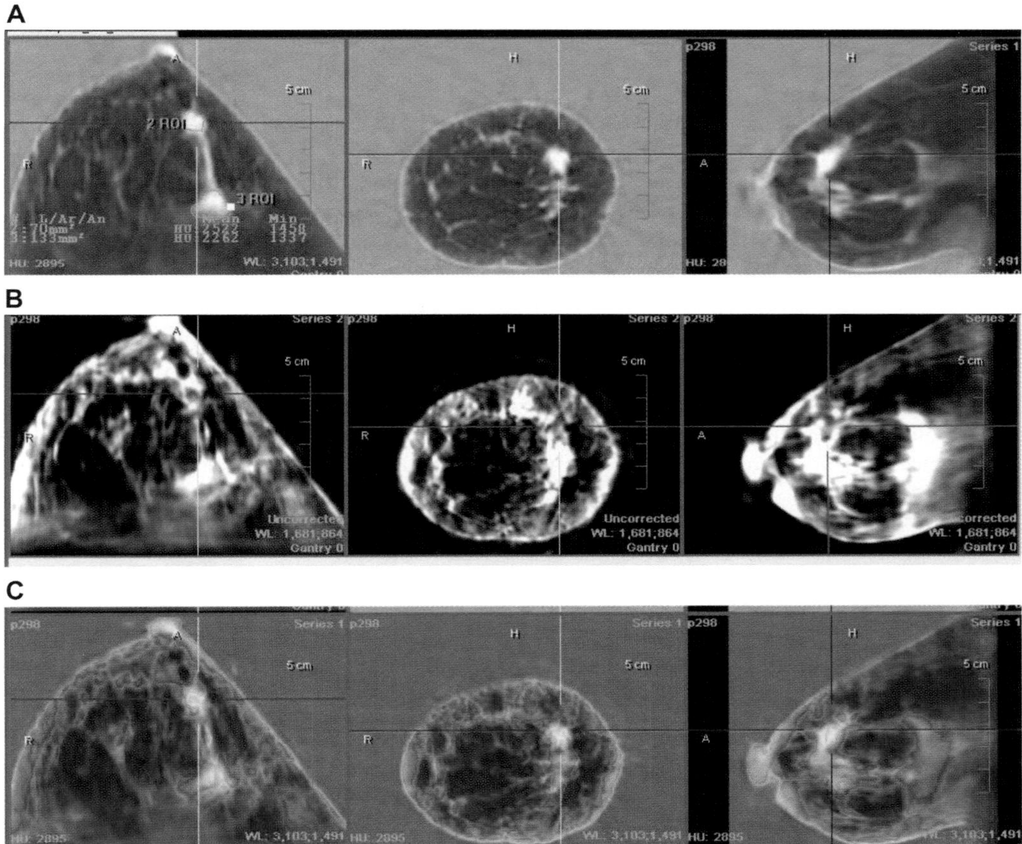

Fig. 4. Ultrasound CT images in a patient who had two lesions that were found to be infiltrating carcinomas when biopsied. (*A*) The images represent speed of sound in three different orientations. The center image is of a single coronal slice and shows an area of high sound (the bright area at the intersection of the vertical and horizontal lines). The other two images are multiplanar reconstructions in two views. The image on the right displays the breast in the sagittal (vertical) plane, whereas the view on the left shows the breast in the axial (horizontal) plane. The reconstruction in the axial view is especially notable as it appears to show tumor in the ductal tissue connecting the two masses, which was not evident on the patient's mammogram. (*B*) Attenuation of sound images in three different orientations. Again, the central image is of the coronal view and the right and left images are multiplanar reconstructions in the sagittal and axial planes, respectively. The two lesions also are distinguishable in these images, although not as clearly as in the speed of sound images. (*C*) Fusion representations of the speed of sound and speed of attenuation images.

mammography results and reported that a 97.1% negative predictive value could be achieved; for lesions less than 1 cm, a 100% negative predictive value was achieved. The investigators advanced the notion that with such results, BI-RADS 4 lesions could be converted safely to BI-RADS 3 and followed at 6-month intervals [86].

Other approaches

Innovation and funding limit the number of ways that the breast can be imaged, either in search of early cancer or to exclude the presence of cancer. Almost the entire nondestructive EM spectrum can be directed into the breast in hopes of finding the right combination of physical properties and energy source to safely and accurately discriminate between benign and malignant breast tissue.

Microwave imaging has been suggested as a means of determining water content in tissue, where discrimination of malignant tissue with higher water content can be discerned from normal breast tissue and fat. Focused low-power microwaves are transmitted into the noncompressed breast and backscattered energy is received by a series of antennas that surround the breast. A three-dimensional image is reconstructed. Early data suggest that tumors as small as 2 mm should be detectable up to a breast depth of 4 cm [87]. Lateral spatial resolution may be limiting, at 0.5 cm.

Early investigative work is being conducted into several new technologies. Pilot studies are examining the tomographic spectroscopic acquisition of three distinct energies within the EM spectrum, in search of the optimal breast adjunctive tool. Near-infrared spectroscopy (NIS), EIS, and microwave imaging spectroscopy (MIS) are being studied, first in normal patients and then in a small series of patients with lesions that provide histologic confirmation of the diagnosis. These technologies use a similar physical design in equipment. The patient lies on a modified stereotactic prone biopsy table, with a modality-specific array of transmit and receive transducers placed circumferentially around the breast. Energy is transmitted into the breast and received raw data are mathematically reconstructed to reflect alteration of propagated energy by the physical properties of the breast and internal pathology. Each modality has specific EM property display-light diffusion for NIS, electrical current flow for EIS, and microwave propagation for MIS. These technologies, in part, have been studied and discussed previously; however, this investigative work allows for the potential of multimodality imaging, perhaps even fusion of the data acquired with other imaging techniques. Evaluating the detection of hemoglobin concentration with NIS and determining electrical permittivity and conductivity with EIS or cellular and tissue water content with MIS are being studied [88].

The introduction of physical energy, coupled with EM energy imaging, to cause physical alteration and alter the propagative characteristics of transmitted energy also is being studied. This principle already is in use, exemplified by fremitus during ultrasound breast imaging to differentiate between the likelihood of benign and malignant solid nodules.

Several of these modalities are in development or the early clinical phase. Thermoacoustic CT exposes the breast to short pulses of externally applied EM energy. The physical alteration of the tissue results in generation of energy upon return to its native state. Generated sound waves can be detected by an array of ultrasound transducers that surround the breast. The absorption and subsequent release of energy are related to tissue type. The generated energy, in the form of ultrasound, is used to reconstruct a three-dimensional image of the breast tissue. The energy applied is 434 MHz radiation. Spatial resolution of 2 to 5 mm to a depth of 40 mm is reported [89].

Similar theoretic principles apply to MR elastography, where introduced acoustic energy, acting as mechanical stress, is detected by motion-sensitive MR imaging techniques. A shear stiffness quantitative map is generated in imaging planes. A differential in stiffness, with tumors exhibiting a shear stiffness increase of an average of 418% more than normal breast tissue, has been demonstrated. This method is proposed for lesion characterization and early detection [90].

Summary

Since Roentgen's identification of the potential of X-ray energies to penetrate the body and be captured on a detector to provide differential transmission information that relates to anatomic structures, the quest to provide anatomic and physiologic information regarding normal and pathologic states by manipulating other forms of energy has invited novel, but not always successful, investigations. Using a wide range of transmission and emission properties derivative to the entire EM spectrum, and coupling such perturbations to sophisticated computer processing, data spectrums and images have been derived that seem to relate to specific disease states. The proprietary nature of such "black box" approaches that presumably rely on experienced-based patterns is not entirely dissimilar to the development of computer-aided detection algorithms, where reconciling results may or may not be subject to a reproducible analysis.

Given the complexity of many of these approaches, the determination of whether theoretic constructs can be translated into clinical applications is dependent on a strict evaluation of empiric results. Like many new ventures, early enthusiasm historically has been tempered by subsequent performance. The essence of clinical trials is to help determine whether proposed applications are valid, and results often are dependent on specific methodologies used. That successful exploitation of certain energy manipulations can improve patient care has been exemplified by the use of diagnostic ultrasound, X-ray, and annihilation reactions, such as fluorodeoxyglucose. Whether or not attempts to identify small physiologic or anatomic disturbances by other means that, for example, are dependent upon the accumulation of deoxyhemoglobin, remain the goal of many of the products and investigations discussed herein.

Almost by definition, nonconventional imaging techniques become conventional when theory can be reconciled with empirically observed results, when clinical trials demonstrate accuracy and reproducibility, and when the cost-effective use of such technologies shows a persuasive impact on patient care. Some breakthroughs in science are not predictable, unlike most physical properties that reflect multiple energy manifestations of the EM spectrum. Familiarity with the approaches discussed here invite review to be familiar with the types of investigations being conducted, to recognize the rationales that underscore such investigations as a reflection of basic science, and to prepare for introducing such technologies into clinical practice, should they reach intended clinical validation.

References

[1] National Institutes of Health. NIH Consensus Conference on the Treatment of Early-Stage Breast Cancer. JAMA 1991;265:391–5.

[2] Warren SL. Roentgenologic study of the breast. AJR Am J Roentgenol 1930;24:113–24.

[3] Beanery RP, Lammerstsma AA, Jones T, et al. Positron emission tomography for in-vivo measurement of regional blood flow, oxygen utilization, and blood volume in patients with breast carcinoma. Lancet 1984;8369:131–4.

[4] Cox PH, Belfer AJ, van der Pompe WB. Thallium 201 chloride uptake in tumours, a possible implication in heart scintigraphy. Br J Radiol 1976;49:767–8.

[5] Hisada K, Tonami N, Miyamae T, et al. Clinical evaluation of tumor imaging with 210Tl chloride. Radiology 1978;129:497–500.

[6] Waxman AD, Ramanna L, Memsic LD, et al. Thallium scintigraphy in the evaluation of mass abnormalities of the breast. J Nucl Med 1993;34:18–23.

[7] Hassan IM, Sahweil A, Constantinides C, et al. Uptake and kinetics of Tc-99m hexakis 2-methoxy isobutyl isonitrile in benign and malignant lesions in the lungs. Clin Nucl Med 1989;14:333–40.

[8] Delmon-Mongeon LI, Piwnica-Worms D, Van de Abbeeloe AD, et al. Uptake of the cation hexakis (2 methosyisobutylisonitriloe)-technisium-99m by human carcinoma cell lines in vitro. Cancer Res 1990;50:2198–202.

[9] Khalkhali I, Mena I, Diggles L. Review of imaging techniques for the diagnosis of breast cancer: a new role of prone scintimammography using technetium-99m sestamibi. Eur J Nucl Med 1994;21:357–62.

[10] Taillifer R, Robidoux A, Lambert R, et al. Technetium-99m-sestamibi prone scintimammography to detect primary breast cancer and axillary lymph node involvement. J Nucl Med 1995;26:1758–65.

[11] Khalkhali I, Cutrone JA, Mena IG, et al. Scintimammography: the complementary role of Tc-99m sestamibi prone breast imaging for the diagnosis of breast carcinoma. Radiology 1995; 196:421–6.

[12] Maffioli L, Agresti R, Chiti A, et al. Prone scintimammography in patients with nonpalpable breast lesions. Anticancer Res 1996;16:1269–73.

[13] Khalkhali I, Villanueva-Meyer J, Edell SL. Diagnostic accuracy of 99m Tc-sestamibi imaging: multicenter trial results. J Nucl Med 2000;41:1973–9.

[14] Polan RL, Klein BD, Richman RH. Scintimammogrphy in patients with minimal mammographic or clinical findings. Radiographics 2001;21:641–53.

[15] Kotlyarov EV. Invited commentary. Radiographics 2001;21:653–5.

[16] Fenlon HM, Phelan NC, O'Sullivan P, et al. Benign versus malignant breast disease: comparison of contrast-enhanced MR imaging and Tc-99m tetrofosmin scintigraphy. Radiology 1997;205:214–20.

[17] Brem RJ, Rapelyea A, Zisman G, et al. Occult breast cancer: scintimammography with high-resolution breast-specific gamma camera in women at high risk for breast cancer. Radiology 2005;232:274–9.

[18] Scopinaro F, Pani R, De Vincentis G, et al. High-resolution scintimammography improves the accuracy of technetium-99m methoxyisobutylisonitrile scintimammography: use of a new dedicated gamma camera. Eur J Nucl Med 1999;26:1279–88.

[19] Brem RJ, Schoonjans JM, Kieper DA, et al. High resolution scintimammography: a pilot study. J Nucl Med 2002;43:909–15.

[20] Mueller B, O'Connor MK, Blevis I, et al. Evaluation of a small CZT detector for scintimammography. J Nucl Med 2003;44:602–9.

[21] Rhodes DJ, O'Connor MK, Phillips SW, et al. Molecular breast imaging: a new technique using Tc-99m scintimammography for the detection of small breast lesions. Mayo Clin Proc 2005;80: 24–30.

[22] Helbich TH, Becherer A, Trattnig S, et al. Differentiation of benign and malignant breast lesions: MR imaging versus Tc-99m sestamibi scintimammography. Radiology 1997;202:421–9.

[23] Mankoff DA, Dunnwald LK, Gralow JR, et al. Monitoring the response of patients with advanced breast cancer to neoadjuvant chemotherapy using [technitium 99m]-sestamibi scintimammography. Cancer 1999;85:240–3.

[24] van den Bossche B, vanBelle S, De Winter F, et al. Early prediction of endocrine therapy effect in advanced breast cancer patients using 99mTc-depreotide scintigraphy. J Nucl Med 2006;47: 6–13.

[25] Kapoor V, McCook BM, Torok FS. An introduction to PET-CT imaging. Radiographics 2004; 24:523–43.

[26] Martin WH, Delbeke D, Patton JA, et al. Detection of malignancies with SPECT versus PET with 2-[fluorine-18]fluro-2-deoxy-D-glucose. Radiology 1996;198:225–31.

[27] Shreve PD, Steventon RS, Deters EC, et al. Oncologic diagnosis with 2-[Fluoro-18] fluoro-2-deoxy-D-glucose imaging: dual head coincidence gamma camera versus positron emission tomographic scanner. Radiology 1998;207:431–7.

[28] Brown RS, Wahl RL. Overexpression of Glut-1 glucose transporter in human breast cancer: an immunohistochemical study. Cancer 1993;72: 2979–85.

[29] Shreve PD, Anzai Y, Wahl R. Pitfalls in oncologic diagnosis with FDG PET imaging: physiologic and benign variants. Radiogrpahics 1999;19:61–77.

[30] Fordon BA, Flanagan FL, Dehdashti F. Whole body positron emission tomography: normal variations, pitfalls and technical considerations. AJR Am J Roentgenol 1997;169:1675–80.

[31] Azasadny KR, Wahl RL. Standardized uptake values of normal tissues in FDG/PET: variations with body weight and a method of correction: "SUV-lean". Radiology 1993;187:743–50.

[32] Smith MF, Majewski S, Weisenberger AG, et al. Analysis of factors affecting positron emission mammography (PEM) image formation. IEEE Trans Nucl Sci 2003;50:53–9.

[33] Murthy KI, Aznar M, Bergman AM, et al. Positron emission mammographic instrument: initial results. Radiology 2000;215:280–5.

[34] Thompson CJ, Murthy K, Weinberg IN, et al. Feasibility study for positron emission mammography. Med Phys 1994;21:529–38.

[35] Rosen EL, Turkington TG, Soo MS, et al. Detection of primary breast carcinoma with a dedicated large-field-of-view FDG PET mammography device: initial experience. Radiology 2005;234:527–34.

[36] Tafra L, Cheng Z, Uddo J. Pilot clinical trial of 18F-fluorodeoxyglucose positron-emission mammography in the surgical management of breast cancer. Am J Surg 2005;190:628–32.

[37] Murthy K, Aznar M, Thompson CJ, et al. Results of preliminary clinical trials of the positron emission mammography system PEM-I: a dedicated breast imaging system producing glucose metabolic images using FDG. J Nucl Med 2000;41:1851–8.

[38] Hoegerle S, Juengling F, Otte A, et al. Combined FD and [F-18]Fluoride whole body PET: a feasible two-in-one approach to cancer imaging. Radiology 1998;209:253–8.

[39] Weir L, Worsley MD, Bernstein V. The value of FDG positron emission tomography in the management of patients with breast cancer. Breast J 2005;11:204–9.

[40] Eubank WB, Mankoff D, Bhattacharya M, et al. Impact of FDG PET on defining the extent of disease and on the treatment of patients with recurrent or metastatic breast cancer. AJR Am J Roentgenol 2004;183:479–86.

[41] Kole AC, Nieweg OE, Pruim J, et al. Detection of unknown occult primary tumors using positron emission tomography. Cancer 1998;82:1160–6.

[42] Brenner RJ, Rothman B. Detection of primary breast cancer in women with known adenocarcinoma metastatic to the axilla: use of magnetic resonance imaging following negative clinical and mammographic examination. J Magn Reson Imaging 1997;7:1153–8.

[43] Smith IC, Welch AE, Hutcheon AW, et al. Positron emission tomography using [F18] fluorodeoxy-D-glucose to predict the pathologic response of breast cancer to primary chemotherapy. J Clin Oncol 2000;18:1676–88.

[44] Inoue T, Koyama K, Oriucdhi N, et al. Detection of malignant tumors: whole body PET with fluorine 18 alfa-methyl tyrosine versus FDG-preliminary study. Radiology 2001;220:54–62.

[45] Yutani K, Tatsumi M, Uehara T, et al. Effects of patients' being prone during FDG PET for the diagnosis of breast cancer. AJR Am J Roentgenol 1999;173:1337–9.

[46] Mintun MA, Welch MJ, Siegel BA, et al. Breast cancer: PET imaging of estrogen receptors. Radiology 1998;169:45–8.

[47] Laronga C. Editorial comment, breast disease: yearbook quarterly. 2004;14:413–4.

[48] Halverson KJ, Taylor ME, Perez CA, et al. Regional nodal management and patterns of failure following conservative surgery and radiation therapy for state I and II breast cancer. Int J Radiat Oncol Biol Phys 1993;26:593–9.

[49] Ivens D, Hoe AL, Podd TJ, et al. Assessment of morbidity from complete axillary dissection. Br J Cancer 1992;66:136–8.

[50] Fisher B, Wolmark W, Bauer M, et al. The accuracy of clinical nodal staging and of limited axillary dissection as a determinant of histologic nodal status in carcinoma of the breast. Surg Gynecol Obstet 1981;152:765–72.

[51] Cabanas RM. An approach for the treatment of penile carcinoma. Cancer 1977;39:456–66.

[52] Morton DL, Wen DR, Wong JH, et al. Technical details of intraoperative lymphatic mapping for early state melanoma. Arch Surg 1992;127:392–9.

[53] Giuliano AE, Krgan DM, Guenther JM, et al. Lymphatic mapping and sentinel lymphadenectomy for breast cancer. Ann Surg 1994;220:391–401.

[54] Krag DN, Weaver DL, Alex JC, et al. Surgical resection and radiolocalization of sentinel lymph node in breast cancer using a gamma probe. Surg Oncol 1993;2:335–9.

[55] Hsueh EC, Turner RR, Glass EC, et al. Sentinel node biopsy in breast cancer. J Am Coll Surg 1999;189:207–12.

[56] Krag D, Weaver D, Ashikaga T, et al. The sentinel node in breast cancer: a multicenter validation study. N Engl J Med 1998;339:941–6.

[57] Chang CHJ, Nesbit DE, Fisher DR, et al. Computed tomographic mammography using a conventional body scanner. AJR Am J Roentgenol 1982;138:553–8.

[58] Gisvold JJ, Reese DF, Karsell PR. Computed tomographic mammography (CTM). AJR Am J Roentgenol 1979;133:1143–9.

[59] Lindfors KK, Boone JM, Nelson TR, et al. Initial clinical evaluation of breast computed tomography. Presented at RSNA.

[60] Ning R, Tang X, Yu R, et al. Flat panel detector-based cone beam volume CT imaging: detector evaluation. Proc Soc Photo Opt Instrum Eng 1999;3659:192–203.

[61] Chen B, Ning R. Cone beam volume CT breast imaging (CBVCTBI): wavelet analysis: based multiresolution reconstruction and de-noise technique. Proc Soc Photo Opt Instrum Eng 2002;4682:218–44.
[62] Brenner RJ. Asymmetric densities of the breast: strategies for imaging evaluation. Semin Roentgenol 2001;36:201–16.
[63] Paulsen KD, Meaney PM, Gilman LC, editors. Alternative breast imaging: four model-based approaches. New York: Springer; 2005.
[64] Mammography and beyond: developing technologies for the early detection of breast cancer by national academy press, national cancer policy board, Institute of Medicine. National Academies Press; 2001.
[65] Lawson R. Implications of surface temperatures in the diagnosis of breast cancer. Can Med Assoc J 1956;75:309.
[66] Myers PC, Barrett AH, Sadowsky NL. Microwave thermography of normal and cancer breast tissue. Ann N Y Acad Sci 1980;335:443–55.
[67] Gautherie M. Temperature and blood flow patterns in breast cancer during natural evolution and following radiotherapy. In: Gautherie M, Albert E, editors. Biomedical thermology. New York: A. Liss; 1982. p. 21–64.
[68] Isard HJ, Becker W, Shilo R, et al. Breast thermography after 4 years and 10,000 studies. AJR Am J Roentgenol 1972;115:811–21.
[69] Moskowitz M, Milbrath J, Gartside P, et al. Lack of efficacy of thermography as a screening tool for minimal and stage I breast cancer. N Engl J Med 1976;295:249–52.
[70] Weidner N, Semple JP, Welch WR, et al. Tumor angiogenesis and metastasis-correlation in invasive breast cancer. N Engl J Med 1991;324:1–8.
[71] Head JF, Wang F, Elliott RL. Breast thermography is a noninvasive prognostic procedure that predicts tumor growth rate in breast cancer patients. Ann N Y Acad Sci 1993;698:153–8.
[72] Yahara T, Koga T, Yoshida S, et al. Relationship between microvessel density and thermographic hot areas in breast cancer. Surg Today 2003; 33(4):243–8.
[73] Isard HJ, Sweitzer CJ, Edelstein GR. Breast thermography: a prognostic indicator for breast cancer survival. Cancer 1988;62:484–8.
[74] Parisky YR, Sardi A, Hamm R, et al. Efficacy of computerized infrared imaging analysis to evaluate mammographically suspicious lesions. AJR Am J Roentgenol 2003;180:263–9.
[75] Arena F, Barone C, DiCicicco T. Use of digital infrared imaging in enhanced breast cancer detection and monitoring of the clinical response to treatment. Presented at the 25th Annual International Conference of the IEEE Engineering in Medicine & Biology Society. Cancun (Mexico), September 17–21, 2003.
[76] National Cancer Institute. Transillumination not effective for early breast cancer detection. Cancer Facts 1990.
[77] McDonald DM, Choyke PL. Imaging of angiogenesis: from microscope to clinic. Nat Med 2003;9:713–25.
[78] Gibson AP, Hebden JC, Arridge SR. Recent advances in diffuse optical imaging. Phys Med Biol 2005;50:R1–43.
[79] Zhu Q, Conant E, Chance B. Optical imaging as an adjunct to sonograph in differentiating benign from malignant breast lesions. J Biomed Opt 2000;5(2):229–36.
[80] Zhang Q, Brukilacchio TJ, Li A, et al. Coregistered tomographic x-ray and optical breast imaging: initial results. J Biomed Opt 2005;10(2):1–9.
[81] Secci Angelo, Sohval Robert, Masyukov Ivan. Dynamic optical breast imaging: preliminary results from two data interpretation methods. White paper. Mahwah (NJ): DOBI Medical International, Inc.; 2004.
[82] Floery D, Helbich T, Riedl C, et al. Characterization of benign and malignant breast lesions with computed tomography laser mammography (CTLM): initial experience. Invest Radiol Breast Imaging Part 1 2005;40(6):328–35.
[83] Johnson SA, Abbott T, Bell R, et al. Non-invasive breast tissue characterization using ultrasound speed and attenuation: in vivo validation. In: Andre MP, editor. Acoustical imaging, vol. 28. the Netherlands: Springer Netherlands; 2007. p. 147–54.
[84] Center for Devices and Radiological Health, FDA, Radiological Devices Panel Meeting, August 17, 1998. Available at: http://www.fda.gov/ohrms/dockets/ac/98/transcpt/3446t1.rtf. Accessed April 3, 2000.
[85] Stojadinovic A, Moskovitz O, Gallimidi Z, et al. Prospective study of electrical impedance scanning for identifying young women at risk for breast cancer. Breast Cancer Res Treat 2006; 97(2):179–89.
[86] Fuchsjaeger MH, Flory D, Reiner CS, et al. The negative predictive value of electrical impedance scanning in BI-RADS category IV breast lesions. Breast Cancer Res Treat 2006;97(2):179–89, Epub 2006 Feb 21.
[87] Hagness SC, Taflove A, Bridges JE. Two-dimensional FDTD analysis of a pulsed microwave confocal system for breast cancer detection: fixed-focus and antenna-array sensors. IEEE Trans Biomed Eng 1998;45(12):1470–9.
[88] Poplack SP, Paulsen KD, Hartor A, et al. Electromagnetic breast imaging: average tissue property values in women with negative clinical findings. Radiology 2004;231:571–80.
[89] Kruger RA, Kiser WL, Reinecke DR, et al. Application of thermoacoustic computed tomography to breast imaging. In: Boone John M, Dobbins James T III, editors. Proceedings of SPIE, medical imaging. Vol 3659. Bellingham (WA): Physics of Medical Imaging; 1999. p. 426–30.
[90] McKnight AL, Kugel JL, Rossman P, et al. MR elastography of breast cancer: preliminary results. AJR Am J Roentgenol 2002;178:1411–7.

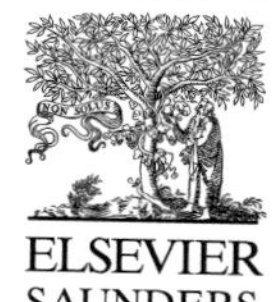

ELSEVIER
SAUNDERS

RADIOLOGIC
CLINICS
OF NORTH AMERICA

Radiol Clin N Am 45 (2007) 925–929

Index

Note: Page numbers of article titles are in **boldface** type.

A

B

doi:10.1016/S0033-8389(07)00152-2

C

D

V